Clinical Echocardiography and Other Imaging Techniques in Cardiomyopathies

Bruno Pinamonti • Gianfranco Sinagra

Editors

Clinical Echocardiography and Other Imaging Techniques in Cardiomyopathies

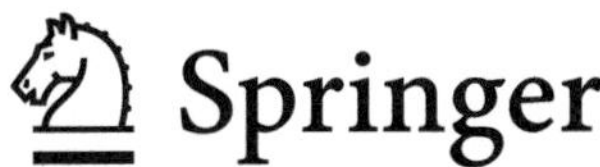 Springer

Editors
Bruno Pinamonti, MD
Cattinara University Hospital
Trieste
Italy

Gianfranco Sinagra, MD, FESC
Cattinara University Hospital
Trieste
Italy

ISBN 978-3-319-34856-8   ISBN 978-3-319-06019-4   (eBook)
DOI 10.1007/978-3-319-06019-4
Springer Cham Heidelberg New York Dordrecht London

Printed on acid-free paper

Springer is part of Springer Science+Business Media (www.springer.com)

Foreword

Thirty years ago cardiomyopathies were defined and classified as heart muscle diseases of unknown etiology. In the following years, great progress has been achieved in the knowledge of such diseases, considered as a true challenge of complexity, with many disciplines called for the understanding of aetiology, pathogenesis, diagnosis and treatment. The integration of clinical cardiology with basic research, the interaction between various medical disciplines, the national and international cooperation as well as a systematic, rigorous collection of data through long-term registries are the main factors that have contributed to this ongoing progress.

In the past, our understanding of these disorders was mainly based on the correlation of clinical findings with postmortem anatomy and long-term follow-up. The irruption and constant development of new technologies have radically changed the general knowledge and our diagnostic and therapeutic approach to patients. This was initially based on electrocardiography, on traditional radiology and later on cardiac catheterization and cardioangiography, an important tool which allows to obtain good morphologic and functional definition. However, the invasiveness of this technique carried some procedural risks for the patients. In the following decades, two-dimensional and Doppler echocardiography became the most important imaging tools for the study of cardiomyopathies, with progressive improvements, such as three-dimensional, contrast and stress echocardiography, which allow a more detailed and dynamic evaluation of myocardial structure and function. Nowadays, echocardiography has a central role in the definition of the phenotype, in the assessment of diffuse and localized abnormalities and of pathophysiology underlying these conditions. In some cases it is the most important clue to diagnosis, as in right ventricular cardiomyopathy, in "infiltrative" diseases of the myocardium or in left ventricular non-compaction. Echocardiography should always be interpreted in the clinical context and integrated with other clinical findings.

In the recent years, cardiac magnetic resonance improved our general understanding and diagnostic assessment of these conditions. When echocardiography is limited in providing an exact diagnosis, cardiac magnetic resonance may have a pivotal role in contributing a detailed assessment and answering many clinical questions. Moreover, by analyzing the late gadolinium enhancement sequences it is possible to identify the pattern of distribution of myocardial fibrosis (that may be helpful in differentiating between ischemic and non-ischemic etiopathogenesis), while T1- and T2-weighted pulse sequences are useful in detecting edema, abnormal fat or amyloid.

Other imaging techniques, such as X-ray computed tomography (CT), positron emission tomography (PET), and single photon emission tomography (SPECT) are less used, but their role may be important in certain situations.

The great amount of data published in recent years about cardiomyopathies, as well as cardiac imaging and its role in diagnosis, prognosis and therapeutic management, have been critically analyzed by the authors of this book, a group historically involved in the study of heart muscle diseases. The authors underscore the importance of a multidisciplinary approach and the need of an imaging interpretation deeply integrated with the clinical information and context.

I am convinced that this book will support clinical cardiologists in a rational use of cardiac imaging and help them in gaining a more comprehensive approach in the diagnosis and treatment of these complex conditions.

Trieste, Italy   Fulvio Camerini, MD, EFESC

Preface

This book was designed by the Editors as a thorough up-to-date review of the role of imaging in cardiomyopathies, based on the existing literature and on the authors' working experience in the tertiary referral center on cardiomyopathies of the University Hospital of Trieste, Italy. Particular attention was given to the clinical significance of echocardiographic findings, as well as those derived from other imaging modalities, in the different groups of cardiomyopathies. Diagnostic, prognostic, and possible therapeutic implications of imaging data are considered. Clinically important information achieved by both basic and advanced echocardiography (e.g. three-dimensional and speckle-tracking echocardiography) are examined. Additionally, the role of magnetic resonance imaging and other radiological and radionuclide cardiac imaging modalities was described.

Relevant data obtained from the published literature and from the authors' experience were presented in a critical way in order to provide the clinician and the imaging cardiologist with valuable support in the appropriate use of imaging techniques for the optimal management of patients affected by cardiomyopathies.

Considering that the main focus of the book is imaging, a significant section was dedicated to imaging examples of typical cases of cardiomyopathies, mainly studied by the authors. Furthermore, echocardiographic video loops of various cases of cardiomyopathies are available online and are extremely useful to fully appreciate the impact of imaging in clinical practice.

The experience of the authors, who come from the same institution (i.e. the Cardiovascular Department of the University Hospital of Trieste, Italy), derives from a 30-year-long work started by the foundation of the Registry of Cardiomyopathies by Prof. Fulvio Camerini. Finally, it is important to remind that, since the initial distinction of the three main groups of cardiomyopathies, significant advances have been made toward a better characterization of distinct subgroups. Nevertheless, areas of overlap in the diagnosis still persist and difficulties in the differential diagnosis are faced in the daily clinical practice.

The authors' hope is that the present book could collect the knowledge of two fields of cardiology, i.e. cardiomyopathies and cardiac imaging, in a clinically meaningful manner.

Trieste, Italy

Bruno Pinamonti, MD
Gianfranco Sinagra, MD, FESC

Contents

Abbreviations

2D	Two-dimensional
3D	Three-dimensional
AF	Atrial fibrillation
ARVC	Arrhythmogenic right ventricular cardiomyopathy
BSA	Body surface area
CA	Cardiac amyloidosis
CMP	Cardiomyopathy
CMR	Cardiac magnetic resonance
CP	Constrictive pericarditis
CRT	Cardiac resynchronization therapy
CT	Computed tomography
CW	Continuous wave
DCM	Dilated cardiomyopathy
ECG	Electrocardiography
EF	Ejection fraction
EMB	Endomyocardial biopsy
EMF	Endomyocardial fibrosis
FAC	Fractional area change
HCM	Hypertrophic cardiomyopathy
HF	Heart failure
ICD	Implantable cardioverter defibrillator
IVS	Interventricular septum
LA	Left atrium
LBBB	Left bundle branch block
LDAC	Left-dominant arrhythmogenic cardiomyopathy
LGE	Late gadolinium enhancement
LV	Left ventricle
LVNC	Left ventricular non-compaction
LVRR	Left ventricular reverse remodeling
MIBG	Metaiodobenzylguanidine
MR	Mitral regurgitation
MV	Mitral valve
NYHA	New York Heart Association
OT	Outflow tract

PCWP	Pulmonary capillary wedge pressure
PET	Positron emission tomography
PISA	Proximal isovelocity surface area
PW	Pulsed wave
RCM	Restrictive cardiomyopathy
RFP	Restrictive filling pattern
RV	Right ventricle
SAM	Systolic anterior motion
SD	Sudden death
SPECT	Single photon emission computed tomography
SSFP	Steady state free precession
TAPSE	Tricuspid annular proximal systolic excursion
TDI	Tissue Doppler imaging
TEE	Trans-esophageal echocardiography
TIC	Tachycardia-induced cardiomyopathy
TR	Tricuspid regurgitation
TTE	Trans-thoracic echocardiography
VT	Ventricular tachycardia
WMA	Wall motion abnormalities

Part I
Cardiomyopathies

Definition, Classification, Epidemiology, and Clinical Relevance of Cardiomyopathies

1

Marco Merlo, Anita Spezzacatene, Francesca Brun, Andrea Di Lenarda, Rossana Bussani, Gianfranco Sinagra, and Fulvio Camerini

1.1 Introduction

Historically , in the first classification [1] the term "Cardiomyopathy" (CMP) was used to describe a heart muscle disease of unknown cause, whereas heart muscle disorders of known etiology (such as coronary artery disease, valvular disease or hypertension) or those associated with systemic diseases were classified as specific CMP. With scientific progress (in particular in genetics and in biotechnology) it became more and more difficult to distinguish between CMP and specific heart muscle diseases (primary and secondary CMP) [2] as it was possible to understand the etiologic basis and pathophysiologic pathways of many so-called "idiopathic" heart muscle disorders. Therefore, in the last years important advances have been made to re-define and re-classify CMP.

M. Merlo (✉) • A. Spezzacatene • F. Brun • G. Sinagra, MD, FESC • F. Camerini
Department of Cardiology, University Hospital of Trieste,
via P. Valdoni 7, Trieste 34139, Italy
e-mail: supermerloo@libero.it; anita.spe@gmail.com;
frabrun77@gmail.com; gianfranco.sinagra@aots.sanita.fvg.it; camerini.cardio@alice.it

A. Di Lenarda
Cardiovascular Center, Azienda per i Servizi Sanitari n°1 di Trieste,
Via Slataper 9, Trieste 34100, Italy
e-mail: andrea.dilenarda@aots.sanita.fvg.it

R. Bussani
Department of Pathology and Morbid Anatomy, University Hospital of Trieste,
via P. Valdoni 7, Trieste 34139, Italy

B. Pinamonti, G. Sinagra (eds.), *Clinical Echocardiography and Other Imaging Techniques in Cardiomyopathies*, DOI 10.1007/978-3-319-06019-4_1,
© Springer International Publishing Switzerland 2014

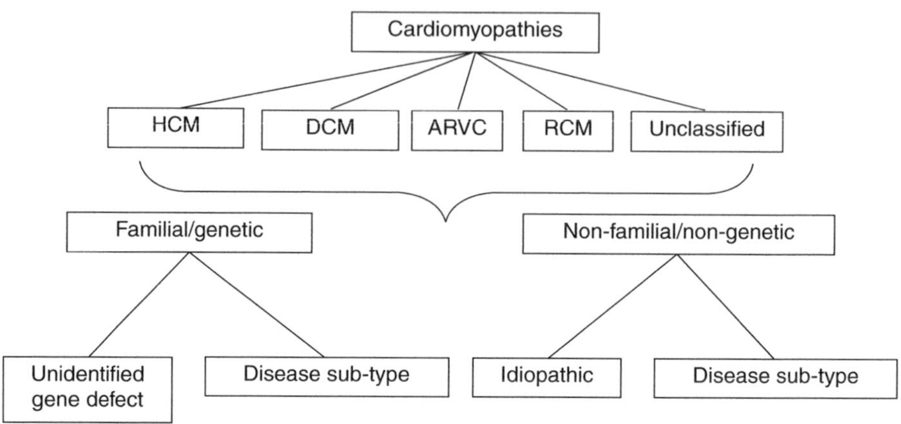

Fig. 1.1 Classification System of Cardiomyopathies proposed by the European Society of Cardiology [4]. *ARVC* arrhythmogenic right ventricular cardiomyopathy, *DCM* dilated cardiomyopathy, *HCM* hypertrophic cardiomyopathy, *RCM* restrictive cardiomyopathy

1.2 Definition and Classification

In spite of the global effort to have a single definition and classification of CMP, to date some controversial and debated issues remain, particularly between the last reports on this topic of American Heart Association and European Society of Cardiology [3, 4].

In their last report, an expert committee of the American Heart Association proposed this definition of CMP: *"cardiomyopathies are a heterogeneous group of diseases of the myocardium associated with mechanical and/or electrical dysfunction that usually (but not invariably) exhibit inappropriate ventricular hypertrophy or dilatation and are due to a variety of causes that frequently are genetic. Cardiomyopathies either are confined to the heart or are part of a generalized systemic disorders, often leading to cardiovascular death or progressive heart failure-related disability"* [3]. In this classification CMP are distinguished in Primary or Secondary, depending on the solely/predominant involvement of the heart or a cardiac manifestation of a systemic disorder, respectively. It has to be noted that this classification is based mainly on etiology, distinguishing CMPs in genetic, acquired and mixed. In addition, other not previously considered heart diseases were included, as the ion channel diseases (primary genetic CMP), and Tako-tsubo and peri-partum diseases (primary mixed CMP).

More recently, the European Society of Cardiology [4] focused its CMP classification predominantly on clinical and morphological features. Therefore, the CMP were defined as a *"myocardial disorder in which structure and function of the myocardium are abnormal, in the absence of coronary artery disease, hypertension, valvular disease and congenital heart disease sufficient to cause the observed myocardial abnormality"* (Fig. 1.1). In this report the CMPs were distinguished into four main specific morphological and functional phenotypes: dilated CMP (DCM) (Fig. 1.2), hypertrophic CMP (HCM) (Fig. 1.3), restrictive CMP (RCM), and

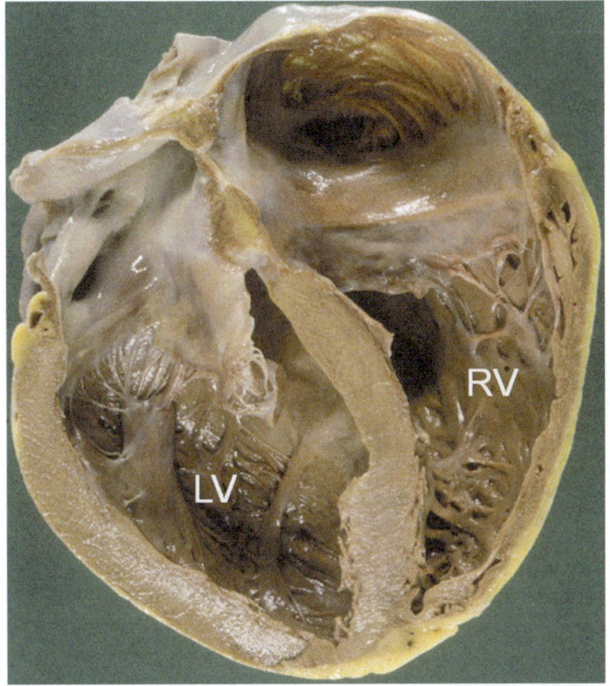

Fig. 1.2 Gross pathologic specimen of a case of Dilated cardiomyopathy who died suddenly. Left ventricle (*LV*) is grossly enlarged, without evident wall hypertrophy. *RV* right ventricle

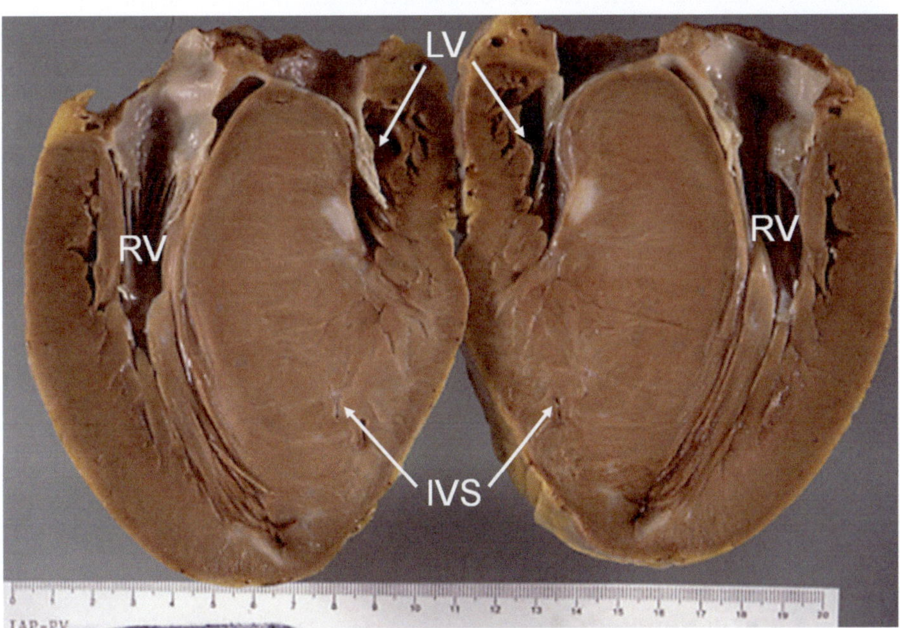

Fig. 1.3 Case of Hypertrophic cardiomyopathy. Severe left ventricular (*LV*) hypertrophy, predominant at the level of interventricular septum (*IVS*) is evident. LV chamber is small. The right ventricle (*RV*) is also hypertrophic

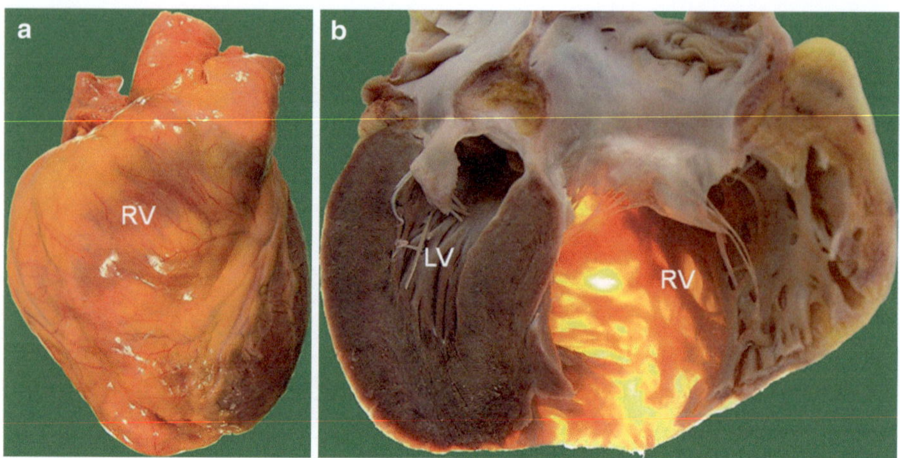

Fig. 1.4 Case of arrhythmogenic right ventricular cardiomyopathy. (**a**): External appearance of anterior aspect of the heart shows an enlarged right ventricle (*RV*) with a yellowish appearance, compatible with fatty infiltration. (**b**): section of the heart (4 chamber view) confirms the severe RV dilatation and shows the extreme wall thinning of RV (note the transillumination of RV thinned wall). *LV* left ventricle

arrhythmogenic right ventricular (RV) CMP (ARVC) (Fig. 1.4). CMPs were further sub-classified in familial and non-familial forms. According to a Consensus statement, a familial CMP can be diagnosed in the presence of two or more affected individuals in a single family, or a first-degree relative with well documented unexplained sudden death (SD) at <35 years of age [5].

Very recently the World Heart Federation published a new comprehensive classification, the so called MOGE(S) classification [6]. This descriptive nosologic system was constructed in a similar manner as the TNM system universally used for staging tumors. Each cardiomyopathy can be defined according to 5 characteristics: M describes the morphofunctional pattern of the CMP, such as HCM, DCM, etc; O the organ involvement; G the genetic/familial inheritance pattern, and E an explicit etiological annotation with details of genetic defect or underlying disease/cause: in addition S as an option describes the functional status using the ACC/AHA stage and NYHA functional class. The MOGE(S) classification can be considered a compromise between the American [3] and European [4] classifications and is expected to be a major advance in the field of CMPs, allowing, as stated by the Authors, "better understanding of the disease, easier communication among physicians and helping to develop multicenter/multinational registries to promote research in diagnosis and management of cardiomyopathies".

1.3   Clinical Relevance

Exceptional progresses of knowledge in the field of CMPs have been done in the last decades. However, despite many causing disease genetic mutations have been found, and some specific or common pathophysiologic pathways have been

Table 1.1 Recruitment rate of patients in Heart Muscle Disease Registry of Trieste (1978–31/12/2013)

	Disease				
Year of recruitment	IDCM	Myocarditis	ARVC	HCM	Total
Before 1979	5		2		7
1979–1980	17		1		18
1981–1982	10	2	3		15
1983–1984	20	15	7	1	43
1985–1986	38	17	6	6	67
1987–1988	41	4	8	12	65
1989–1990	60	4	5	13	82
1991–1992	80	4	7	7	98
1993–1994	99	7	13	22	141
1995–1996	89	7	10	16	122
1997–1998	62	3	6	10	81
1999–2000	74	2	5	12	93
2001–2002	69	2	5	8	84
2003–2004	71	4	7	11	93
2005–2006	80	9	4	22	115
2007–2008	75	7	15	45	142
2009–2010	51	8	7	43	109
2011–2013	90	11	8	48	157
Total n° of patients	**1,031**	**106**	**119**	**276**	**1,532**

ARVC arrhythmogenic right ventricular cardiomyopathy, *HCM* hypertrophic cardiomyopathy, *IDCM* idiopathic dilated cardiomyopathy

hypothesized, controversial and open issues are still present that should be faced by future basic and clinical research.

Some important points of clinical relevance in CMPs have to be mentioned, as the role of familial/genetic screening, and the importance of systematic follow-up and specific registries.

The ongoing evidence of the relevance and frequency of genetic CMPs [7] should indicate a systematic familial screening in all 1st degree family members of probands. In fact, familial screening can provide an earlier diagnosis with a subsequent better long-term outcome [8].

Moreover, patients affected by CMPs require a regular long-term follow-up for continuous monitoring of the evolution of disease, better assessment of the effects of treatment, and risk re-stratification [9]. An important point to remember is that the familial and genetic screenings and the regular long-term follow-up have important costs in terms of human and economic resources. CMPs also set important ethical issues – such as the implications of the identification at genetic screening of apparently non affected family members with presence of gene mutation [7], potential risk of pregnancy, and employment or sport activity in young patients without other associated diseases – that the clinical cardiologist has to face often without specific guidelines. Thus, in absence of specific clinical trials, the presence of registries enrolling clinical, instrumental and prognostic data of large cohorts of patients affected by CMPs and systematically followed in the long-term has a paramount relevance for the correct management of these diseases by clinical cardiologists. In Tables 1.1 and 1.2 are respectively reported the recruitment rate and the summary of enrolled patients and length and number of follow-up evaluation of the Heart Muscle Disease Registry of Trieste, active from 1978.

Table 1.2 Update of Heart Muscle Disease Registry of Trieste (1978–31/12/2013)

	IDCM	HCM	ARVD	Myocarditis	Others
N° of pts	1,031	276	119	106	230
Mean age (years)	45±15	45±20	34±15	38±16	50±14
Males (%)	73	64	70	70	66
Mean follow-up (months)	133±88	104±86	128±92	97±67	44±20
Years of enrolment	1978–2013	1983–2013	1976–2013	1981–2013	1980–2013
N° follow-up (approx.)	6,000	800	500	520	300

ARVC arrhythmogenic right ventricular cardiomyopathy, *HCM* hypertrophic cardiomyopathy, *IDCM* idiopathic dilated cardiomyopathy

1.4 Epidemiology and Definition of Different Cardiomyopathies

1.4.1 Dilated Cardiomyopathy

Dilated Cardiomyopathy (DCM) is defined by the presence of left ventricular (LV) dilatation and systolic dysfunction – genetic or not genetic – in the absence of abnormal loading conditions or coronary artery disease sufficient to cause the LV systolic impairment (Fig. 1.2). RV dilation and dysfunction may also be present but are not required for the diagnosis. DCM represents the third most common cause of heart failure (HF) and the most frequent cause of heart transplantation in western world. The estimated prevalence is 1:2,500 subjects [10, 11]. Familial forms account for 30–48 % of cases and autosomal dominant is the main pattern of inheritance [12]. Autosomal dominant forms of the disease are caused by mutations in cytoskeletal, sarcomeric protein/ Z-band, nuclear membrane and intercalated disc protein genes. X-linked diseases associated with DCM include muscular dystrophies (e.g. Becker and Duchenne) and X-linked DCM. However, about 60 % of DCM remains idiopathic. There are some particular forms of DCM, such as "Mildly Dilated CMP", characterized by advanced HF and severe LV systolic dysfunction occurring without significant LV dilatation [13]. Although some pathological findings differ, the clinical picture and prognosis of mildly dilated CMP are very similar to those of typical DCM [13]. Inflammatory aetiology of DCM has also been described, in particular as a specific evolution of active myocarditis. It is known that active myocarditis, clinically manifested with HF and mostly with LV systolic dysfunction, shows particularly severe prognosis with possible evolution in DCM [14], even though systolic dysfunction is potentially reversible and the natural history is therefore variable [15].

Other peculiar forms of DCM partially or totally reversible are peri-partum CMP and tachycardia-induced CMP (TIC) (see Sect. 1.4.6).

1.4.2 Hypertrophic Cardiomyopathy

Historically, Hypertrophic Cardiomyopathy (HCM) is defined as the presence of myocardial hypertrophy in the absence of abnormal loading conditions (valvular disease or hypertension) sufficient to cause the observed abnormality, and of systemic diseases such as infiltrative or storage diseases [16] (Fig. 1.3).

HCM is the most frequent CMP occurring in approximately 1:500 of the general population [16]. Many individuals have familial disease with an autosomal dominant pattern of inheritance caused by mutations in genes which encode for proteins of cardiac sarcomere. Usual characteristics of HCM are small sized LV cavity and normal to increased ejection fraction (EF). Some patients with HCM develop LV dilatation and systolic failure in the end-stage of the disease. In the young, HCM can be often associated with congenital syndromes, inherited metabolic disorders, and neuromuscular diseases.

1.4.3 Arrhythmogenic Right Ventricular Cardiomyopathy

Arrhythmogenic Right Ventricular Cardiomyopathy (ARVC) is a peculiar CMP characterized by progressive dystrophy and replacement of RV myocardium with adipose and fibrous tissue often confined to a 'triangle of dysplasia' comprising the RV inflow, outflow, and apex (Fig. 1.4). This disease can be diagnosed clinically, in accordance with published criteria [17] by the presence of RV dysfunction (global or regional), associated with histological evidence for the disease and/or electrocardiographic abnormalities,. Pathologic abnormalities predominantly affect morphology and function of the RV, but they also occur in the LV or can be present in the absence of clinically detectable structural changes in either ventricle. The estimated prevalence of ARVC is 1:5,000 and it is a frequent cause of SD in young people, particularly in some areas of Europe. Autosomal recessive forms of ARVC – e.g. Naxos and Carvajal syndromes caused by mutations in genes encoding plakoglobin and desmoplakin, respectively – were described, but the majority of cases are caused by autosomal dominantly inherited mutations in genes encoding proteins of the desmosome complex of cardiomyocytes. Moreover, mutations in TGF-ß, Ryanodine receptor and also Titin [18] genes may be associated with an ARVC phenotype.

1.4.4 Restrictive Cardiomyopathy

Restrictive Cardiomyopathy (RCM) is characterized by a pattern of ventricular filling in which increased stiffness of the myocardium causes an increase in ventricular diastolic pressure with only small increases in volume. Typically, the restrictive physiology is associated with normal or reduced ventricular volumes, and normal wall thickness. Although ventricular systolic pump function, as expressed by EF, is usually preserved in RCM, LV contractility is frequently abnormal.

RCM is the least common type of CMP. It may be idiopathic, familial, secondary to mediastinal radiation, or to various systemic disorders, as cardiac amyloidosis (CA) and Fabry's disease, more appropriately considered infiltrative (storage CMPs; see below). Familial RCM is often characterized by autosomal dominant inheritance, which sometimes is caused by mutations in the troponin I gene; another related gene is that for desmin protein (usually associated with skeletal myopathy).

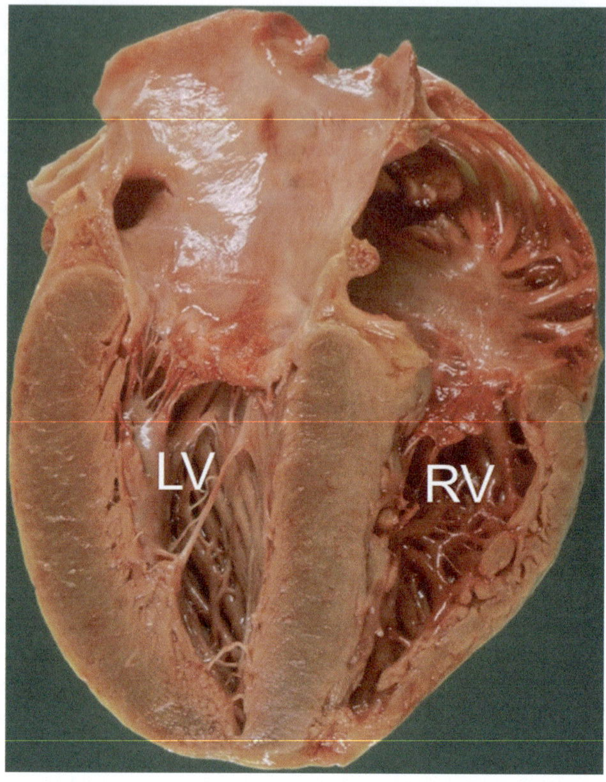

Fig. 1.5 Case of cardiac amyloidosis. Diffuse thickening of ventricular walls with pink coloration is evident, in absence of chamber dilatation. *LV* left ventricle, *RV* right ventricle

RCM can also be the result of endomyocardial pathology (fibrosis, fibro-elastosis, and thrombosis) that impairs diastolic function. These disorders can be sub-classified according to the presence or absence of hypereosinophilia.

1.4.5 Infiltrative and Storage Cardiomyopathies

Infiltrative and Storage CMP are characterized by intercellular or intracellular deposition of various substances within the myocardium that can result in LV hypertrophy and/or restrictive phenotype. Genetic and acquired forms can be observed. CA (Fig. 1.5), sarcoidosis, Fabry's disease, and glycogen storage diseases are some examples. Mytochondrial CMP were also included in this chapter, considering that the cardiac involvement is usually characterized by increased myocardial thickness and accumulation of abnormal mytochondria.

1.4.6 Other Cardiomyopathies

In the last classifications there is still doubt on the correct classification of some forms of CMP, in particular left ventricular non-compaction (LVNC) and Tako-tsubo CMP.

Concerning LVNC, it is not clear whether this is a separate CMP, or a congenital or acquired morphological trait shared by many phenotypically distinct CMP. It is characterized by prominent LV trabeculae and deep inter-trabecular recesses [19]. In some patients, LVNC is associated with LV dilatation and systolic dysfunction, which can be transient in neonates. LVNC is frequently familial, with at least 25 % of asymptomatic relatives having a range of echocardiographic abnormalities. Tako-tsubo CMP is characterized by transient regional systolic dysfunction involving the LV apex ("apical ballooning") and/or mid-ventricle in the absence of obstructive coronary disease on coronary angiography. Patients frequently present with an abrupt onset of angina-like chest pain, and have diffuse T-wave inversion, sometimes preceded by ST segment elevation, and mild cardiac enzymes elevation [20]. Most reported cases occur in post-menopausal women. Symptoms are often preceded by emotional or physical stress and LV function usually normalizes over a period of days to weeks and recurrence is rare.

Another relevant CMP is tachycardia-induced CMP (TIC), defined as ventricular dysfunction resulting from a prolonged increase of heart rate (generally a tachyarrhythmia) which is reversible upon control of the arrhythmia or the heart rate [21]. TIC may present itself at any age mimicking DCM or myocarditis. Supraventricular tachycardias are more frequently involved than ventricular arrhythmias. Furthermore, under this section we mentioned myocarditis as an acute or a chronic inflammatory process affecting the myocardium produced by a wide variety of toxins and drugs or infectious agents which, in some cases, can evolve in chronic inflammation and DCM. In particular DCM secondary to myocarditis is more frequent in viral etiology as it constitutes a trigger toward an autoimmune reaction that causes immunologic damage to the myocardium, culminating in DCM with LV dysfunction.

Peri-partum CMP is characterized by signs of HF and LV systolic dysfunction occurring during the last month of pregnancy or within 5 months of delivery [22]. It seems to be linked with several risk factors such as one or more prior pregnancies, multi-fetal pregnancy, older maternal age, high blood pressure.

Finally, CMP secondary to antineoplastic drugs (principally antracyclines) presents with a mixed hypokinetic-restrictive pattern.

References

1. Report of the WHO/ISFC task force on the definition and classification of cardiomyopathies (1980) Br Heart J 44:672–673
2. Report of the 1995 World Health Organization/International Society and Federation of Cardiology Task Force on the Definition and Classification of Cardiomyopathies (1996) Circulation 93:841–842
3. Maron BJ, Towbin JA, Thiene G, Antzelevitch C, Corrado D, Arnett D, Moss AJ, Seidman CE, Young JB, American Heart Association; Heart Failure and Transplantation Committee Council on Clinical Cardiology; Quality of Care and Outcomes Research and Functional Genomics and Translational Biology Interdisciplinary Working Groups; Council on Epidemiology and Prevention (2006) Contemporary definitions and classification of the cardiomyopathies: an American Heart Association Scientific Statement from the Council on Clinical Cardiology, Heart Failure and Transplantation Committee; Quality of Care and Outcomes Research and Functional Genomics and Translational Biology Interdisciplinary Working Groups; and Council on Epidemiology and Prevention. Circulation 113:1807–1816

4. Elliott P, Andersson B, Arbustini E, Bilinska Z, Cecchi F, Charron P, Dubourg O, Kuhl U, Maisch B, McKenna WJ, Monserrat L, Pankuweit S, Rapezzi C, Seferovic P, Tavazzi L, Keren A (2008) Classification of the cardiomyopathies: a position statement from the European Society of Cardiology Working Group on Myocardial and Pericardial Diseases. Eur Heart J 29:270–276

5. Mestroni L, Maisch B, McKenna WJ, Schwartz K, Charron P, Rocco C, Tesson F, Richter A, Wilke A, Komajda M (1999) Guidelines for the study of familial dilated cardiomyopathies. Collaborative Research Group of the European Human and Capital Mobility Project on Familial Dilated Cardiomyopathy. Eur Heart J 20:93–102

6. Arbustini E, Narula N, Dec W, et al (2013) The MOGE(S) classification for a phenotype-genotype nomenclature of cardiomyopathy. J Am Coll Cardiol 62:2046–2072

7. Camerini F, Sinagra G, Mestroni L (eds) (2013) Genetic cardiomyopathies. Springer, Milano

8. Moretti M, Merlo M, Barbati G, Di Lenarda A, Brun F, Pinamonti B, Gregori D, Mestroni L, Sinagra G (2010) Prognostic impact of familial screening in dilated cardiomyopathy. Eur J Heart Fail 12:922–927

9. Merlo M, Pyxaras SA, Pinamonti B, Barbati G, Di Lenarda A, Sinagra G (2011) Prevalence and prognostic significance of left ventricular reverse remodeling in dilated cardiomyopathy receiving tailored medical treatment. J Am Coll Cardiol 57:1468–1476

10. Codd MB, Sugrue DD, Gersh BJ, Melton LJ 3rd (1989) Epidemiology of idiopathic dilated and hypertrophic cardiomyopathy. A population-based study in Olmsted County, Minnesota, 1975-1984. Circulation 80:564–572

11. Rakar S, Sinagra G, Di Lenarda A, Poletti A, Bussani R, Silvestri F, Camerini F (1997) Epidemiology of dilated cardiomyopathy. A prospective post-mortem study of 5252 necropsies. The Heart Muscle Disease Study Group. Eur Heart J 18:117–123

12. Mestroni L, Rocco C, Gregori D, Sinagra G, Di Lenarda A, Miocic S, Vatta M, Pinamonti B, Muntoni F, Caforio AL, McKenna WJ, Falaschi A, Giacca M, Camerini F (1999) Familial dilated cardiomyopathy: evidence for genetic and phenotypic heterogeneity. Heart Muscle Disease Study Group. J Am Coll Cardiol 34:181–190

13. Keren A, Gottlieb S, Tzivoni D, Stern S, Yarom R, Billingham ME, Popp RL (1990) Mildly dilated congestive cardiomyopathy. Use of prospective diagnostic criteria and description of the clinical course without heart transplantation. Circulation 81:506–517

14. Anzini M, Merlo M, Sabbadini G, Barbati G, Finocchiaro G, Pinamonti B, Salvi A, Perkan A, Di Lenarda A, Bussani R, Bartunek J, Sinagra G (2013) Long-term evolution and prognostic stratification of biopsy-proven active myocarditis. Circulation 128:2384–2394

15. Quigley PJ, Richardson RP, Meany BT (1987) Long-term follow-up of acute myocarditis. Correlation of ventricular function and outcome. Eur Heart J 8(Suppl J):39–42

16. Elliott P, McKenna WJ (2004) Hypertrophic cardiomyopathy. Lancet 363:1881–1891

17. Rowland E, McKenna WJ, Sugrue D, Barclay R, Foale RA, Krikler DM (1984) Ventricular tachycardia of left bundle branch block configuration in patients with isolated right ventricular dilatation. Clinical and electrophysiological features. Br Heart J 51:15–24

18. Taylor M, Graw S, Sinagra G, Barnes C, Slavov D, Brun F, Pinamonti B, Salcedo EE, Sauer W, Pyxaras S, Anderson B, Simon B, Bogomolovas J, Labeit S, Granzier H, Mestroni L (2011) Genetic variation in titin in arrhythmogenic right ventricular cardiomyopathy-overlap syndromes. Circulation 124:876–885

19. Jenni R, Oechslin EN, van der Loo B (2007) Isolated ventricular non-compaction of the myocardium in adults. Heart 93:11–15

20. Gianni M, Dentali F, Grandi AM, Sumner G, Hiralal R, Lonn E (2006) Apical ballooning syndrome or takotsubo cardiomyopathy: a systematic review. Eur Heart J 27:1523–1529

21. Pèrez-Silva A, Merino JL (2009) Tachycardia-induced cardiomyopathy. E-J ESC Counc Cardiol Pract 7(16)

22. Elkayam U, Akhter MW, Singh H, Khan S, Bitar F, Hameed A, Shotan A (2005) Pregnancy-associated cardiomyopathy: clinical characteristics and a comparison between early and late presentation. Circulation 111:2050–2055

Genetics: Genotype/Phenotype Correlations in Cardiomyopathies

2

Francesca Brun, Concetta Di Nora, Michele Moretti, Anita Spezzacatene, Luisa Mestroni, and Fulvio Camerini

2.1 Introduction

When considering etiology, many cardiomyopathies (CMP) have a genetic origin; some are acquired (inflammation, alcohol, drugs, etc.), whereas others may have a mixed origin [1]. The relationships between gene mutations and phenotype are complex and not always clear. One challenging point is the observation that mutations in the same gene may cause different types of CMP; moreover, the various CMP are characterized by great heterogeneity in clinical phenotypes. The key features to note for different inheritance patterns are as follows:

- Autosomal dominant inheritance is characterized by the presence of affected individuals in every generation, with the possibility of male-to-male transmission and a 50 % risk to offsprings of affected parents.
- Autosomal recessive inheritance is the least common pattern in heart-muscle diseases. It should be suspected when both parents of the proband are unaffected and consanguineous. Males and females are equally affected. Parents of an affected child are obligate carriers, with a 25 % risk of having a carrier son/daughter in each pregnancy.

F. Brun (⊠) • C. Di Nora • M. Moretti • A. Spezzacatene • F. Camerini, MD, EFESC
Department of Cardiology, University Hospital of Trieste,
Via P Valdoni, No 7, Trieste 34149, Italy
e-mail: frabrun77@gmail.com; concetta.dinora@gmail.com; michele.moretti@gmail.com; anita.spe@gmail.com

L. Mestroni, MD, FACC, FESC
Cardiovascular Institute, University of Colorado,
Molecular Genetics Program,
12700 E. 19th Ave F442, Denver, CO 80045-2507, USA
e-mail: luisa.mestroni@ucdenver.edu

B. Pinamonti, G. Sinagra (eds.), *Clinical Echocardiography and Other Imaging Techniques in Cardiomyopathies*, DOI 10.1007/978-3-319-06019-4_2,
© Springer International Publishing Switzerland 2014

- X-linked inheritance should be suspected if males are the only or most severely affected individuals. In X-linked inheritance, all daughters of an affected father will be carriers and no male–male transmission is observed. A female carrier has a 50 % risk of having affected sons and a 50 % risk of daughters that carry the gene defect. In some X-linked disorders, such as Anderson–Fabry disease, female carriers can develop milder and later disease because of unfavorable inactivation of the X-chromosome (lionization) [2].
- Matrilineal (or mitochondrial) inheritance in which women but not men transmit the disease to offspring (male and female) is typical of mutations in mitochondrial DNA.

Although differences exist in the classification of major cardiac organizations, genetic CMP have historically been broken down into several major phenotypic categories: hypertrophic, dilated, arrhythmogenic, and restrictive [3].

2.2 Genetic Approach: From Genotype to Phenotype

2.2.1 Dilated Cardiomyopathy

Most genetic dilated cardiomyopathy (DCM) inheritance follows an autosomal dominant pattern, although X-linked, recessive, and mitochondrial patterns of inheritance occur as well. At least 30–50 % of DCM cases are familial, suggesting the involvement of a defective gene [4]. X-linked DCM results from mutations in the dystrophin gene. It may be clinically indistinguishable from idiopathic DCM (IDCM) [5]. Creatine kinase levels are usually (but not always) elevated.

DCM is characterized by a high level of genetic complexity and involvement of different structures of myocytes. Initially, DCM was considered to be a disease of the cytoskeleton; later, it was demonstrated that other structures may be involved, such as sarcomere, Z-disc, nucleoskeleton, mitochondria, desmosomes, sodium and potassium channels, and lysosomal membrane [4, 6]. Mutations in >30 genes across a wide variety of cellular components and pathways have been associated with DCM. The most common sarcomeric mutations are reported in *MYH7*, in *TNNT2*, in *MYBPC3* [7, 8] and alpha-myosin heavy chain (*MYH6*). Hershberger et al. also found rare variants in genes of the sarcomeric complex that "likely" or "possibly" caused the disease in their study population [4]. Herman et al. reported a high frequency of "deleterious variants" in the titin gene in a large, multicenter DCM cohort [9]. Among known sarcomeric genes involved in DCM pathogenesis, some, when mutated, can cause hypertrophic cardiomyopathy (HCM), restrictive cardiomyopathy (RCM), and left ventricular (LV) noncompaction (LVNC). An inevitable limitation is the considerable overlap encountered between categories into which diseases have been segregated (overlap phenotypes). Merlo et al. found that carriers of rare sarcomeric gene variants represented a subgroup of DCM patients with a particularly severe phenotype characterized by a high frequency of ventricular arrhythmias, a high incidence of cardiovascular events, and pump failure [10]. Furthermore, in lamin A/C (*LMNA*) gene mutation carriers, up to ten different phenotypes (laminopathies) have been described, with variable involvement of skeletal and/or cardiac muscle and also of white fat, peripheral nerves, bones, or premature aging [11]. In this peculiar CMP, conduction disease can precede development of DCM in some families, whereas in other families, DCM occurs first. The practical significance is that individuals who may have mild DCM caused by *LMNA* mutations may be at risk of sudden death (SD), whereas this scenario is highly unlikely with most sarcomeric and all cytoskeletal abnormalities. Therefore, when SD is seen in a family with mild DCM, testing for *LMNA* mutations may be helpful and lead to early consideration for implanted cardiac defibrillator (ICD) therapy [12]. Reports of increased arrhythmogenicity in *SCN5A-associated* [13] and desmosomal-associated [14] DCM indicate that a similar approach may be taken when these mutations are identified.

2.2.2 Hypertrophic Cardiomyopathy

HCM is a genetic disease usually caused by mutations in genes encoding sarcomeric and nonsarcomeric proteins. HCM is usually inherited as an autosomal dominant trait; de novo mutations are rare. The major group includes sarcomeric mutations (up to 90 %), in which 15 different genes have been identified [15]; nonsarcomeric (Z-disc or calcium-handling proteins) account for <1 % of cases, and a further 5 % of patients have metabolic disorders, neuromuscular disease, chromosome abnormalities, and genetic malformation syndromes [16].

After two decades of molecular research, the relationship between sarcomere mutations and clinical outcome in patients with HCM has proven to be unreliable, largely attributable to phenotypic heterogeneity, highly variable intra- and interfamily expressivity, and incomplete penetrance. Among several sarcomeric genes identified, defects of beta-myosin heavy-chain (*MYH7*) and myosin-binding protein C (*MYBPC3*) account for up to 70 % of HCM, followed by troponin T gene defects (*TNNI3, TNNT2*) and other less commonly involved genes (*ACTC1, CSRP3, CRYAB, CAV3, MYH6, MYL2, MYL, TNNC1, TCAP, MYOZ1, MYOZ2*) [17].

Specific mutations in *MYH7* (*Arg403Gln, Arg453Cys, and Arg719Trp*) appear convincingly associated with adverse outcomes; however, data suggests that at-risk patients carrying these mutations also display clinical risk factors at the time of events, limiting the added prognostic benefit of genetic diagnosis [18].

An exception to this is HCM caused by mutations in cardiac *TNNT2*, which may cause ventricular arrhythmias and SD in the absence of impressive morphological (mild LV hypertrophy) or hemodynamic features (obstruction, diastolic dysfunction) [19]. Moreover, possible exceptions are emerging, including preliminary data suggesting that double, triple, or compound sarcomere mutations (evident in 5 % of patients with HCM) [20] could be associated with greater disease severity, including SD, also in the absence of conventional risk factors [21]. In addition, complicating the scenario, some HCM phenocopies, characterized by infiltrative and storage CMP, can be caused by disorders of different genetic origin; for example, those resulting from mutations in genes encoding protein kinase adenosine monophosphate (AMP)-activated, gamma-2 noncatalytic subunit (*PRKAG2*) [22], lysosome-associated membrane protein 2 (*LAMP2*) (Danon disease), alpha-galactosidase deficiency (Fabry disease), and transthyretin (TTR) protein (familial amyloid TTR CMP). Moreover, an HCM phenotype may be present in other congenital diseases, such as Noonan syndrome and mitochondrial syndromes. Finally, several studies have shown the important influences exerted by modifying genes and lifestyle in HCM expression. Indeed, in some cases, modifier genes are neither necessary nor sufficient to cause HCM because environmental influences, such as diet, lifestyle, and exercise, can have a predominant role [23].

2.2.3 Arrhythmogenic Right Ventricular Cardiomyopathy

Arrhythmogenic right ventricular cardiomyopathy (ARVC) is another disease of genetic origin and is usually characterized by mutations in genes encoding different proteins mainly involving intercellular junctions (see Chaps. 19, 20, 21, 22, and 23). These proteins (plakoglobin, desmoplakin, plakophilin, desmoglein, desmocollin) are localized in the desmosomes and are important for maintaining tissue architecture and integrity. In addition, nondesmosomal genes are described and include transforming growth factor beta 3 (TGFβ3) and transmembrane protein 43 (TMEM43). Inheritance patterns are mainly autosomal dominant, but rare recessive forms (Naxos disease and Carvajal syndrome) are also observed and well described. In this disease, a high genetic complexity is suggested by the fact that ARVC may be linked to genes related (or not) to the cell-adhesion complex: for example, genes encoding cardiac ryanodine receptor 2 (*RYR2*) and transforming growth factor β3 (*TGFB3*). Furthermore, in ARVC5, *TMEM43* gene mutation causes a fully penetrant disease variant with lethal arrhythmic outcome [24]. In a large ARVC cohort, Rigato et al confirmed that carriers of more than one gene mutation (compound-digenic heterozygosity) have a high risk factor for lifetime major arrhythmic events and *SD* [25]. Moreover, Taylor et al provide evidence that titin mutations can also cause ARVC, given that structural impairment of the titin spring constitutes a novel mechanism underlying myocardial remodelling and SD [26].

2.2.4 Other Cardiomyopathies

RCM and LVNC have been classified individually, but evidence exists for considerable overlap between these syndromes and HCM and DCM. Familial RCM is increasingly recognized as a specific phenotype within the HCM spectrum [27]. Similarly, LVNC is an imaging diagnosis with profound overlap with both DCM and HCM phenotypes and their disease-causing mutations [28]. For LVNC, the definition of the clinical phenotype remains under debate, and population prevalence varies widely depending on the cohort examined and the diagnostic criteria utilized [29].

In conclusion, genetic testing is becoming an important tool for a personalized medical approach to CMP. However, it must not be viewed as a simple blood test: a negative genetic test can never, by itself, rule out the presence of the CMP. Likewise, a positive genetic test must be carefully considered as only one component of a comprehensive cardiogenetic evaluation, together with an accurate clinical diagnosis, an understanding of the probabilistic nature of genetic testing, and an accurate family history [30].

2.3 Clinical Approach: From Phenotype to Genotype

The clinical approach should define the characteristics of CMP and should also explore, when present, the characteristics of involvement of other organs and systems. This approach does not necessarily involve the use of novel or particularly sophisticated tests; however, it requires a detailed analysis of the proband and an in-depth assessment of family background. The construction of a three- four-generation family pedigree must record not only the presence or absence of CMP in relatives, but also other features that support the diagnosis of a genetic cardiovascular disorder (SD, heart failure, cardiac transplantation, insertion of pacemakers or ICD, and stroke at a young age). Noncardiac manifestations in relatives, such as neuromuscular disease, osteoarticular disorder, mental retardation, abnormal craniofacial features, sensorineural hearing loss, visual impairment, skin and hair abnormalities, chronic kidney disease, hematopoietic, endocrine, and genital disorders, also provide diagnostic clues (Tables 2.1 and 2.2).

CMP may also be a feature of rare congenital dysmorphic syndromes that are diagnosed during infancy and childhood [31]. A detailed description of these disorders is outside of the aim of this chapter. It is evident that CMP are a common feature of multisystem diseases. The mechanisms of multiorgan involvement are heterogeneous, and a complete evaluation includes researching red flags, such as the following [32, 33]:

- Physical examination (Tables 2.1 and 2.2)
- Electrocardiogram abnormalities (Table 2.3)
- Laboratory tests (Table 2.4)
- Echocardiography/cardiac magnetic resonance: hypertrophy pattern, pericardial effusion, valve thickening, bulging, sacculations, sparkling myocardium texture, late gadolinium enhancement (LGE) (Table 2.5). Some typical features are described, such as LGE localized to the inferolateral wall in patients with Anderson–Fabry disease or dystrophinopathies and to the circumferential subendocardial wall in cardiac amyloidosis. The echocardiogram remains the first-line imaging tool in patients with suspected CMP. It has a central role in defining the morphological and functional phenotype and in guiding treatment decisions.

Table 2.1 Examples of signs and symptoms that should raise suspicion of specific diagnoses grouped according to the main cardiac features

Phenotypic finding	Cardiac features	Diseases to consider
Sensorineural deafness	HCM	Mitochondrial diseases
		Anderson–Fabry disease
		LEOPARD syndrome
	DCM	Epicardin mutation
		Mitochondrial diseases
Muscle weakness	HCM	Mitochondrial diseases
		Glycogenosis
	DCM	Dystrophinopathies
		Sarcoglycanopathies
		Laminopathies
		Myotonic dystrophy
		Desminopathies
	RCM	Desminopathies
Learning difficulties, mental retardation	HCM	Mitochondrial diseases
		Noonan Syndrome
		Danon disease
	DCM	Dystrophinopathies
		Mitochondrial diseases
		Myotonic dystrophy
		FKTN mutations
	RCM	Noonan syndrome
Myotonia (involuntary muscle contraction with delayed relaxation)		Myotonic dystrophy (type 1 and type 2)
Paraesthesia/sensory abnormalities/ neuropathic pain	HCM	Amyloidosis
		Anderson–Fabry disease
	RCM	Amyloidosis

HCM hypertrophic cardiomyopathy, *DCM* dilated cardiomyopathy, *RCM* restrictive cardiomyopathy, *LEOPARD syndrome* lentigines, echocardiograph conduction abnormalities, ocular hypertelorism, pulmonary stenosis, abnormal genitalia, retardation of growth, and sensorineural deafness, *FKTN* fukutin

As with all imaging modalities, echocardiography rarely suggests a specific etiology, but it can be helpful in the context of a number of features in directing further investigation.

- Others: exercise test, nuclear imaging, endomyocardial biopsy

The key to diagnostic success is, therefore, a CMP-centered approach to clinical assessment coupled with a systematic stepwise use of cardiac and noncardiac diagnostic tests. The comparative diagnosis between different forms is also important from a prognostic and sometimes therapeutic point of view. Some clinical features of CMP can also vary within the same family, a phenomenon that indicates that sometimes there is not a clear-cut relationship between the mutation and its clinical consequences [34, 35].

Table 2.2 Examples of skin/eyes signs that should raise suspicion of specific cardiac features

Phenotypic finding	Cardiac features	Disease to be considered
Visual impairment	HCM	TTR-related amyloidosis (vitreous opacities, cotton wool type)
		Danon disease (retinitis pigmentosa)
		Anderson–Fabry disease (cataracts, corneal opacities)
	DCM	*CRYAB* (polar cataract) type 2 myotonic dystrophy (subcapsular cataract)
Carpal tunnel syndrome (bilateral)	HCM	TTR-related amyloidosis
	RCM	Amyloidosis
Lentigines/café au lait spots	HCM	LEOPARD syndrome
Angiokeratoma hypohidrosis	HCM	Anderson–Fabry disease
Palmoplantar keratoderma, woolly hair	ARVC	Naxos and Carvajal syndromes

HCM hypertrophic cardiomyopathy, *DCM* dilated cardiomyopathy, *RCM* restrictive cardiomyopathy, *ARVC* arrhythmogenic right ventricular cardiomyopathy, *TTR* transthyretin protein, *LEOPARD syndrome* lentigines, echocardiograph conduction abnormalities, ocular hypertelorism, pulmonary stenosis, abnormal genitalia, retardation of growth, and sensorineural deafness

Table 2.3 Laboratory findings that should raise the suspicion of specific cardiac features

High serum creatine kinase (CK)	HCM	Mitochondrial diseases
		Glycogenosis
		Danon disease
	DCM	Dystrophinopathies
		Sarcoglycanopathies
		Zaspopathies (*LDB3* gene)
		Laminopathies
		Myotonic dystrophy
		FKTN mutations
	RCM	Desminopathies
		Myofibrillar myopathies
Proteinuria with/without low glomerular filtration rate	HCM	Anderson–Fabry disease
	RCM	Amyloidosis
High transaminase	HCM	Mitochondrial diseases
		Glycogenosis
		Danon disease
High transferrin saturation/ hyperferritinemia	DCM	Hemochromatosis
	RCM	
Lactic acidosis	HCM	Mitochondrial diseases
	DCM	
Myoglobinuria	HCM	Mitochondrial diseases
	DCM	
Leukocytopenia	HCM	Mitochondrial diseases (*TAZ* gene/Barth syndrome)
	DCM	

HCM hypertrophic cardiomyopathy, *DCM* dilated cardiomyopathy, *RCM* restrictive cardiomyopathy, *ARVC* arrhythmogenic right ventricular cardiomyopathy, *TTR* transthyretin protein, *LEOPARD syndrome* lentigines, echocardiograph conduction abnormalities, ocular hypertelorism, pulmonary stenosis, abnormal genitalia, retardation of growth, and sensorineural deafness, *FKTN* fukutin, *TAZ* tafazzin

Table 2.4 Examples of electrocardiographic (ECG) abnormalities that should raise the suspicion of specific diagnoses grouped according to the main cardiac features

Phenotypic finding	Cardiac features	Diseases to be considered
Short PR/pre-excitation (WPW like)	HCM	Glycogenosis
		Danon
		PRKAG2
		Anderson–Fabry
		Mitochondrial disease
AV block	HCM	Amyloidosis
		Danon disease
	DCM	Laminopathy
		Emery Dreifuss
		Sarcoidosis
		Desminopathy
	RCM	Desmin-related cardiomyopathy
		Amyloidosis
Extreme LV hypertrophy (Sokolow criteria)	HCM	Danon disease
		Pompe disease
Low QRS voltage	HCM	Amyloidosis
Low P wave amplitude atrial standstill	DCM	Emery Dreifuss
Q waves in posterolateral leads	DCM	Dystrophin-related cardiomyopathy
		Limb-girdle muscular dystrophy
		Sarcoidosis
Inverted T waves in inferolateral leads Epsilon waves in inferolateral leads	ARVC	ARVC with biventricular involvement

WPW Wolff-Parkinson-White syndrome, *AV* arteriovenous, *LV* left ventricular, *HCM* hypertrophic cardiomyopathy, *DCM* dilated cardiomyopathy, *RCM* restrictive cardiomyopathy, *ARVC* arrhythmogenic right ventricular cardiomyopathy, *PRKAG2* protein kinase, AMP-activated, gamma 2 noncatalytic subunit

Table 2.5 Echocardiographic diagnostic clues grouped according to main morphological phenotype

Phenotypic findings	Cardiac features	Diseases to be considered
Increased interatrial septum thickness	HCM	Amyloidosis
Increased atrioventricular valve thickness		Amyloidosis; Anderson–Fabry disease
Increased RV free-wall thickness		Amyloidosis, myocarditis, Anderson–Fabry disease
Mild–moderate pericardial effusion		Amyloidosis, myocarditis
Ground-glass appearance of ventricular myocardium		Amyloidosis
Concentric LVH		Glycogenosis, Anderson–Fabry disease
Extreme concentric LVH		Danon disease, Pompe disease
Global hypokinesia (with/without LV dilatation)		Anderson–Fabry; mitochondrial disease; TTR-related amyloidosis; *PRKAG2* mutations; Danon disease; myocarditis; end-stage sarcomeric HCM

Table 2.5 (continued)

Phenotypic findings	Cardiac features	Diseases to be considered
LV noncompaction	DCM	Genetic DCM (more frequently sarcomeric mutations)
Posterolateral akinesia/dyskinesia		Dystrophin-related cardiomyopathy
Mild (absent) dilatation + akinetic/ dyskinetic segments with noncoronary distribution		Myocarditis; sarcoidosis
Coexistent LV segmental dysfunction	ARVC	Biventricular ARVC
Partial LV or RV apical obliteration	RCM	Endomyocardial fibrosis/ hypereosinophilia

LVH left ventricular hypertrophy, *LV* left ventricle, *RV* right ventricle, *HCM* hypertrophic cardiomyopathy, *DCM* dilated cardiomyopathy, *RCM* restrictive cardiomyopathy, *ARVC* arrhythmogenic right ventricular cardiomyopathy, *PRKAG2* protein kinase

Conclusions

Genotype–phenotype relationships are not always simple and clear, and diagnostic approach and possible interpretations may be complex. Different mutations in the same gene can cause apparently identical phenotypes as well as be associated with phenotypes that are radically different one from the other. It is necessary to bring genetics closer to clinical practice, to create a bridge between clinical observation and molecular genetics, thus helping identify a possible specific genetic background. Clinical assessment should not be restricted to cardiological examinations; indeed, CMP represent a challenging interface between cardiology and many other medical specialties. Another important aspect is recognizing red flags, which guide rational selection of further diagnostic tests, including genetic analysis, and thereby identification of specific CMP subtypes. Arbustini et al. proposed a descriptive nosology that combines morphofunctional traits and organ-system involvement with familial inheritance patterns, identified genetic defects, or other etiologies [36]. The current body of knowledge suggests a genetic basis for understanding CMP pathophysiology, provides potential targets for therapeutic intervention, contributes to diagnosis, allows for cascade screening, and occasionally informs prognosis [33].

References

1. Maron BJ, Towbin JA, Thiene G, Antzelevitch C, Corrado D, Arnett D, Moss AJ, Seidman CE, Young JB (2006) Contemporary definitions and classification of the cardiomyopathies: an American Heart Association Scientific Statement from the Council on Clinical Cardiology, Heart Failure and Transplantation Committee; Quality of Care and Outcomes Research and Functional Genomics and Translational Biology Interdisciplinary Working Groups; and Council on Epidemiology and Prevention. Circulation 113(14):1807–1816. doi:10.1161/CIRCULATIONAHA.106.174287

2. Wang RY, Lelis A, Mirocha J, Wilcox WR (2007) Heterozygous Fabry women are not just carriers, but have a significant burden of disease and impaired quality of life. Genet Med 9(1):34–45. doi:10.1097/GIM.0b013e31802d8321

3. Elliott P, Andersson B, Arbustini E, Bilinska Z, Cecchi F, Charron P, Dubourg O, Kuhl U, Maisch B, McKenna WJ, Monserrat L, Pankuweit S, Rapezzi C, Seferovic P, Tavazzi L, Keren A (2008) Classification of the cardiomyopathies: a position statement from the European Society Of Cardiology Working Group on Myocardial and Pericardial Diseases. Eur Heart J 29(2):270–276. doi:10.1093/eurheartj/ehm342

4. Hershberger RE, Cowan J, Morales A, Siegfried JD (2009) Progress with genetic cardiomyopathies: screening, counseling, and testing in dilated, hypertrophic, and arrhythmogenic right ventricular dysplasia/cardiomyopathy. Circ Heart Fail 2(3):253–261. doi:10.1161/CIRCHEARTFAILURE.108.817346

5. Arbustini E, Diegoli M, Morbini P, Dal Bello B, Banchieri N, Pilotto A, Magani F, Grasso M, Narula J, Gavazzi A, Vigano M, Tavazzi L (2000) Prevalence and characteristics of dystrophin defects in adult male patients with dilated cardiomyopathy. J Am Coll Cardiol 35(7): 1760–1768

6. Sinagra G, Di Lenarda A, Moretti M, Mestroni L, Pinamonti B, Perkan A, Salvi A, Pyxaras S, Bussani R, Silvestri F, Camerini F (2008) The challenge of cardiomyopathies in 2007. J Cardiovasc Med (Hagerstown) 9(6):545–554. doi:10.2459/JCM.0b013e3282f2c9f9

7. Chang AN, Potter JD (2005) Sarcomeric protein mutations in dilated cardiomyopathy. Heart Fail Rev 10(3):225–235. doi:10.1007/s10741-005-5252-6

8. Moller DV, Andersen PS, Hedley P, Ersboll MK, Bundgaard H, Moolman-Smook J, Christiansen M, Kober L (2009) The role of sarcomere gene mutations in patients with idiopathic dilated cardiomyopathy. Eur J Hum Genet 17(10):1241–1249. doi:10.1038/ejhg.2009.34

9. Herman DS, Lam L, Taylor MR, Wang L, Teekakirikul P, Christodoulou D, Conner L, DePalma SR, McDonough B, Sparks E, Teodorescu DL, Cirino AL, Banner NR, Pennell DJ, Graw S, Merlo M, Di Lenarda A, Sinagra G, Bos JM, Ackerman MJ, Mitchell RN, Murry CE, Lakdawala NK, Ho CY, Barton PJ, Cook SA, Mestroni L, Seidman JG, Seidman CE (2012) Truncations of titin causing dilated cardiomyopathy. N Engl J Med 366(7):619–628. doi:10.1056/NEJMoa1110186

10. Merlo M, Sinagra G, Carniel E, Slavov D, Zhu X, Barbati G, Spezzacatene A, Ramani F, Salcedo E, Di Lenarda A, Mestroni L, Taylor MR (2013) Poor prognosis of rare sarcomeric gene variants in patients with dilated cardiomyopathy. Clin Transl Sci. doi:10.1111/cts.12116

11. Sylvius N, Tesson F (2006) Lamin A/C and cardiac diseases. Curr Opin Cardiol 21(3): 159–165. doi:10.1097/01.hco.0000221575.33501.58

12. Taylor MR, Fain PR, Sinagra G, Robinson ML, Robertson AD, Carniel E, Di Lenarda A, Bohlmeyer TJ, Ferguson DA, Brodsky GL, Boucek MM, Lascor J, Moss AC, Li WL, Stetler GL, Muntoni F, Bristow MR, Mestroni L (2003) Natural history of dilated cardiomyopathy due to lamin A/C gene mutations. J Am Coll Cardiol 41(5):771–780

13. McNair WP, Ku L, Taylor MR, Fain PR, Dao D, Wolfel E, Mestroni L (2004) SCN5A mutation associated with dilated cardiomyopathy, conduction disorder, and arrhythmia. Circulation 110(15):2163–2167. doi:10.1161/01.CIR.0000144458.58660.BB

14. Elliott P, O'Mahony C, Syrris P, Evans A, Rivera Sorensen C, Sheppard MN, Carr-White G, Pantazis A, McKenna WJ (2010) Prevalence of desmosomal protein gene mutations in patients with dilated cardiomyopathy. Circ Cardiovasc Genet 3(4):314–322. doi:10.1161/CIRCGENETICS.110.937805

15. Watkins H, Ashrafian H, McKenna WJ (2008) The genetics of hypertrophic cardiomyopathy: teare redux. Heart 94(10):1264–1268. doi:10.1136/hrt.2008.154104

16. Millat G, Bouvagnet P, Chevalier P, Dauphin C, Jouk PS, Da Costa A, Prieur F, Bresson JL, Faivre L, Eicher JC, Chassaing N, Crehalet H, Porcher R, Rodriguez-Lafrasse C, Rousson R (2010) Prevalence and spectrum of mutations in a cohort of 192 unrelated patients with hypertrophic cardiomyopathy. Eur J Med Genet 53(5):261–267. doi:10.1016/j.ejmg.2010.07.007

17. Maron BJ, Maron MS, Semsarian C (2012) Genetics of hypertrophic cardiomyopathy after 20 years: clinical perspectives. J Am Coll Cardiol 60(8):705–715. doi:10.1016/j.jacc.2012.02.068

18. Saltzman AJ, Mancini-DiNardo D, Li C, Chung WK, Ho CY, Hurst S, Wynn J, Care M, Hamilton RM, Seidman GW, Gorham J, McDonough B, Sparks E, Seidman JG, Seidman CE, Rehm HL (2010) Short communication: the cardiac myosin binding protein C Arg502Trp mutation: a common cause of hypertrophic cardiomyopathy. Circ Res 106(9):1549–1552. doi:10.1161/CIRCRESAHA.109.216291
19. Watkins H, McKenna WJ, Thierfelder L, Suk HJ, Anan R, O'Donoghue A, Spirito P, Matsumori A, Moravec CS, Seidman JG et al (1995) Mutations in the genes for cardiac troponin T and alpha-tropomyosin in hypertrophic cardiomyopathy. N Engl J Med 332(16):1058–1064. doi:10.1056/NEJM199504203321603
20. Girolami F, Ho CY, Semsarian C, Baldi M, Will ML, Baldini K, Torricelli F, Yeates L, Cecchi F, Ackerman MJ, Olivotto I (2010) Clinical features and outcome of hypertrophic cardiomyopathy associated with triple sarcomere protein gene mutations. J Am Coll Cardiol 55(14):1444–1453. doi:10.1016/j.jacc.2009.11.062
21. Maron BJ, Maron MS, Semsarian C (2012) Double or compound sarcomere mutations in hypertrophic cardiomyopathy: a potential link to sudden death in the absence of conventional risk factors. Heart Rhythm 9(1):57–63. doi:10.1016/j.hrthm.2011.08.009
22. Fabris E, Brun F, Porto AG, Losurdo P, Vitali Serdoz L, Zecchin M, Severini GM, Mestroni L, Di Chiara A, Sinagra G (2013) Cardiac hypertrophy, accessory pathway, and conduction system disease in an adolescent: the PRKAG2 cardiac syndrome. J Am Coll Cardiol 62(9):e17. doi:10.1016/j.jacc.2013.02.099
23. Alcalai R, Seidman JG, Seidman CE (2008) Genetic basis of hypertrophic cardiomyopathy: from bench to the clinics. J Cardiovasc Electrophysiol 19(1):104–110. doi:10.1111/j.1540-8167.2007.00965.x
24. Merner ND, Hodgkinson KA, Haywood AF, Connors S, French VM, Drenckhahn JD, Kupprion C, Ramadanova K, Thierfelder L, McKenna W, Gallagher B, Morris-Larkin L, Bassett AS, Parfrey PS, Young TL (2008) Arrhythmogenic right ventricular cardiomyopathy type 5 is a fully penetrant, lethal arrhythmic disorder caused by a missense mutation in the TMEM43 gene. Am J Hum Genet 82(4):809–821. doi:10.1016/j.ajhg.2008.01.010
25. Rigato I, Bauce B, Rampazzo A, Zorzi A, Pilichou K, Mazzotti E, Migliore F, Perazzolo Marra M, Lorenzon A, De Bortoli M, Calore M, Nava A, Daliento L, Gregori D, Iliceto S, Thiene G, Basso C, Corrado D (2013) Compound and digenic heterozygosity predicts life-time arrhythmic outcome and sudden cardiac death in desmosomal gene-related arrhythmogenic right ventricular cardiomyopathy. Circ Cardiovasc Genet. doi:10.1161/CIRCGENETICS.113.000288
26. Taylor M, Graw S, Sinagra G, Barnes C, Slavov D, Brun F, Pinamonti B, Salcedo EE, Sauer W, Pyxaras S, Anderson B, Simon B, Bogomolovas J, Labeit S, Granzier H, Mestroni L (2011) Genetic variation in titin in arrhythmogenic right ventricular cardiomyopathy-overlap syndromes. Circulation 124(8):876–885. doi:10.1161/CIRCULATIONAHA.110.005405
27. Sen-Chowdhry S, Syrris P, McKenna WJ (2010) Genetics of restrictive cardiomyopathy. Heart Fail Clin 6(2):179–186. doi:10.1016/j.hfc.2009.11.005
28. Pantazis AA, Elliott PM (2009) Left ventricular noncompaction. Curr Opin Cardiol 24(3):209–213. doi:10.1097/HCO.0b013e32832a11e7
29. Kohli SK, Pantazis AA, Shah JS, Adeyemi B, Jackson G, McKenna WJ, Sharma S, Elliott PM (2008) Diagnosis of left-ventricular non-compaction in patients with left-ventricular systolic dysfunction: time for a reappraisal of diagnostic criteria? Eur Heart J 29(1):89–95. doi:10.1093/eurheartj/ehm481
30. Ackerman MJ, Priori SG, Willems S, Berul C, Brugada R, Calkins H, Camm AJ, Ellinor PT, Gollob M, Hamilton R, Hershberger RE, Judge DP, Le Marec H, McKenna WJ, Schulze-Bahr E, Semsarian C, Towbin JA, Watkins H, Wilde A, Wolpert C, Zipes DP (2011) HRS/EHRA expert consensus statement on the state of genetic testing for the channelopathies and cardiomyopathies: this document was developed as a partnership between the Heart Rhythm Society (HRS) and the European Heart Rhythm Association (EHRA). Europace 13(8):1077–1109. doi:10.1093/europace/eur245
31. Pettersen MD (2014) Cardiomyopathies encountered commonly in the teenage years and their presentation. Pediatr Clin North Am 61(1):173–186. doi:10.1016/j.pcl.2013.09.017

32. Rapezzi C, Arbustini E, Caforio AL, Charron P, Gimeno-Blanes J, Helio T, Linhart A, Mogensen J, Pinto Y, Ristic A, Seggewiss H, Sinagra G, Tavazzi L, Elliott PM (2013) Diagnostic work-up in cardiomyopathies: bridging the gap between clinical phenotypes and final diagnosis. A position statement from the ESC Working Group on Myocardial and Pericardial Diseases. Eur Heart J 34(19):1448–1458. doi:10.1093/eurheartj/ehs397
33. Sinagra G, Mestroni L, Camerini F (2013) Genetic cardiomyopathies: a clinical approach, 1st edn. Springer, Milan. doi:10.1007/978-88-470-2757-2
34. Watkins H, Ashrafian H, Redwood C (2011) Inherited cardiomyopathies. N Engl J Med 364(17):1643–1656. doi:10.1056/NEJMra0902923
35. Lopes LR, Elliott PM (2013) New approaches to the clinical diagnosis of inherited heart muscle disease. Heart 99(19):1451–1461. doi:10.1136/heartjnl-2012-301995
36. Arbustini E, Narula N, Dec GW, Reddy KS, Greenberg B, Kushwaha S, Marwick T, Pinney S, Bellazzi R, Favalli V, Kramer C, Roberts R, Zoghbi WA, Bonow R, Tavazzi L, Fuster V, Narula J (2013) The MOGE(S) classification for a phenotype-genotype nomenclature of cardiomyopathy: endorsed by the World Heart Federation. J Am Coll Cardiol 62(22):2046–2072. doi:10.1016/j.jacc.2013.08.1644

Role of Basic and Advanced Imaging in Cardiomyopathies

3

Elena Abate, Bruno Pinamonti, Laura Massa, Giancarlo Vitrella, Giorgio Faganello, Manuel Belgrano, and Lorenzo Pagnan

3.1 Introduction

Basic and advanced imaging plays a pivotal role in cardiomyopathies (CMP), not only for determining the diagnosis but also for assessing prognosis, guiding patient management, detecting disease progression, evaluating treatment, and screening asymptomatic relatives of individuals affected by familial forms of the disease (Table 3.1).

3.2 Diagnosis

Transthoracic echocardiography (TTE) is an optimal, low-cost, highly reproducible, noninvasive diagnostic tool that can often provide a comprehensive evaluation of the typical morphological and functional characteristics of CMP. However, different CMP can share common echocardiographic features, and differential diagnosis among the specific types of CMP can be particularly difficult. For example, left ventricular (LV) dilation and systolic dysfunction can be found not only in idiopathic dilated cardiomyopathy (DCM) but also in advanced hypertrophic cardiomyopathy

E. Abate, MD (✉) • B. Pinamonti, MD • L. Massa, MD (✉) • G. Vitrella, MD
Department of Cardiology, University Hospital of Trieste,
via P. Valdoni 7, Trieste 34139, Italy
e-mail: abate.elena@gmail.com; bruno.pinamonti@gmail.com;
laura.massa@aots.sanita.fvg.it; giancarlo.vitrella@gmail.com

G. Faganello, MD
Cardiovascular Center, Azienda per i Servizi Sanitari n° 1, via Slataper, 9,
Trieste 34125, Italy
e-mail: giorgio.faganello@libero.it

M. Belgrano, MD • L. Pagnan, MD
Radiology Unit, University Hospital of Trieste, via P. Valdoni 7, Trieste 34139, Italy
e-mail: belgranom@gmail.com; pagny@inwind.it

B. Pinamonti, G. Sinagra (eds.), *Clinical Echocardiography and Other Imaging Techniques in Cardiomyopathies*, DOI 10.1007/978-3-319-06019-4_3,
© Springer International Publishing Switzerland 2014

Table 3.1 Main objectives of imaging studies in cardiomyopathies (CMP)

Objectives	
Diagnosis	Evaluate typical morphological and functional characteristics of CMP and differential diagnosis (red flags)
Prognosis	Imaging indices with prognostic value: LV dilation and systolic/diastolic dysfunction (RFP), LV remodeling and dyssynchrony, LV viability, RV involvement, functional MR and TR, intracavitary thrombosis, LA dilation, pulmonary hypertension, LV OT gradient, LGE, abnormal MIBG uptake
Follow-up	Detect changes in functional cardiac parameters
	Evaluate reversible forms of CMP
Treatment	Measure LV EF for indication to ICD or CRT
	Detect valvulopathy for correction (percutaneous vs. surgical)
	Detect ischemia for revascularization
	Detect intracavitary thrombosis for anticoagulation
	Role in the evaluation for heart transplantation
	LV OT obstructive gradient for septal reduction
	Indicate pericardial resection in CP
Screening	Familial disease forms

CP constrictive pericarditis, *CRT* cardiac resynchronization therapy, *EF* ejection fraction, *ICD* implantable cardioverter defibrillator, *LA* left atrial, *LGE* late gadolinium enhancement, *LV* left ventricular, *MIBG* 123-metaiodobenzylguanidine, *MR* mitral regurgitation, *OT* outflow tract, *RFP* restrictive filling pattern, *RV* right ventricular, *TR* tricuspid regurgitation

(HCM), arrhythmogenic right ventricular cardiomyopathy (ARVC) with biventricular involvement, myocarditis, and – more commonly – in ischemic, hypertensive, or valvular heart diseases [1]. Some authors have therefore suggested the search for diagnostic clues (red flags) to identify specific pathologies and discriminate among the various diseases [2]: namely, in the presence of a hypertrophic phenotype, a ground-glass appearance of the myocardium associated with increased thickness of interatrial septum, atrioventricular valves, and right ventricular (RV) wall, as well as mild pericardial effusion, are imaging clues suggesting the diagnosis of cardiac amyloidosis (CA). Furthermore, transesophageal echocardiography (TEE) and stress echocardiography can add some information in specific patients. In particular, TEE can better assess the mechanism and severity of valvular diseases; dobutamine stress echocardiography can detect a biphasic response typical of ischemic heart disease and distinguish between true aortic valve stenosis and pseudostenosis associated with DCM.

Advanced noninvasive imaging techniques, such as cardiac magnetic resonance (CMR) imaging, computed tomography (CT), and nuclear imaging, can be useful in selected and more challenging cases in which echocardiography does not provide a definite diagnosis. CMR, in particular, permits a highly accurate measure of LV and RV volumes, ejection fraction (EF), wall thickness, and mass; moreover, it is considered the diagnostic method of choice for anatomical and functional RV evaluation in suspected ARVC [3] and for distinguishing between LV noncompaction versus DCM with prominent apical trabeculations or apical HCM [4]. The presence and distribution pattern of late gadolinium enhancement (LGE) is paramount in differentiating ischemic heart disease from other forms of CMP [5]. In case of suspected myocarditis, CMR can provide additional information, detecting myocardial edema in the acute phase of the disease [6]. Moreover, thanks to its high negative predictive value for coronary artery disease diagnosis, coronary angio-CT is useful to distinguish between ischemic and nonischemic CMP [7]. Nuclear imaging can add important information regarding myocardial perfusion and viability. Furthermore, sympathetic cardiac imaging is now employed to study myocardial intake of 123-metaiodobenzylguanidine (MIBG), which is significantly reduced in idiopathic DCM [8].

3.3   Prognosis

The major prognostic echocardiographic markers in DCM patients are the amount of LV dilation and systolic dysfunction, LV remodeling and dyssynchrony [9], RV involvement [10], functional mitral regurgitation (MR) [11], intracavitary thrombosis [12], and a restrictive filling pattern (RFP) of the LV [13]. A previous study demonstrated the value of monitoring the LV filling pattern with TTE during invasive treatment: reversibility of the RFP was correlated with better long-term outcome [14]. Also, reassessment of the LV filling pattern after optimal medical therapy is essential, given the fact that a persistent RFP denotes a worse prognosis [15]. Finally, the presence of viability shown on a dobutamine stress test is correlated with better survival and higher likelihood of improved LV function in DCM patients [16].

Regarding HCM, several echocardiographic parameters have demonstrated prognostic value: a maximum wall thickness >30 mm is considered one of the major risk factors for sudden death (SD); moreover, a resting LV outflow tract (OT) gradient >30 mmHg, presence of LV systolic dysfunction, apical aneurysms, increased LV mass, and left atrial (LA) dilation denote a worse prognosis [17–19]. As in DCM, evidence of diastolic dysfunction has clinical and prognostic value also in HCM: the presence or persistence of RFP identifies more symptomatic patients with a significantly worse prognosis and with increased risk of evolution to end-stage HCM [17, 20].

In restrictive cardiomyopathy (RCM), transmitral- and pulmonary-vein-flow Doppler imaging patterns not only allow assessment of hemodynamic severity of the disease but also have prognostic value [13]. Furthermore, LA diameter >60 mm is a negative prognostic factor, especially in older patients with advanced New York Heart Association (NYHA) class [21]. In ARVC, evidence of severe RV dilation and dysfunction, as well as LV involvement, portends a worse prognosis [22, 23]. In CA, LV wall thickness ≥15 mm, LV fractional shortening ≤20 %, and presence of RFP characterize patients with lower survival potential [24, 25].

Studies on myocarditis show that LV dysfunction at diagnosis indicates a worse outcome even in the absence of clinical signs of heart failure (HF) [26, 27]. Other authors demonstrated that RV systolic dysfunction is an independent predictor of adverse outcome in these patients [28].

Also CMR provides important information when risk stratifying patients with CMP, particularly by detecting LGE, which is consistent with fibrosis. In DCM patients, baseline presence and transmurality of LGE in a myocardial segment are inversely related to its functional improvement at follow-up, even in optimal medical therapy [29], and are markers of diastolic dysfunction [30]. Presence and extent of LGE also demonstrate an association with adverse outcome [31]. Therefore, according to some authors, LGE might help in the arrhythmic risk stratification of patients, indicating use of an implantable cardioverter defibrillator (ICD) [31].

LGE, particularly in the lateral and posterior LV wall, is also inversely related to functional improvement after cardiac resynchronization therapy (CRT) [32].

In HCM, the evidence of myocardial ischemia (in the absence of epicardial disease) and abnormal myocardial blood flow reserve (compatible with microvascular dysfunction) detected with CMR and positron emission tomography (PET) is associated with arrhythmias, LV remodeling, systolic dysfunction, and risk of cardiovascular mortality [33]. Moreover, presence of diffuse LGE at CMR is a risk factor for SD in HCM, in association with maximal LV wall thickness and evidence of LV OT obstruction [34]. The presence of LGE denotes an increased mortality risk also in patients with myocarditis [35, 36]. Finally, analysis of sympathetic cardiac innervation with MIBG may be prognostically useful in HF patients and may help in selecting patients for ICD therapy: preliminary data indicate that abnormal MIBG uptake is a predictor for ventricular arrhythmia recurrence [37], increased incidence of SD, and appropriate ICD discharges [38]. Also, it is independently related to HF progression and cardiac mortality risk [39].

3.4 Follow-up

TTE is the imaging approach of choice for the follow-up of patients with CMP. Serial TTE evaluations during disease course demonstrate incremental prognostic value compared with the single basal TTE assessment [26, 27]. Furthermore, medical treatment must be adjusted according to clinical parameters as well as to echocardiographic data at follow-up [40]. Additionally, TTE examinations are pivotal for detecting deterioration as well as improvement in functional cardiac parameters, considering the fact that initial indications for aggressive and invasive treatments might no longer persist after optimal medical therapy [41].

In DCM, detecting LV systolic function improvement [42], reverse LV remodeling, and RFP reversibility [15] allows identification of patients with excellent long-term outcome [41].

Furthermore, a subgroup of HCM patients (~5 %) can present evolution with LV remodeling and progressive LV dilation and dysfunction, with wall thinning and diffuse LV hypokinesis resembling DCM. In this phase, a differential diagnosis between the two CMP is particularly difficult; serial imaging evaluation is therefore important to detect disease evolution [43].

Finally, TTE assessment at follow-up is important in assessing the evolution of the reversible forms of CMP (inflammatory, alcoholic, tachy-induced, stress-induced, chemotherapy-induced, hypertensive, peripartum): normalization of echocardiographic parameters once the etiological factor is removed denotes an excellent prognosis [26, 27].

3.5 Treatment

Imaging has an important role in managing patients with CMP and provides useful information necessary for choosing the best treatment option. Accurate imaging assessment of LV EF is important for indicating ICD and CRT. Furthermore, evaluation of mechanical dyssynchrony demonstrates potential value for selecting patients for CRT. Detecting valvulopathy associated with LV dysfunction has important therapeutic consequences: functional MR in DCM can be treated with mitral annuloplasty [44] and percutaneous mitral valve (MV) repair with MitraClip implantation [45]. Echocardiography plays an important role in patient selection, during the procedure, and in the follow-up of these patients. Diagnosing ischemic CMP has potential therapeutic implications such as percutaneous or surgical revascularization, particularly if reversibility of LV dysfunction is demonstrated at dobutamine stress test. Identifying intracavitary thrombosis or spontaneous echocontrast in association with severe LV systolic dysfunction might indicate the need for anticoagulation therapy.

Patients with DCM and severe HF refractory to medical therapy are usually referred to heart transplantation. Indications do not include echocardiographic data. However, a complete echo-Doppler study is helpful in excluding potential contraindications (severe pulmonary hypertension), in selecting alternative treatment strategies, and in supporting prognostic assessment; for instance, persistent RFP might have an additional incremental value in patient selection for this treatment [46].

Detection of a significant LV intraventricular obstructive gradient at rest or during echo stress in HCM patients suggests the possible indication for surgical or percutaneous septal reduction [47]. Contrast echocardiography (with contrast injection in septal coronary vessels during coronary angiography) provides guidance during percutaneous alcohol septal ablation by identifying the vessel that supplies the targeted myocardial territory [48]. Intraoperative TEE offers important information during surgical septal myectomy. In addition, MV abnormalities are rather common in HCM: evaluation of MV anatomical features predictive of successful valve repair therefore seems important [49].

Finally, distinguishing between RCM and constrictive pericarditis (CP) by imaging pericardial thickening using CMR or CT, and studying respiratory variations of transmitral and tricuspid velocities by Doppler TTE have important therapeutic implications given the possibility of surgical treatment with pericardial resection in CP.

3.6 Screening

Imaging plays a role also in screening asymptomatic relatives of individuals affected by familial forms of the disease. TTE is the most feasible technique in this setting. CMR should be considered in selected patients with equivocal TTE.

References

1. Pinamonti B, Cacciatore G (2002) Dilated cardiomyopathy: indication and role of non-invasive instrumental evaluation. Ital Heart J Suppl 3:405–411
2. Rapezzi C, Arbustini E, Caforio AL et al (2013) Diagnostic work-up in cardiomyopathies: bridging the gap between clinical phenotypes and final diagnosis. A position statement from the ESC Working Group on Myocardial and Pericardial Diseases. Eur Heart J 34:1448–1458

3. Blake LM, Scheinman MM, Higgins CB (1994) MR features of arrhythmogenic right ventricular dysplasia. AJR Am J Roentgenol 162:809–812
4. Cheng H, Zhao S, Jiang S et al (2011) Comparison of cardiac magnetic resonance imaging features of isolated left ventricular non-compaction in adults versus dilated cardiomyopathy in adults. Clin Radiol 66:853–860
5. McCrohon JA, Moon JC, Prasad SK et al (2003) Differentiation of heart failure related to dilated cardiomyopathy and coronary artery disease using gadolinium-enhanced cardiovascular magnetic resonance. Circulation 108:54–59
6. Friedrich MG, Strohm O, Schulz-Menger J et al (1998) Contrast media-enhanced magnetic resonance imaging visualizes myocardial changes in the course of viral myocarditis. Circulation 97:1802–1809
7. Budoff MJ, Shavelle DM, Lamont DH et al (1998) Usefulness of electron beam computed tomography scanning for distinguishing ischemic from nonischemic cardiomyopathy. J Am Coll Cardiol 32:1173–1178
8. Glowniak JV, Turner FE, Gray LL et al (1989) Iodine-123 metaiodobenzylguanidine imaging of the heart in idiopathic congestive cardiomyopathy and cardiac transplants. J Nucl Med 30:1182–1191
9. Douglas PS, Morrow R, Ioli A et al (1989) Left ventricular shape, afterload and survival in idiopathic dilated cardiomyopathy. J Am Coll Cardiol 13:311–315
10. Ghio S, Recusani F, Klersy C et al (2000) Prognostic usefulness of the tricuspid annular plane systolic excursion in patients with congestive heart failure secondary to idiopathic or ischemic dilated cardiomyopathy. Am J Cardiol 85:837–842
11. Junker A, Thayssen P, Nielsen B et al (1993) The hemodynamic and prognostic significance of echo-Doppler-proven mitral regurgitation in patients with dilated cardiomyopathy. Cardiology 83:14–20
12. Faris R, Coats AJ, Henein MY (2002) Echocardiography-derived variables predict outcome in patients with nonischemic dilated cardiomyopathy with or without a restrictive filling pattern. Am Heart J 144:343–350
13. Pinamonti B, Di Lenarda A, Sinagra G et al (1993) Restrictive left ventricular filling pattern in dilated cardiomyopathy assessed by Doppler echocardiography: clinical, echocardiographic and hemodynamic correlations and prognostic implications. Heart Muscle Disease Study Group. J Am Coll Cardiol 22:808–815
14. Pozzoli M, Traversi E, Cioffi G et al (1997) Loading manipulations improve the prognostic value of Doppler evaluation of mitral flow in patients with chronic heart failure. Circulation 95:1222–1230
15. Pinamonti B, Zecchin M, Di Lenarda A et al (1997) Persistence of restrictive left ventricular filling pattern in dilated cardiomyopathy: an ominous prognostic sign. J Am Coll Cardiol 29:604–612
16. Pinamonti B, Perkan A, Di Lenarda A et al (2002) Dobutamine echocardiography in idiopathic dilated cardiomyopathy: clinical and prognostic implications. Eur J Heart Fail 4:49–61
17. Pinamonti B, Di Lenarda A, Nucifora G et al (2008) Incremental prognostic value of restrictive filling pattern in hypertrophic cardiomyopathy: a Doppler echocardiographic study. Eur J Echocardiogr 9:466–471
18. Thaman R, Gimeno JR, Murphy RT et al (2005) Prevalence and clinical significance of systolic impairment in hypertrophic cardiomyopathy. Heart 91:920–925
19. Yang H, Woo A, Monakier D et al (2005) Enlarged left atrial volume in hypertrophic cardiomyopathy: a marker for disease severity. J Am Soc Echocardiogr 18:1074–1082
20. Pinamonti B, Merlo M, Nangah R et al (2010) The progression of left ventricular systolic and diastolic dysfunctions in hypertrophic cardiomyopathy: clinical and prognostic significance. J Cardiovasc Med (Hagerstown) 11:669–677
21. Ammash NM, Seward JB, Bailey KR et al (2000) Clinical profile and outcome of idiopathic restrictive cardiomyopathy. Circulation 101:2490–2496
22. Pinamonti B, Dragos AM, Pyxaras SA et al (2011) Prognostic predictors in arrhythmogenic right ventricular cardiomyopathy: results from a 10-year registry. Eur Heart J 32:1105–1113

23. Sen-Chowdhry S, Morgan RD, Chambers JC et al (2010) Arrhythmogenic cardiomyopathy: etiology, diagnosis, and treatment. Annu Rev Med 61:233–253
24. Buja LM, Khoi NB, Roberts WC (1970) Clinically significant cardiac amyloidosis. Clinicopathologic findings in 15 patients. Am J Cardiol 26:394–405
25. Klein AL, Hatle LK, Taliercio CP et al (1991) Prognostic significance of Doppler measures of diastolic function in cardiac amyloidosis. A Doppler echocardiography study. Circulation 83:808–816
26. Anzini M, Moretti M, Merlo M et al (2013) Controversial issues and working practice in myocarditis: from scientific data to clinical grounds. G Ital Cardiol (Rome) 14:504–516
27. Anzini M, Merlo M, Sabbadini G et al (2013) Long-term evolution and prognostic stratification of biopsy-proven active myocarditis. Circulation 128:2384–2394
28. Mendes LA, Dec GW, Picard MH et al (1994) Right ventricular dysfunction: an independent predictor of adverse outcome in patients with myocarditis. Am Heart J 128:301–307
29. Leong DP, Chakrabarty A, Shipp N et al (2012) Effects of myocardial fibrosis and ventricular dyssynchrony on response to therapy in new-presentation idiopathic dilated cardiomyopathy: insights from cardiovascular magnetic resonance and echocardiography. Eur Heart J 33:640–648
30. Moreo A, Ambrosio G, De Chiara B et al (2009) Influence of myocardial fibrosis on left ventricular diastolic function: noninvasive assessment by cardiac magnetic resonance and echo. Circ Cardiovasc Imaging 2:437–443
31. Iles L, Pfluger H, Lefkovits L et al (2011) Myocardial fibrosis predicts appropriate device therapy in patients with implantable cardioverter-defibrillators for primary prevention of sudden cardiac death. J Am Coll Cardiol 57:821–828
32. Chalil S, Foley PW, Muyhaldeen SA et al (2007) Late gadolinium enhancement-cardiovascular magnetic resonance as a predictor of response to cardiac resynchronization therapy in patients with ischaemic cardiomyopathy. Europace 9:1031–1037
33. Maron MS, Olivotto I, Maron BJ et al (2009) The case for myocardial ischemia in hypertrophic cardiomyopathy. J Am Coll Cardiol 54:866–875
34. Olivotto I, Gistri R, Petrone P et al (2003) Maximum left ventricular thickness and risk of sudden death in patients with hypertrophic cardiomyopathy. J Am Coll Cardiol 41:315–321
35. Grun S, Schumm J, Greulich S et al (2012) Long-term follow-up of biopsy-proven viral myocarditis: predictors of mortality and incomplete recovery. J Am Coll Cardiol 59:1604–1615
36. Mahrholdt H, Wagner A, Deluigi CC et al (2006) Presentation, patterns of myocardial damage, and clinical course of viral myocarditis. Circulation 114:1581–1590
37. Akutsu Y, Kaneko K, Kodama Y et al (2008) Cardiac sympathetic nerve abnormality predicts ventricular tachyarrhythmic events in patients without conventional risk of sudden death. Eur J Nucl Med Mol Imaging 35:2066–2073
38. Nagahara D, Nakata T, Hashimoto A et al (2008) Predicting the need for an implantable cardioverter defibrillator using cardiac metaiodobenzylguanidine activity together with plasma natriuretic peptide concentration or left ventricular function. J Nucl Med 49:225–233
39. Kasama S, Toyama T, Sumino H et al (2008) Prognostic value of serial cardiac 123I-MIBG imaging in patients with stabilized chronic heart failure and reduced left ventricular ejection fraction. J Nucl Med 49:907–914
40. Merlo M, Pyxaras SA, Pinamonti B et al (2011) Prevalence and prognostic significance of left ventricular reverse remodeling in dilated cardiomyopathy receiving tailored medical treatment. J Am Coll Cardiol 57:1468–1476
41. Zecchin M, Merlo M, Pivetta A et al (2012) How can optimization of medical treatment avoid unnecessary implantable cardioverter-defibrillator implantations in patients with idiopathic dilated cardiomyopathy presenting with "SCD-HeFT criteria?". Am J Cardiol 109:729–735
42. Cintron G, Johnson G, Francis G et al (1993) Prognostic significance of serial changes in left ventricular ejection fraction in patients with congestive heart failure. The V-HeFT VA Cooperative Studies Group. Circulation 87(6 Suppl):VI17–VI23
43. Olivotto I, Cecchi F, Gistri R et al (2006) Relevance of coronary microvascular flow impairment to long-term remodeling and systolic dysfunction in hypertrophic cardiomyopathy. J Am Coll Cardiol 47:1043–1048

44. Bolling SF, Pagani FD, Deeb GM et al (1998) Intermediate-term outcome of mitral reconstruction in cardiomyopathy. J Thorac Cardiovasc Surg 115:381–388
45. Franzen O, van der Heyden J, Baldus S et al (2011) MitraClip(R) therapy in patients with end-stage systolic heart failure. Eur J Heart Fail 13:569–576
46. Hansen A, Haass M, Zugck C et al (2001) Prognostic value of Doppler echocardiographic mitral inflow patterns: implications for risk stratification in patients with chronic congestive heart failure. J Am Coll Cardiol 37:1049–1055
47. Olivotto I, Montereggi A, Mazzuoli F et al (1999) Clinical utility and safety of exercise testing in patients with hypertrophic cardiomyopathy. G Ital Cardiol 29:11–19
48. Faber L, Seggewiss H, Gleichmann U (1998) Percutaneous transluminal septal myocardial ablation in hypertrophic obstructive cardiomyopathy: results with respect to intraprocedural myocardial contrast echocardiography. Circulation 98:2415–2421
49. Kaple RK, Murphy RT, DiPaola LM et al (2008) Mitral valve abnormalities in hypertrophic cardiomyopathy: echocardiographic features and surgical outcomes. Ann Thorac Surg 85(5):1527–1535

Part II

Dilated Cardiomyopathy

Dilated Cardiomyopathy: Clinical Assessment and Differential Diagnosis

Marco Merlo, Anita Spezzacatene, Davide Stolfo, Francesca Brun, and Gianfranco Sinagra

4.1 Introduction

Dilated cardiomyopathy (DCM) is a heart-muscle disorder characterized by systolic dysfunction and dilatation of the left ventricular (LV) cavity, with normal LV wall thickness. Sometimes, both ventricles are dilated and dysfunctional, but the involvement of the right ventricle (RV) is neither necessary nor sufficient for the diagnosis of DCM. This disease represents a relevant health problem in adult and pediatric populations, as it is associated with important morbidity and mortality rates and with frequent hospital admissions. Moreover, it is the third cause of heart failure (HF) and the first cause of heart transplant.

The estimated prevalence of DCM is about 1:2,500 of the general population, whereas the incidence is about 7:100,000 inhabitants per year [1]. However, due to the fact that many patients remain asymptomatic for a very long period until the onset of a marked ventricular dysfunction, the real incidence and prevalence of DCM could be significantly higher than the reported.

Males are more frequently affected than females, with an ~3:1 ratio [1], and symptoms tend to be age related, as they appear more frequently around the fourth to fifth decade of life, even though pediatric onset is not so rare. Familial/genetic forms are usually characterized by incomplete penetrance and variable age-related expression.

M. Merlo (✉) • A. Spezzacatene • D. Stolfo • F. Brun • G. Sinagra, MD, FESC
Department of Cardiology, University Hospital of Trieste,
via P. Valdoni 7, Trieste 34139, Italy
e-mail: supermerloo@libero.it; anita.spe@gmail.com; davide.stolfo@gmail.com;
frabrun77@gmail.com; gianfranco.sinagra@aots.sanita.fvg.it

B. Pinamonti, G. Sinagra (eds.), *Clinical Echocardiography and Other Imaging Techniques in Cardiomyopathies*, DOI 10.1007/978-3-319-06019-4_4,
© Springer International Publishing Switzerland 2014

4.2   Etiology

DCM can be familial or nonfamilial. Familial DCM accounts for only 30–48 % of cases of DCM, and the main pattern of inheritance is autosomal dominant (56 %). Autosomal recessive pattern accounts for 16 % of cases with genetic characterization, followed by X-linked forms (10 %), autosomal dominant forms associated with subclinical skeletal muscle disease (7.7 %), and nonclassifiable forms (7.7 %) [2].

The majority of nonfamilial forms have an acquired etiology, such as cardiotoxic drugs, alcohol abuse, heavy metals, autoimmune disorders, neuromuscular diseases, or infective agents, such as viral (coxsackievirus, adenovirus, parvovirus, HIV), bacterial (Borrelia, Rickettsia), mycobacterial, and fungal or parasitic (*Trypanosoma cruzi*). However, a genetic cause can be found in some apparently sporadic cases (new mutation, incomplete penetrance). Finally, a consistent group of DCM has no apparent cause and must be classified as idiopathic.

4.3   Clinical Phenotype

In DCM, the phenotype is widely heterogeneous: age of onset, clinical characteristics, and severity vary not only among different families, but also among members of the same family. Affected patients usually present signs and symptoms of HF associated with other cardiac manifestations, such as conduction disturbances [left bundle branch block (LBBB) or atrioventricular blocks], arrhythmias, and/or valvular diseases, such as functional mitral or tricuspid regurgitation. Complications, such as thromboembolism, and sudden death (SD) are not rare. A typical pattern of onset is characterized by a long clinically silent period of many years, and then the disease can become evident after a flu-like syndrome: during a prolonged recovery period, the patient suffers from dyspnea, extreme fatigue, and signs of HF-like edema. A study conducted in Trieste [3] reported the clinical/instrumental characteristics of DCM patients at first presentation according to the decade of enrolment (from 1978 to 2007) (Table 4.1). Progressive earlier diagnosis over time is clear: patients enrolled in the most recent decades had a progressively shorter history of HF, were less symptomatic for HF, and had less severe heart disease. Furthermore, patients with a previous history of HF episodes at enrolment progressively decreased in number, probably as an effect of systematic familial screening. Familial screening in DCM facilitates diagnosis in nonprobands at an early stage of disease, which is characterized by a less compromised LV and lower prevalence of LBBB, thus favorably impacting on the long-term prognosis [4].

4.4   Diagnostic Criteria

After clinical suspicion or screening, DCM is diagnosed by demonstration at imaging (typically 2D echocardiography) of LV dilatation and systolic dysfunction after excluding specific causes sufficient to determine the degree of myocardial

Table 4.1 Baseline clinical–instrumental characteristics of idiopathic dilated cardiomyopathy (DCM) patients according to decade of enrolment in the Heart Muscle Diseases Registry of Trieste

	First decade, 1978–1987; 110 (12.8 %)	Second decade, 1988–1997; 376 (44.1 %)	Third decade, 1998–2007; 367 (43.1 %)	P value
Age (years)	46±17	44±15	45±14	0.425
Male gender (%)	74	73	71	0.856
Familial IDCM (%)	12	18	15	0.197
Duration of HF (months) [range]	2 [0–17][c]	3 [0–13][e]	0 [0–5]	**<0.001[g]**
SBP (mmHg)	126±14	124±16[e]	127±19	**0.020**
NYHA III–IV (%)	36[c, d]	23	25	**0.029**
Patients with previous episodes of HF (%)	87	79	66	<0.001
Anemia[a] (%)	9	12	10	0.456
GFR ≤60 ml/min (%)	15	8	11	0.336
Sinus rhythm (%)	84	90	89	0.222
LBBB (%)	26	32	30	0.464
LVEF (%)	29±9[c]	31±11[e]	33±11	**<0.001**
LVEDD-I (mm/m^2)	39±7[c,d]	37±6[e]	34±5	**<0.001**
LVEDV-I (ml/m^2)	114±60[c]	107±41[e]	91±34	**<0.001**
Restrictive filling pattern (%)		37[e]	17	**<0.001[f]**
Moderate–severe MR (%)[b]		39	34	0.157[f]
Beta-blockers after first evaluation (%)	11[c, d]	82	86	**<0.001**
ACE inhibitors or ARBs after first evaluation (%)	34[c, d]	93	93	**<0.001**
Digitalis after first evaluation (%)	66[c, d]	79[e]	38	**<0.001**
Aldosterone antagonists after first evaluation (%)	8	5[e]	18	**0.001**
ICD implantation during follow-up (%)	1[c, d]	14	13	**0.002**
Time from diagnosis to implantation (months) [range]	268	129 [99–165]	22 [2–47]	**<0.001[g]**
CRT implantation during follow-up (%)	0	6	6	0.301[f]
Time from diagnosis to implantation (months) [range]		151 [129–206]	23 [10–82]	**<0.001[f, g]**

Bold data *p* values <0.05

ARBs angiotensin receptor blockers, *BMI* body mass index, *CRT* cardiac resynchronization therapy, *GFR* glomerular filtration rate, *HF* heart failure, *ICD* implantable cardioverter defibrillator, *IDCM* idiopathic dilated cardiomyopathy, *LBBB* left bundle branch block, *LVEDD*-I indexed left ventricular end-diastolic diameter, *LVEDV-I* indexed left ventricular end-diastolic volume, *LVEF* left ventricular ejection fraction, *MR* mitral regurgitation, *SBP* systolic blood pressure

[a]Anemia: hemoglobin <13 g/dl for males, <12 g/dl for females
[b]MR with a jet area >4 cm^2 at color Doppler was classified as moderate or severe
[c]*P*<0.05 between first and third decades
[d]*P*<0.05 between first and second decades
[e]*P*<0.05 between second and third decades
[f]*P* value computed only between second and third decades
[g]Kruskal–Wallis *p* value

Table 4.2 Major and minor criteria for diagnosing DCM

Major criteria

1   LVEF 45 % (>2 SD) and/or FS <25 % (>2 SD), as ascertained by echocardiography, radionuclide scanning or angiography

2   LVEDD >117 % of the predicted value corrected for age and body surface area, which corresponds to 2 SD of the predicted normal limit +5 %

Minor criteria

1   Unexplained supraventricular (atrial fibrillation or sustained arrhythmias) or ventricular arrhythmias, frequent (>1,000 . 24 h^{-1}) or repetitive (three or more beats with >120 beats/min^{-1}) before the age of 50

2   LVEDD >112 % of predicted value

3   Left ventricular dysfunction: LVEF <50 % or FS <28 %

4   Unexplained conduction disease: 2 or 3 atrioventricular conduction defects, complete LVBBB, sinus nodal dysfunction

5   Unexplained sudden death or stroke before 50 years of age

6   Segmental wall-motion abnormalities (<1 segment, or 1 if not previously present) in the absence of intraventricular conduction defect or ischemic heart disease

Adapted from Mestroni et al. [5]

DCM dilated cardiomyopathy, *SD* standard deviation, *LVEF* left ventricular ejection fraction, *LVEDD* left ventricular end diastolic diameter, *FS* fractional shortening, *LVBBB* left ventricular bundle branch block

dysfunction and dilatation, such as systemic arterial hypertension (>160/100 mmHg), coronary heart disease (stenosis >50 % of the luminal diameter in a major branch), chronic excessive alcohol consumption (>100 g/day), rapid and sustained supraventricular arrhythmias, systemic diseases, pericardial diseases, congenital heart diseases, and cor pulmonale. Clinical examination, electrocardiography (ECG) and chest X-ray radiography are not specific for DCM, whereas on echocardiography, it is possible to evaluate disease criteria.

In 1999 a collaborative European study proposed a standardization of diagnostic criteria and methods of enrollment in familial DCM. Inclusion criteria were a LV ejection fraction (EF) <45 % documented at 2D echocardiography or angiography and/or a fractional shortening <25 % at M-mode echocardiography and an LV end-diastolic diameter >117 % of the predicted value corrected for age and body surface area (BSA). Familial DCM was diagnosed in the presence of two or more affected individuals in a single family or in the presence of a first-degree relative of a DCM patient, with well-documented, unexplained SD at <35 years of age. Moreover, major and minor criteria were formulated to distinguish affected, possibly affected, and nonaffected family members (Table 4.2) [5].

4.5   Prognostic Stratification and Therapy

Prognosis of patients with DCM has significantly improved compared to the past, when ~50 % of affected patients died within 2 years of diagnosis [6]. In the last decade, in particular, an 8-year survival rate of >85 % was estimated in DCM, with an incidence

Table 4.3 Occurrence of major events in the study population according to decade of enrolment in the Heart Muscle Diseases Registry of Trieste

	First decade, 1978–1987; 110 patients	Second decade, 1988–1997; 376 patients	Third decade, 1998–2007; 367 patients	P value, first vs. second decade	P value, first vs. third decade	P value, second vs. third decade
Mean follow-up (months)	151±29	153±82	93±41	0.389	**0.03**	**<0.001**
All-cause mortality/ heart transplant, n (%)	77 (70)	178 (47)	53 (14)	**<0.001**	**<0.001**	**<0.001**
Incidence (events/100 patients/years)	5.6	3.9	1.9			
Heart transplant, n (%)	6 (6)	51 (14)	17 (5)	**0.02**	0.724	**<0.001**
Incidence (events/100 patients/years)	0.4	1.1	0.6			
Cardiovascular death, n (%)	57 (52)	91 (24)	18 (5)	**<0.001**	**<0.001**	**<0.001**
Incidence (events/100 patients/years)	4.1	2.0	0.6			
Pump failure death, n (%)	38 (35)	32 (9)	6 (2)	**<0.001**	**<0.001**	**<0.001**
Incidence (events/100 patients/years)	2.8	0.7	0.2			
Unexpected sudden death, n (%)	16 (15)	51 (14)	9 (3)	0.793	**<0.001**	**<0.001**
Incidence (events/100 patients/years)	1.2	1.1	0.3			
Unknown cause death, n (%)	13 (12)	31 (9)	16 (4)	0.338	**0.004**	**0.014**
Incidence (events/100 patients/years)	1.0	0.7	0.6			
Appropriate intervention of ICD (% of implanted patients)	0	32	38	NC	NC	0.499
Incidence (events/100 implanted patients/ years)		2.4	4.8		NC	0.499

Bold data p values <0.05

ICD implantable cardioverter defibrillator, *NC* p value not calculated, only two patients implanted with ICD in the first decade

of fewer than two major events per 100 patients per year, significantly higher than in the previous two decades [3] (Table 4.3). Many factors contributed to the improvement during this time. First is earlier diagnosis, especially when the disease is diagnosed while still in the asymptomatic phase [7]. In this sense, familial screening is an important instrument for the early diagnosis of DCM in asymptomatic patients and can impact long-term survival [4]. Therefore, a systematic familial screening with clinical interview, physical examination, ECG, and echocardiography should be performed on all probands (even in sporadic cases) and their first-degree relatives from puberty to 50 years of age.

Another important factor that influences the better prognosis in DCM is evidence-based optimal medical treatment: many clinical trials demonstrated the beneficial role of angiotensin-converting enzyme (ACE) inhibitors (Enalapril) and beta-blockers (metoprolol, carvedilol, and bisoprolol) [8–11]. Also, nonpharmacological treatments, such as implantable cardioverter defibrillators (ICD) and cardiac resynchronization therapy (CRT) with a biventricular pacemaker impact favorably on DCM prognosis [12, 13].

Response to medical treatment can vary; it is estimated that cardiac function is normalized in one third of patients, one third remains stable, and one third worsens despite optimal medical treatment. Reasons for these differences are unknown, but probably, there is a genetic predisposition.

However, the role of follow-up over time should be considered essential, especially when considering LV reverse remodeling, which is associated with an impressively better outcome in terms of survival free from heart transplant and SD [14]. Therefore, an individualized, regular, long-term follow-up represents the cornerstone of good management of this disease due to the lack of prognostic models identifying precise subgroups of patients suitable for more aggressive and earlier therapies.

To date, the principal aims of therapy in DCM are to treat HF and prevent malignant arrhythmias and SD. Due to the fact that DCM is a rare disease, there are no specific randomized trials oriented specifically to treatment but only to HF in general.

Many studies demonstrated the efficacy of different drugs in alleviating symptoms and improving prognosis in patients with HF. ACE inhibitors [8], angiotensin receptor antagonists, beta-blockers [10], and antialdosterone agents (spironolactone and eplerenone) [15, 16] clearly impact survival, whereas diuretics such as furosemide relieve symptoms (they could also influence prognosis, but their role in this context has not yet been demonstrated). Anticoagulants can be used in select cases at higher risk of thromboembolism, especially in patients with LVEF <30 % and in those with atrial fibrillation. Not only drug type but also dosage optimization is fundamental in order to improve symptoms and positively impact on morbidity and mortality. Indeed, optimal medical therapy, defined as administration of evidence-based therapy at target dosages or maximum tolerated dosages, improves DCM prognosis, significantly increasing the survival-free from pump failure death. Moreover, CRT is useful in preventing HF death in patients with low LVEF (i.e., <35 %) and prolonged QRS mostly in advanced New York Heart Association (NYHA) classes, and lower functional classes [13, 17].

Concerning SD prevention, despite the proven effect of medical treatment with beta-blockers [18], ICD implantation proves to be the most valid therapeutic tool, as it dramatically decreased the incidence of SD in the past decade [3]. The device should be implanted at least 3 months after optimization of medical treatment [19], even though the related drawback could be loss of a nonnegligible proportion of patients in the meantime. The challenge is to identify which patients could benefit from an early ICD independent of optimized medical treatment [20].

New therapeutic options for HF are taking place. One is percutaneous mitral leaflet repair (MitraClip) in patients with severe functional mitral regurgitation (MR) at high risk of surgery. It is safe and effective in reducing MR, improving symptoms, and promoting reverse remodeling, with a reduction in LV volumes [21]. Another option in end-stage HF is implantation of a ventricular-assist device, which can support either LV or RV or both. It can be implanted as bridge to recovery or to heart transplantation or as destination therapy [22]. In case of refractory HF, when pharmacological and nonpharmacological treatment is no longer efficacious, the final option is heart transplant.

4.6 Problems in Differential Diagnosis

Ventricular dysfunction at imaging is not sufficient for the diagnosis of DCM as an exclusion diagnosis and represents a challenge for clinical cardiologists. In fact, many other conditions display the same abnormal pattern (Chaps. 5, 6 and 7).

Hypertensive heart disease in the dilated-hypokinetic stage [23] and ischemic heart disease with multivessel involvement are the most common examples encountered in clinical practice and should be excluded before establishing a diagnosis of idiopathic DCM. In the first case, LV dilatation and systolic dysfunction – frequently accompanied by overt HF – are present in patients with a long history of moderate to severe systemic hypertension. Previous documentation of LV hypertrophy with preserved LVEF can be present. LV hypertrophy usually remains evident, even if apparently reduced, in the overt HF hypokinetic phase, showing ECG and echocardiographic signs (i.e., LV eccentric hypertrophy with increased LV mass). On the other hand, chronic coronary artery disease may manifest as progressive HF without history of myocardial infarction or chest pain. This ischemic cardiomyopathy (CMP) is characterized by LV dilatation and systolic dysfunction and usually by segmental wall motion abnormalities (WMA) corresponding to ischemic ECG changes and coronary distribution. Also, some valvular diseases should be considered in the differential diagnosis of DCM. In fact, both severe MR and aortic stenosis (and, less frequently, aortic regurgitation or mitral stenosis) can lead to ventricular dysfunction due to severe volume or pressure overload, respectively. In this case, clinical and echocardiographic findings are fundamental in the differential diagnosis, and in selected cases, prompt surgical treatment could be decisive and can improve ventricular function.

When we excluded secondary causes of ventricular dysfunction, differential diagnosis of DCM remains necessary in the field of CMP. In fact, mild LV dilatation and ventricular WMA can be the result of active myocarditis that could mimic DCM, presenting frequently with HF or ventricular arrhythmias. Suggestive clinical history (i.e., new-onset HF in the absence of risk factors, recent flu-like syndrome), ECG (i.e., in some cases, low QRS voltage), echocardiography (i.e., ventricular dysfunction in the absence of severe dilatation, possible hypertrophic walls due to interstitial edema, WMA not corresponding to coronary distribution, intraventricular thrombi), and cardiac magnetic resonance (CMR) can orient treatment toward endomyocardial biopsy, the gold standard for diagnosis of myocarditis, and may guide correct patient management.

Other CMP could manifest with the dilated pattern and should be considered in the differential diagnosis [24]. For instance, sometimes it is difficult to distinguish DCM and arrhythmogenic right ventricular cardiomyopathy (ARVC) with biventricular involvement [25]. However, the presence of RV dysfunction, WMA with multiple aneurysms in the right or both ventricles at echocardiography, and the presence of specific diagnostic ARVC criteria [26], can lead to a correct diagnostic classification. Even hypertrophic cardiomyopathy (HCM) could represent an issue in the differential diagnosis of DCM, as the echocardiographic pattern could be similar to DCM if the patient is evaluated for the first time in the advanced hypokinetic stage. Furthermore, it is noteworthy that amyloidosis and hemochromatosis with systolic dysfunction, dilatation, and normal wall thickness could be confused with DCM [27, 28].

A final issue in the differential diagnosis is the effect of alcohol on myocardial dilatation. The phenotype of alcoholic CMP is variable but usually manifests as DCM, even though LV hypertrophy is possible in initial stages of the disease [29]. Appropriate focused patient history is fundamental, and alcohol abstinence is frequently associated with marked functional improvement.

Conclusion

In conclusion, once differential diagnosis has been formulated through first-level exams [clinical, ECG, laboratory findings, echocardiography (*see* Chap. 5)], efforts should be directed toward more specific investigations, such as cardiac computed tomography, CMR, positron emission tomography, coronary angiography, right ventricle catheterization, and endomyocardial biopsy, to better and more precisely define the diagnosis and choose the correct treatment in selected cases. If DCM remains idiopathic, genetic screening should be performed, even though genetic DCM accounts for only 30–48 % of cases. It must be noted that, at present, the role of genetics in clinical management of DCM has not been clarified and must be considered a research tool.

References

1. Codd MB, Sugrue DD, Gersh BJ et al (1989) Epidemiology of idiopathic dilated and hypertrophic cardiomyopathy. A population-based study in Olmsted County, Minnesota, 1975-1984. Circulation 80:564–572
2. Mestroni L, Rocco C, Gregori D et al (1999) Familial dilated cardiomyopathy: evidence for genetic and phenotypic heterogeneity. Heart Muscle Disease Study Group. J Am Coll Cardiol 34:181–190
3. Merlo M, Pivetta A, Pinamonti B, Zecchin M et al (2013) Long-term prognostic impact of therapeutic strategies in patients with idiopathic dilated cardiomyopathy: changing mortality over the last 30 years. Eur J Heart Fail 16(3):317–24
4. Moretti M, Merlo M, Barbati G et al (2010) Prognostic impact of familial screening in dilated cardiomyopathy. Eur J Heart Fail 12:922–927

5. Mestroni L, Maisch B, McKenna WJ et al (1999) Guidelines for the study of familial dilated cardiomyopathies. Collaborative Research Group of the European Human and Capital Mobility Project on Familial Dilated Cardiomyopathy. Eur Heart J 20:93–102
6. Franciosa JA, Wilen M, Ziesche S et al (1983) Survival in men with severe chronic left ventricular failure due to either coronary heart disease or idiopathic dilated cardiomyopathy. Am J Cardiol 51:831–836
7. Aleksova A, Sabbadini G, Merlo M et al (2009) Natural history of dilated cardiomyopathy: from asymptomatic left ventricular dysfunction to heart failure–a subgroup analysis from the Trieste Cardiomyopathy Registry. J Cardiovasc Med (Hagerstown) 10:699–705
8. The SOLVD Investigators (1991) Effect of enalapril on survival in patients with reduced left ventricular ejection fractions and congestive heart failure. N Engl J Med 325:293–302
9. Effect of metoprolol CR/XL in chronic heart failure: Metoprolol CR/XL Randomised Intervention Trial in Congestive Heart Failure (MERIT-HF) (1999). Lancet 353:2001–2007
10. Packer M, Bristow MR, Cohn JN et al (1996) The effect of carvedilol on morbidity and mortality in patients with chronic heart failure. U.S. Carvedilol Heart Failure Study Group. N Engl J Med 334:1349–1355
11. The Cardiac Insufficiency Bisoprolol Study II (CIBIS-II): a randomised trial (1999). Lancet 353:9–13
12. Bardy GH, Lee KL, Mark DB et al (2005) Amiodarone or an implantable cardioverter-defibrillator for congestive heart failure. N Engl J Med 352:225–237
13. Cleland JG, Daubert JC, Erdmann E et al (2005) The effect of cardiac resynchronization on morbidity and mortality in heart failure. N Engl J Med 352:1539–1549
14. Merlo M, Pyxaras SA, Pinamonti B et al (2011) Prevalence and prognostic significance of left ventricular reverse remodeling in dilated cardiomyopathy receiving tailored medical treatment. J Am Coll Cardiol 57:1468–1476
15. Pitt B, Zannad F, Remme WJ et al (1999) The effect of spironolactone on morbidity and mortality in patients with severe heart failure. Randomized Aldactone Evaluation Study Investigators. N Engl J Med 341:709–717
16. Zannad F, McMurray JJ, Krum H et al (2011) Eplerenone in patients with systolic heart failure and mild symptoms. N Engl J Med 364:11–21
17. Moss AJ, Hall WJ, Cannom DS et al (2009) Cardiac-resynchronization therapy for the prevention of heart-failure events. N Engl J Med 361:1329–1338
18. Grimm W, Christ M, Bach J et al (2003) Noninvasive arrhythmia risk stratification in idiopathic dilated cardiomyopathy: results of the Marburg Cardiomyopathy Study. Circulation 108:2883–2891
19. McMurray JJ, Adamopoulos S, Anker SD et al (2012) ESC Guidelines for the diagnosis and treatment of acute and chronic heart failure 2012: The Task Force for the Diagnosis and Treatment of Acute and Chronic Heart Failure 2012 of the European Society of Cardiology. Developed in collaboration with the Heart Failure Association (HFA) of the ESC. Eur Heart J 33:1787–1847
20. Zecchin M, Merlo M, Pivetta A et al (2012) How can optimization of medical treatment avoid unnecessary implantable cardioverter-defibrillator implantations in patients with idiopathic dilated cardiomyopathy presenting with "SCD-HeFT criteria?". Am J Cardiol 109:729–735
21. Whitlow PL, Feldman T, Pedersen WR et al (2012) Acute and 12-month results with catheter-based mitral valve leaflet repair: the EVEREST II (Endovascular Valve Edge-to-Edge Repair) High Risk Study. J Am Coll Cardiol 59:130–139
22. Osaki S, Edwards NM, Velez M et al (2008) Improved survival in patients with ventricular assist device therapy: the University of Wisconsin experience. Eur J Cardiothorac Surg 34:281–288
23. Iorio A, Pinamonti B, Bobbo M et al (2013) Characterization and long-term outcome of Hypertensive Dilated Cardiomyopathy. A distinct phenotype of hypertensive heart disease? J Am Coll Cardiol 61:10-S. doi:10.1016/S0735-1097(13)60595-1
24. Rapezzi C, Arbustini E, Caforio AL et al (2013) Diagnostic work-up in cardiomyopathies: bridging the gap between clinical phenotypes and final diagnosis. A position statement from the ESC Working Group on Myocardial and Pericardial Diseases. Eur Heart J 34:1448–1458

25. Pinamonti B, Sinagra G, Salvi A et al (1992) Left ventricular involvement in right ventricular dysplasia. Am Heart J 123:711–724
26. Marcus FI, McKenna WJ, Sherrill D et al (2010) Diagnosis of arrhythmogenic right ventricular cardiomyopathy/dysplasia: proposed modification of the task force criteria. Eur Heart J 31:806–814
27. Finocchiaro G, Pinamonti B, Merlo M et al (2013) Focus on cardiac amyloidosis: a single-center experience with a long-term follow-up. J Cardiovasc Med (Hagerstown) 14:281–288
28. Lj O (1987) Echocardiographic features of idiopathic emochromatosis. Am J Cardiol 60:885–889
29. Tobin JR Jr, Driscoll JF, Lim MT et al (1967) Primary myocardial disease and alcoholism. The clinical manifestations and course of the disease in a selected population of patients observed for three or more years. Circulation 35:754–764

Basic Echocardiography in Dilated Cardiomyopathy

5

Elena Abate, Bruno Pinamonti, and Andrea Porto

5.1　Introduction

Basic echocardiography has an important role in establishing the diagnosis and assessing the severity of dilated cardiomyopathy (DCM) [1, 2]. It also provides useful information regarding prognosis and helps guide treatment (*see* Chap. 8). The main echocardiographic characteristics of DCM are left ventricular (LV) dilation and systolic dysfunction [1]. Other features include LV diastolic dysfunction with elevated LV filling pressure, LV dyssynchrony, functional mitral regurgitation (MR) and tricuspid regurgitation (TR), right ventricular dysfunction, atrial dilatation [2], and secondary pulmonary hypertension (Table 5.1). All echocardiographic measurements are important at diagnosis as well as during follow-up in order to identify disease progression and treatment effects.

5.2　Left Ventricular Dimensions, Geometry, and Systolic Function

The LV is typically globally dilated and dysfunctioning, with diffuse hypokinesis (Clip 5.1). LV dilation may precede LV dysfunction in some cases [1]. It is therefore crucial to precisely assess LV dimensions and index the measurements according to body surface area (BSA). The standard measures include LV end-diastolic diameter, assessed from the parasternal long-axis view (Clip 5.2, diagnostic criteria for DCM

Electronic supplementary material The online version of this chapter (doi: 10.1007/978-3-319-06019-4_5) contains supplementary material, which is available to authorized users. Videos can also be accessed at http://www.springerimages.com/videos/978-3-319-06018-7.

E. Abate, MD (✉) • B. Pinamonti, MD • A. Porto, MD
Department of Cardiology, University Hospital of Trieste,
via P. Valdoni 7, Trieste 34139, Italy
e-mail: abate.elena@gmail.com; bruno.pinamonti@gmail.com

B. Pinamonti, G. Sinagra (eds.), *Clinical Echocardiography and Other Imaging Techniques in Cardiomyopathies*, DOI 10.1007/978-3-319-06019-4_5,
© Springer International Publishing Switzerland 2014

Table 5.1 Echocardiographic features of dilated cardiomyopathy

	Characteristics
Left ventricle	Dimensions: globally dilated (LV end-diastolic diameter >117 % predicted value corrected for age and BSA) Wall thickness: normal or mildly increased with eccentric hypertrophy Geometry: increased sphericity Systolic function: reduced (LV EF <45 % and/or fractional shortening <25 %) with diffuse hypokinesis Diastolic function: frequently impaired; RFP Dyssynchrony: present, especially if severe LV dysfunction and LBBB
Right ventricle	In case of biventricular involvement, RV dilation and dysfunction are possible
Atria	Bi-atrial dilation is frequent
Mitral valve	Functional MR is frequent and due to annular dilation and apical tethering
Tricuspid valve	Functional TR is frequent, with pulmonary hypertension and RV dilation and/or dysfunction

BSA body surface area, *EF* ejection fraction, *LBBB* left bundle branch block, *LV* left ventricle, *MR* mitral regurgitation, *RFP* restrictive filling pattern, *RV* right ventricle, *TR* tricuspid regurgitation

is LV end-diastolic diameter >117 % predicted value corrected for age and BSA), and LV volumes from apical four- and two-chamber views [1].

Patients with hypokinetic LV without severe dilation (i.e., LV end-diastolic diameter within 15 % of normal values) are defined as having mildly dilated cardiomyopathy (CMP) [3, 4] (Clip 5.3) and are considered to be within the spectrum of DCM. In advanced cases with severe LV dilation and systolic dysfunction, the LV geometry is altered, becoming more spherical (Figs. 5.1 and 5.2; Clips 5.4a, 5.4b, and 5.5). The so-called LV remodeling is characterized by an increased short-axis/long-axis ratio (sphericity index) [5]. This geometric abnormality contributes to LV systolic dysfunction by increasing LV wall stress and reducing contractility, and it can worsen functional MR.

LV wall thickness is usually normal or only mildly increased in DCM. Severe LV hypertrophy excludes the diagnosis of DCM and suggests the presence of other types of CMP, such as hypertrophic, infiltrative, or hypertensive CMP with hypokinetic evolution (Table 5.2). However, even in the presence of normal LV wall thickness, LV mass is often increased due to LV dilation (eccentric hypertrophy with increase in volume/mass ratio and radius/thickness ratio) [6].

An essential echocardiographic feature for the diagnosis of DCM is global LV systolic dysfunction, i.e., a significantly depressed LV ejection fraction (EF) (usual diagnostic cutoff <45 %) [1]. Accurate measurement of LV systolic function is pivotal in DCM patients given the fact that many therapeutic decisions rely on this parameter, such as the indication for implantable cardioverter defibrillator (ICD) or cardiac resynchronization therapy (CRT). In case of bad image quality, when <80 % of the endocardial border is visualized (or more than two contiguous segments are not visualized), the use of contrast agents is indicated for LV opacification and better evaluation of LV volumes and EF (Clip 5.6) [7].

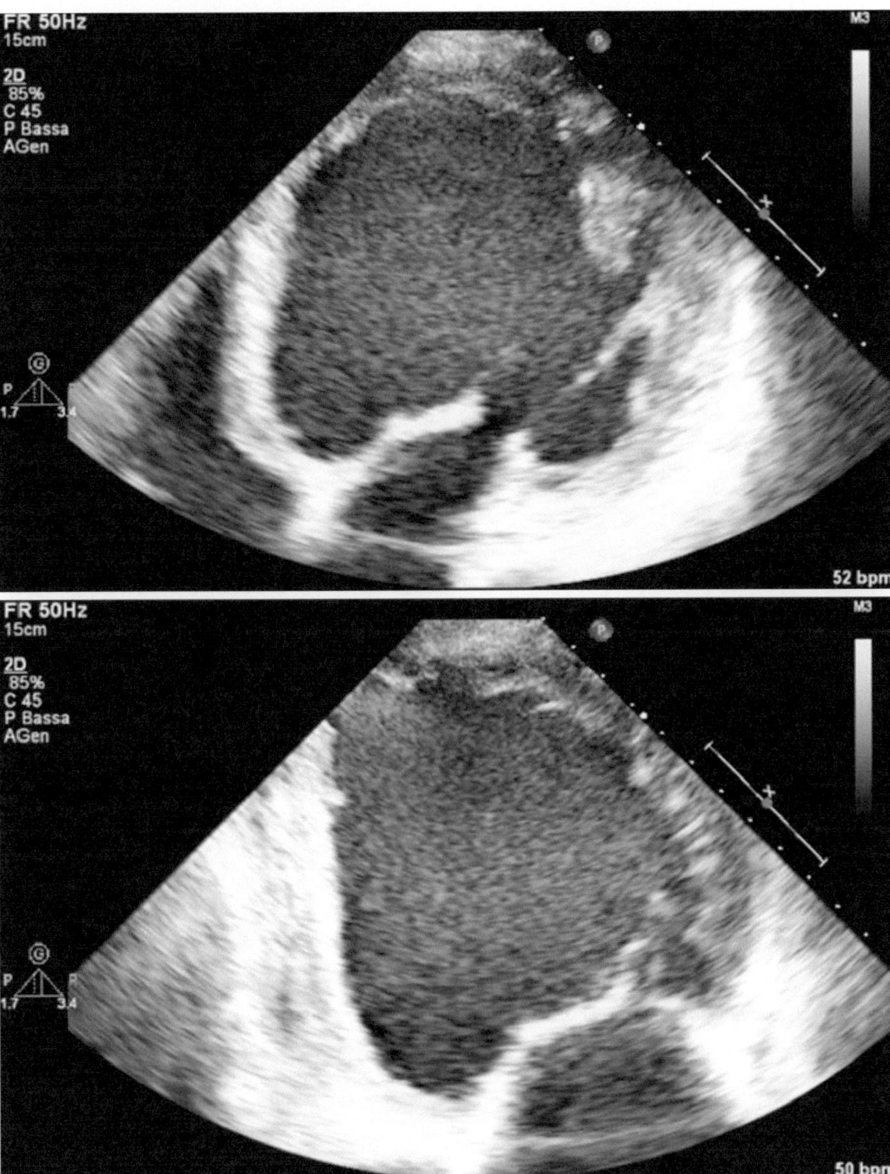

Fig. 5.1 Apical four-chamber (*upper panel*) and two-chamber (*lower panel*) views – end-diastolic frames – of a patient with advanced dilated cardiomyopathy with severe left ventricular (LV) dilation and systolic dysfunction and LV remodeling, resulting in a spherical LV geometry

Another useful index for LV function assessment in this population is the myocardial performance index, or Tei index – i.e., the ratio of the LV isovolumic contraction + relaxation times and ejection time. This is a Doppler parameter that

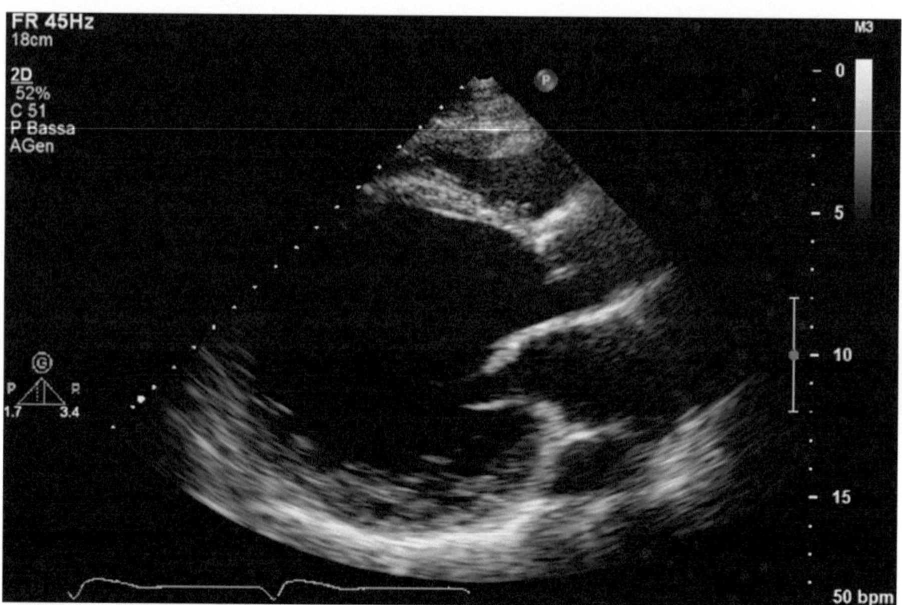

Fig. 5.2 Parasternal long-axis view showing a severely remodeled left ventricle

Table 5.2 Echocardiographic features useful in the differential diagnosis of dilated cardiomyopathy

	LVH	WMA/aneurysm	RV dysfunction	Mild LV dilatation
Hypertensive CMP	+	−	−	+
End-stage HCM	+	−	±	+
Myocarditis	±	+	±	+
ARVC (bi-ventricular)	−	+	+	+
Ischemic CMP	−	+	±	−
Tako-tsubo CMP	−	+	±	±
TIC	−	−	±	+
Infiltrative/storage CMP	+	−	±	+

ARVC arrhythmogenic right ventricular cardiomyopathy, *CMP* cardiomyopathy, *HCM* hypertrophic cardiomyopathy, *LV* left ventricle, *LVH* left ventricular hypertrophy, *RV* right ventricle, *TIC* tachycardia-induced cardiomyopathy, *WMA* wall motion abnormalities

provides a global evaluation of systolic and diastolic function of both ventricles [8]. Furthermore, stroke volume (and cardiac output) can be derived either from LV end-diastolic and end-systolic volumes or from the area of the LV outflow tract (OT) × OT velocity time integral from pulsed-wave (PW) Doppler recordings. This parameter can be useful in selected patients to noninvasively identify a low output state. Finally, dP/dt is an additional index of systolic function that measures the rise in intraventricular pressure during early systole in patients with MR. It appears less dependent on loading conditions than LV EF. However, its usefulness in DCM is not yet defined.

Considering regional wall motion assessment, DCM is usually characterized by global hypokinesis. Regional wall motion abnormalities (WMA) with coronary artery distribution suggest the presence of coronary artery disease (Table 5.2). However, in some DCM cases, regional wall motion is heterogeneous, with akinetic or dyskinetic segments (more frequently anterior or apical) and better contractility usually in the posterior and lateral segments [9]. In rare cases, the presence of LV aneurysm can be found, generally in association with global hypokinesis and significant LV dysfunction. These forms are called idiopathic LV aneurysms and are considered to be within the spectrum of DCM, although without a clear etiopathogenic explanation (Clips 5.7a and 5.7b) [10]. The possibility of previous myocarditis or left-dominant arrhythmogenic CMP must be considered (Table 5.2).

In the presence of severe LV dilation and dysfunction, there is a high probability of spontaneous echocontrast and intracavitary thrombi formation, with risk of embolization (Clips 5.8a and 5.8b). Contrast agents can be useful in this setting, particularly in differentiating thrombi from artefacts.

Finally, in muscular dystrophies associated with DCM, such as Duchenne and Becker types, echocardiography can be normal in the initial phase of the disease, or there can be regional WMA, typically located in the posterolateral and posterobasal regions. With disease progression and fibrosis extension, LV dilation and dysfunction become manifest and can be associated with MR owing to involvement of the posterior papillary muscle. An early diagnosis of cardiac involvement has been reported using dobutamine stress echocardiography [11], tissue Doppler imaging (TDI) [12], and tissue characterization [13].

5.3   Left Ventricular Diastolic Function

LV diastolic dysfunction is often present in DCM. Evaluation of diastolic function is complex as it is influenced by many variables [14]. It is therefore important to consider various indices of diastolic function.

It is well known that diastolic dysfunction stages begin with impaired relaxation at Doppler interrogation of transmitral flow and progress to a restrictive filling pattern (RFP) that denotes high LV filling pressure and LV stiffness (Fig. 5.3) [15]. In DCM, high diastolic pressure and LV stiffness may be due to several factors [16], such as structural myocardial alterations (LV fibrosis), LV cavity dilatation, and ventricular interdependence, with pericardial restraint in case of biventricular involvement and biatrial dilatation [17]. The pseudonormal pattern is an intermediate stage that can represent a worsening from impaired relaxation or an improvement of reversible RFP after optimal treatment [14]. It can be identified by the response of the mitral flow pattern to Valsalva maneuver [18] and the pattern of the pulmonary venous Doppler curve [14, 19].

Other evaluations comprise the study of blood flow propagation velocity in the LV cavity using color-M-mode, left atrial (LA) dimensions and TDI (*see* Chap. 6) [14].

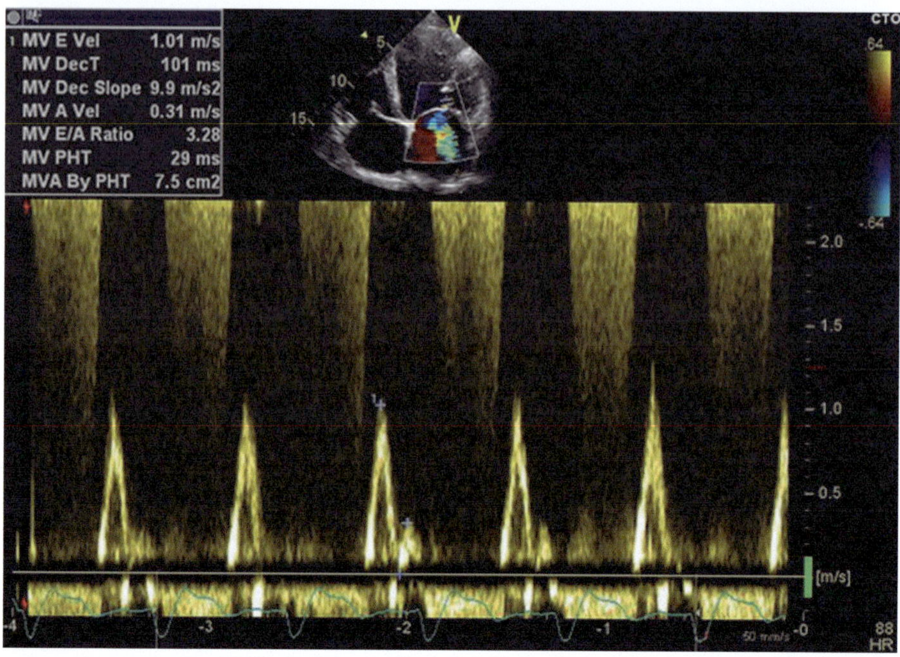

Fig. 5.3 Pulsed-wave Doppler interrogation of transmitral flow showing a restrictive filling pattern (E-wave velocity 1 m/s, A-wave velocity 0.31 m/s, E/A ratio 3.3, E-wave deceleration time 101 ms)

5.4 Left Ventricular Dyssynchrony

Evaluation of LV mechanical dyssynchrony in DCM patients with heart failure (HF), severe LV dysfunction, and left bundle branch block (LBBB) has been widely studied and principally applied to identify potential responders to CRT (Clip 5.9). LV dyssynchrony (i.e., uncoordinated LV wall contraction) results in further reduction of LV function and other negative consequences, such as worsening of functional MR. Therefore, several echocardiographic indices of intraventricular dyssynchrony have been studied, the earliest based on 2D echocardiography and M-mode imaging [20].

Visual estimation of the rocking motion of the apex (apical rocking) is a simple LV mechanical dyssynchrony marker that combines both functional and temporal myocardial inhomogeneities [21]. Moreover, septal flash, defined as an abnormal septal motion on M-mode imaging traces that occurs during the preejection period, has been used as a sign of LBBB-induced dyssynchrony [22]. Another simple M-mode index of LV dyssynchrony is the septal to posterior wall motion delay, which is measured in the parasternal long-axis view at the papillary muscle level (Fig. 5.4).

However, these indices have demonstrated low feasibility, particularly in severely dilated and dysfunctional LV with extensive areas of akinesis. Consequently, other echocardiographic markers of LV dyssynchrony have been proposed based on TDI,

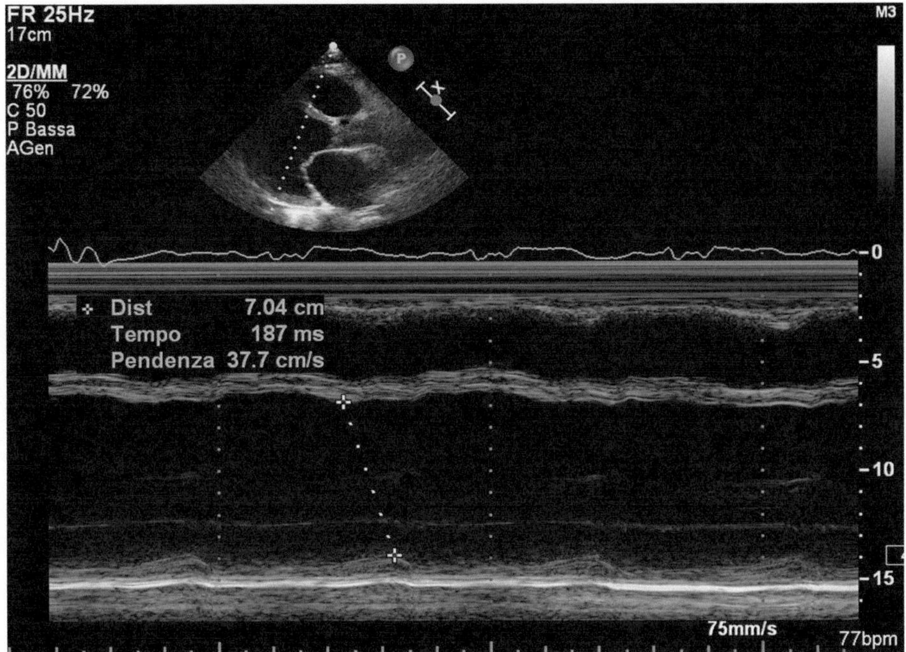

Fig. 5.4 Patient with left ventricular dyssynchrony: there is a septal-to-posterior wall motion delay of 187 ms measured at M-mode imaging in the parasternal long-axis view

speckle tracking, and 3D echocardiography (*see* Chap. 6) [20]. It seems, however, that there is no perfect marker for intraventricular mechanical dyssynchrony evaluation, and it is preferable to use a combination of several indices rather than a single marker [23].

Interventricular dyssynchrony is quantified by measuring the time delay between LV and RV preejection intervals at PW Doppler echocardiography (interventricular mechanical delay). Results of the CArdiac REsynchronization-Heart Failure (CARE-HF) trial demonstrated that the presence of significant interventricular dyssynchrony was related to higher likelihood of favorable response to CRT [24].

Also, evaluation of atrioventricular dyssynchrony can be useful, especially for optimizing atrioventricular delay for atrioventricular pacing. In fact, some DCM patients might have a reduced diastolic filling period, a marker of atrioventricular dyssynchrony, causing reduced stroke volume, increased LA pressure, and diastolic MR.

5.5   Functional Mitral Regurgitation

Functional MR, without structural alterations of mitral valve (MV) leaflets, is frequent in DCM [25]. It is a ventricular rather than valvular disorder. In fact, LV dilation and remodeling is a key determinant of functional MR, leading to mitral annular

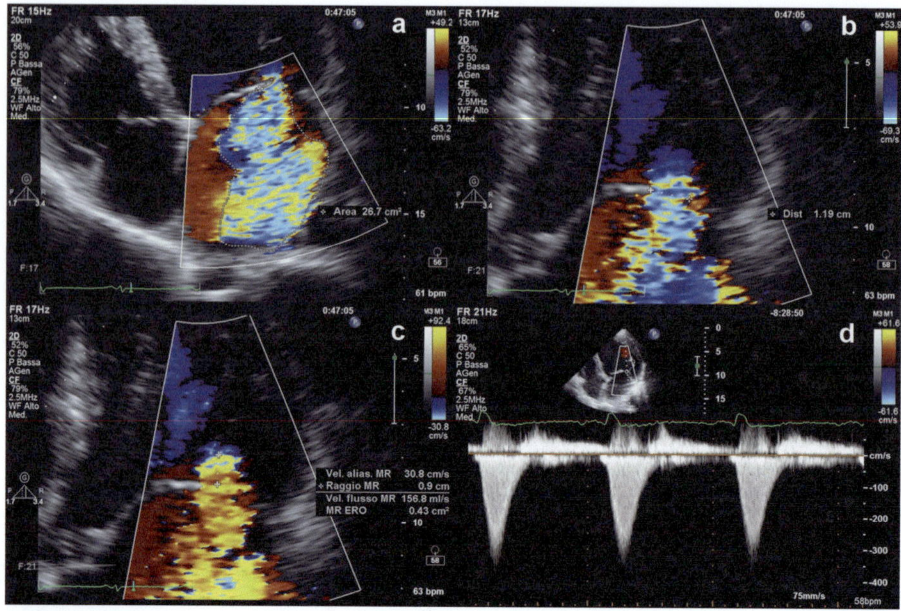

Fig. 5.5 Color-Doppler evaluation of mitral regurgitation severity in a patient with dilated cardiomyopathy and severe functional mitral regurgitation. Jet area is 26.7 cmq (**a**), and *vena contracta* is 1.19 cm (**b**). Proximal isovelocity surface area method was applied to calculate the effective regurgitant orifice area, which is 0.43 cmq (**c**). Continuous-wave Doppler examination of the mitral regurgitation jet shows low velocity and triangular morphology (**d**)

dilatation and papillary muscle displacement, with systolic retraction toward the apex and MV leaflet malcoaptation (Clips 5.10a, 5.10b, and 5.10c). This process is intensified by the reduced LV contractility, further impairing MV closing forces and increasing the degree of MR. MR contributes to reduced forward stroke volume and to increased LV filling pressure and LA and pulmonary artery pressures [25]. Moreover, MR causes LV and LA volume overload and further LV enlargement over time, which in turn impairs mitral leaflet coaptation, thus increasing the degree of MR in a vicious cycle.

The complete echocardiographic evaluation of functional MR in DCM starts from analysis of MV morphology and quantification of annulus dimensions and systolic leaflet retraction (Clips 5.11a and 5.11b). The mitral annulus is saddle shaped and cannot be entirely visualized on 2D echocardiography. Therefore, transesophageal echocardiography (in particular, 3D) can be useful to better evaluate annulus dimensions and valvular morphology and rule out structural mitral leaflet pathology. Furthermore, accurate evaluation of valvular morphology, combined with a poliparametric evaluation of MR severity, is essential for selecting potential candidates for percutaneous edge-to-edge repair with MitraClip implantation [26].

In functional MR, jet direction is usually central but in some cases can be eccentric, with posterior and lateral direction, due to prevalent posterior leaflet tethering (Clip 5.12) [27]. In these cases, it is important to rule out the presence of leaflet prolapse. Color-Doppler measurement of the jet area and *vena contracta* provides a semiquantitative assessment of MR severity (Fig. 5.5, Clips 5.13a and 5.13b) [28]. These evaluations have some limitations in MR quantitation, in particular in the presence of eccentric jets that cannot be entirely visualized in standard planes. Therefore, quantitative methods are recommended, such as calculating the regurgitant volume and regurgitant fraction from mitral and aortic stroke volumes, and the effective regurgitant orifice area with proximal isovelocity surface area (PISA) method (Fig. 5.5). It is important to keep in mind that severity cutoff values are lower in functional MR compared with organic MR: severe functional MR is defined by the effective regurgitant orifice area >0.20 cmq and regurgitant volume >30 ml [26].

In case of severe MR, the continuous wave Doppler of the MR jet has low velocity and a triangular morphology, secondary to high LA pressure and prominent v waves (Fig. 5.5). From the peak velocity it is possible to calculate the systolic pressure gradient between LV and LA, and the LA pressure with the simplified Bernouilli equation.

5.6 Right Ventricular Dilation and Dysfunction

In 30 % of DCM cases, RV function is impaired, with biventricular dysfunction (Clip 5.14). Biventricular involvement is rather frequent in necropsy studies [29]. Conversely, it is unusual to observe prevalent RV dilation and dysfunction, and in these cases, the presence of an arrhythmogenic RV CMP with biventricular involvement must be suspected [30] (Table 5.2). RV dysfunction in DCM could be due to a biventricular involvement of the CMP and/or can be secondary to pressure overload due to pulmonary hypertension [31].

5.7 Atrial Dilation

Atrial dimensions are influenced by several factors, such as LV filling pressure, MR and TR, and the presence of atrial fibrillation (AF) [32]. LA or biatrial dilation is frequent in DCM patients. In fact, significant LA dilation was present in 54 % of DCM patients in our experience (Clip 5.15) [33]. Furthermore, in case of severe LA dilation and AF, there can be spontaneous echo contrast and thrombosis formation [29].

5.8 Functional Tricuspid Regurgitation

Functional TR is quite frequent in DCM patients (40 % of our patients), especially if there is RV dilation and dysfunction and pulmonary hypertension (Clips 5.16a and 5.16b). Although it rarely has hemodynamic importance, it is significantly related with worse prognosis [34].

5.9 Stress Echocardiography

Low-dose dobutamine stress test has been used to evaluate the contractile reserve, which has prognostic value (*see* Chap. 8). Moreover, LV elastance is a load-independent index of LV contractility and can be calculated as end-systolic blood pressure/LV end-systolic volume index ratio (also called Suga index). It can be assessed during dobutamine stress echocardiography to estimate the inotropic reserve, providing prognostically useful information [35].

Furthermore, coronary flow reserve can be evaluated by PW Doppler in the left anterior descending coronary artery during dipyridamole stress echocardiography. Coronary flow reserve is defined as the ratio of maximal vasodilation to rest peak diastolic coronary flow velocity. This index is reduced not only in patients with coronary artery disease but also in most patients with nonischemic DCM. In the latter, severity of this impairment is correlated with clinical and/or hemodynamic severity of the disease [36].

Dobutamine stress echocardiography can also be useful for the differential diagnosis between DCM (sustained improvement) and ischemic disease (biphasic response) [37]. Furthermore, dobutamine stress test can be helpful to unmask a significant LV intraventricular dyssynchrony, as identified by septal flash, which could not be identified at baseline because of the severe hypokinesis. A recent study demonstrated that the degree of LV dyssynchrony during dobutamine stress test, as identified by the extent of peak septal flash, correlated with the degree of LV remodeling and clinical response after CRT [22].

Finally, it is common practice to perform dobutamine stress echocardiography to differentiate true aortic valve stenosis from pseudostenosis associated with DCM; conversely, there is still no clear evidence regarding the role of exercise stress echocardiography for evaluating functional MR in idiopathic DCM patients [38, 39].

References

1. Mestroni L, Maisch B, McKenna WJ et al (1999) Guidelines for the study of familial dilated cardiomyopathies. Collaborative Research Group of the European Human and Capital Mobility Project on Familial Dilated Cardiomyopathy. Eur Heart J 20:93–102
2. Pinamonti B, Cacciatore G (2002) Dilated cardiomyopathy: indication and role of non-invasive instrumental evaluation. Ital Heart J Suppl 3:405–411
3. Gavazzi A, De Maria R, Renosto G et al (1993) The spectrum of left ventricular size in dilated cardiomyopathy: clinical correlates and prognostic implications. SPIC (Italian Multicenter Cardiomyopathy Study) Group. Am Heart J 125(2 Pt 1):410–422
4. Kurozumi H, Hayakawa M, Kajiya T et al (1992) Clinical evaluation of observations in poorly contracting and nondilated left ventricles (nondilated cardiomyopathy). Am J Cardiol 69:1367–1370
5. Douglas PS, Morrow R, Ioli A et al (1989) Left ventricular shape, afterload and survival in idiopathic dilated cardiomyopathy. J Am Coll Cardiol 13:311–315
6. Wong M, Johnson G, Shabetai R et al (1993) Echocardiographic variables as prognostic indicators and therapeutic monitors in chronic congestive heart failure. Veterans Affairs cooperative studies V-HeFT I and II. V-HeFT VA Cooperative Studies Group. Circulation 87(6 Suppl):VI65–VI70

7. Senior R, Becher H, Monaghan M et al (2009) Contrast echocardiography: evidence-based recommendations by European Association of Echocardiography. Eur J Echocardiogr 10:194–212

8. Tei C, Ling LH, Hodge DO et al (1995) New index of combined systolic and diastolic myocardial performance: a simple and reproducible measure of cardiac function–a study in normals and dilated cardiomyopathy. J Cardiol 26:357–366

9. Wallis DE, O'Connell JB, Henkin RE et al (1984) Segmental wall motion abnormalities in dilated cardiomyopathy: a common finding and good prognostic sign. J Am Coll Cardiol 4:674–679

10. Mestroni L, Morgera T, Miani D et al (1994) Idiopathic left ventricular aneurysm: a clinical and pathological study of a new entity in the spectrum of cardiomyopathies. Postgrad Med J 70(Suppl 1):S13–S20

11. Wong BL, Mukkada VA, Markham LW et al (2005) Depressed left ventricular contractile reserve diagnosed by dobutamine stress echocardiography in a patient with Duchenne muscular dystrophy. J Child Neurol 20:246–248

12. Meune C, Pascal O, Becane HM et al (2004) Reliable detection of early myocardial dysfunction by tissue Doppler echocardiography in Becker muscular dystrophy. Heart 90:947–948

13. Giglio V, Pasceri V, Messano L et al (2003) Ultrasound tissue characterization detects preclinical myocardial structural changes in children affected by Duchenne muscular dystrophy. J Am Coll Cardiol 42:309–316

14. Nishimura RA, Tajik AJ (1997) Evaluation of diastolic filling of left ventricle in health and disease: Doppler echocardiography is the clinician's Rosetta Stone. J Am Coll Cardiol 30:8–18

15. Little WC, Ohno M, Kitzman DW et al (1995) Determination of left ventricular chamber stiffness from the time for deceleration of early left ventricular filling. Circulation 92:1933–1939

16. Grossman W, McLaurin LP, Rolett EL (1979) Alterations in left ventricular relaxation and diastolic compliance in congestive cardiomyopathy. Cardiovasc Res 13:514–522

17. Atherton JJ, Moore TD, Thomson HL et al (1998) Restrictive left ventricular filling patterns are predictive of diastolic ventricular interaction in chronic heart failure. J Am Coll Cardiol 31:413–418

18. Hurrell DG, Nishimura RA, Ilstrup DM et al (1997) Utility of preload alteration in assessment of left ventricular filling pressure by Doppler echocardiography: a simultaneous catheterization and Doppler echocardiographic study. J Am Coll Cardiol 30:459–467

19. Dini FL, Michelassi C, Micheli G et al (2000) Prognostic value of pulmonary venous flow Doppler signal in left ventricular dysfunction: contribution of the difference in duration of pulmonary venous and mitral flow at atrial contraction. J Am Coll Cardiol 36:1295–1302

20. Bax JJ, Abraham T, Barold SS et al (2005) Cardiac resynchronization therapy: part 1–issues before device implantation. J Am Coll Cardiol 46:2153–2167

21. Szulik M, Tillekaerts M, Vangeel V et al (2010) Assessment of apical rocking: a new, integrative approach for selection of candidates for cardiac resynchronization therapy. Eur J Echocardiogr 11:863–869

22. Parsai C, Bijnens B, Sutherland GR et al (2009) Toward understanding response to cardiac resynchronization therapy: left ventricular dyssynchrony is only one of multiple mechanisms. Eur Heart J 30:940–949

23. Lafitte S, Reant P, Serri K et al (2008) Echocardiographic algorithm for cardiac resynchronization. Echocardiography 25:1040–1046

24. Richardson M, Freemantle N, Calvert MJ et al (2007) Predictors and treatment response with cardiac resynchronization therapy in patients with heart failure characterized by dyssynchrony: a pre-defined analysis from the CARE-HF trial. Eur Heart J 28:1827–1834

25. Junker A, Thayssen P, Nielsen B et al (1993) The hemodynamic and prognostic significance of echo-Doppler-proven mitral regurgitation in patients with dilated cardiomyopathy. Cardiology 83:14–20

26. Vahanian A, Alfieri O, Andreotti F et al (2012) Guidelines on the management of valvular heart disease (version 2012). Eur Heart J 33:2451–2496

27. Kwan J, Shiota T, Agler DA et al (2003) Geometric differences of the mitral apparatus between ischemic and dilated cardiomyopathy with significant mitral regurgitation: real-time three-dimensional echocardiography study. Circulation 107:1135–1140
28. Roberts BJ, Grayburn PA (2003) Color flow imaging of the vena contracta in mitral regurgitation: technical considerations. J Am Soc Echocardiogr 16:1002–1006
29. Roberts WC, Siegel RJ, McManus BM (1987) Idiopathic dilated cardiomyopathy: analysis of 152 necropsy patients. Am J Cardiol 60:1340–1355
30. Pinamonti B, Sinagra G, Salvi A et al (1992) Left ventricular involvement in right ventricular dysplasia. Am Heart J 123:711–724
31. Enriquez-Sarano M, Rossi A, Seward JB et al (1997) Determinants of pulmonary hypertension in left ventricular dysfunction. J Am Coll Cardiol 29:153–159
32. Douglas PS (2003) The left atrium: a biomarker of chronic diastolic dysfunction and cardiovascular disease risk. J Am Coll Cardiol 42:1206–1207
33. Di Lenarda A, Pinamonti B, Mestroni L et al (2004) How the natural history of dilated cardiomyopathy has changed. Review of the Registry of Myocardial Diseases of Trieste. Ital Heart J Suppl 5:253–266
34. Hung J, Koelling T, Semigran MJ et al (1998) Usefulness of echocardiographic determined tricuspid regurgitation in predicting event-free survival in severe heart failure secondary to idiopathic-dilated cardiomyopathy or to ischemic cardiomyopathy. Am J Cardiol 82: 1301–1303, A1310
35. Grosu A, Bombardini T, Senni M et al (2005) End-systolic pressure/volume relationship during dobutamine stress echo: a prognostically useful non-invasive index of left ventricular contractility. Eur Heart J 26:2404–2412
36. Santagata P, Rigo F, Gherardi S et al (2005) Clinical and functional determinants of coronary flow reserve in non-ischemic dilated cardiomyopathy: an echocardiographic study. Int J Cardiol 105:46–52
37. Pinamonti B, Perkan A, Di Lenarda A et al (2002) Dobutamine echocardiography in idiopathic dilated cardiomyopathy: clinical and prognostic implications. Eur J Heart Fail 4:49–61
38. Ennezat PV, Marechaux S, Huerre C et al (2008) Exercise does not enhance the prognostic value of Doppler echocardiography in patients with left ventricular systolic dysfunction and functional mitral regurgitation at rest. Am Heart J 155:752–757
39. Yamano T, Nakatani S, Kanzaki H et al (2008) Exercise-induced changes of functional mitral regurgitation in asymptomatic or mildly symptomatic patients with idiopathic dilated cardiomyopathy. Am J Cardiol 102:481–485

Advanced Echocardiographic Technologies in Dilated Cardiomyopathy

6

Elena Abate and Bruno Pinamonti

6.1 Introduction

Advanced echocardiographic techniques, such as 3D echocardiography, tissue Doppler imaging (TDI), and speckle-tracking strain imaging, have recently been introduced for the echocardiographic evaluation of patients with dilated cardiomyopathy (DCM) and have demonstrated significant incremental value over basic echocardiography.

6.2 Left Ventricular Dimensions and Systolic Function

Accurate left ventricular (LV) volumes and ejection fraction (EF) quantitation is crucial in the echocardiographic evaluation of patients with DCM. For instance, improved accuracy of LV volumes and EF assessment might play a substantial role in helping physicians select candidates for implantable cardioverter defibrillator or cardiac resynchronization therapy (CRT). However, it is well known that M-mode and 2D evaluations of LV volumes and EF have limitations [1]. Conversely, 3D echocardiography has been recently validated with cardiac magnetic resonance (CMR) for quantification of ventricular volumes in various cardiomyopathies, including DCM, and demonstrated a higher accuracy and lower inter- and intraobserver variability compared with 2D echocardiography [2, 3]. Some advantages of 3D echocardiography include independence from geometric assumptions, semiautomatic delineation of the endocardial border, and absence of errors deriving from "foreshortening" of the LV apex (Fig. 6.1, Clip 6.1) [4]. Three-dimensional

Electronic supplementary material The online version of this chapter (doi: 10.1007/978-3-319-06019-4_6) contains supplementary material, which is available to authorized users. Videos can also be accessed at http://www.springerimages.com/videos/978-3-319-06018-7.

E. Abate, MD (✉) • B. Pinamonti, MD
Department of Cardiology, University Hospital of Trieste,
via P. Valdoni 7, Trieste 34139, Italy
e-mail: abate.elena@gmail.com; bruno.pinamonti@gmail.com

B. Pinamonti, G. Sinagra (eds.), *Clinical Echocardiography and Other Imaging Techniques in Cardiomyopathies*, DOI 10.1007/978-3-319-06019-4_6,
© Springer International Publishing Switzerland 2014

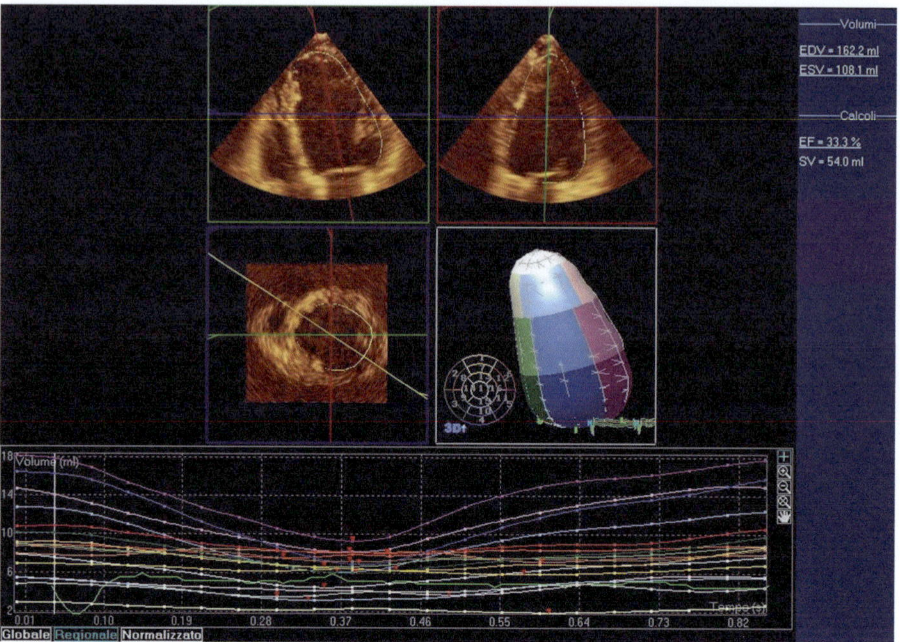

Fig. 6.1 Left ventricular (LV) volumes and ejection fraction (EF) quantification with 3D echocardiography in a patient with dilated cardiomyopathy (DCM) with severe LV dilatation and dysfunction. The endocardial border is manually traced in the apical four-chamber (*upper left panel*), two-chamber (*upper right panel*), and short-axis (*mid left panel*) views, and a 3D LV model is automatically generated (*mid right panel*); subsequently, 3D LV volumes and EF are measured, and a time–volume change curve of all segments during the cardiac cycle is provided (*lower panel*). *EDV* end-diastolic volume, *ESV* end-systolic volume, *SV* stroke volume

echocardiography also provides the possibility for quantitative assessment of LV regional wall motion by measuring the volume change of each segment in the cardiac cycle. This technique demonstrated high feasibility in DCM patients [5] and provided good correlation with CMR [6]. Finally, 3D echocardiography has also been applied in DCM patients and validated against CMR for LV mass assessment, showing excellent correlation with CMR, significant superiority over 2D echocardiography, and low inter- and intraobserver variability [7, 8].

Technological advances in the field of cardiac ultrasound have lead to further new noninvasive techniques, such as TDI and speckle-tracking strain imaging, for assessing cardiac mechanics and segmental and global LV function. The peak systolic myocardial velocity S', a simple TDI index of systolic longitudinal function, is a marker of impaired subendocardial fiber contraction and correlates with myocardial fibrosis [9]. In addition, strain evaluation (by TDI, 2D and 3D speckle-tracking echocardiography) allows discrimination between active and passive movement of all myocardial segments and permits separate assessments of distinct components of myocardial deformation (i.e., longitudinal versus circumferential shortening and radial thickening) [10]. Also, all myocardial deformation

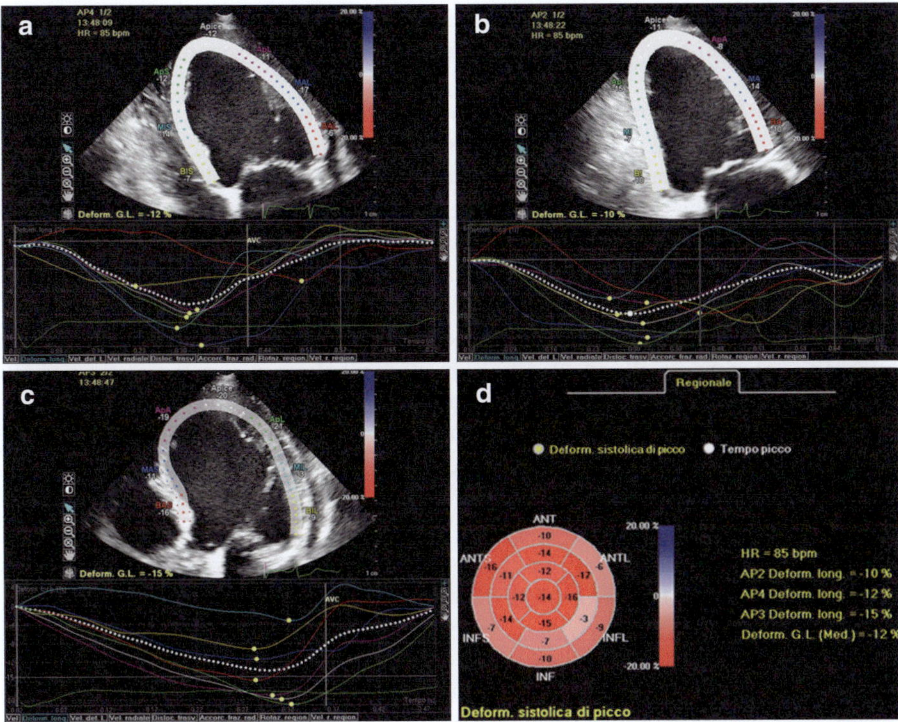

Fig. 6.2 Left ventricular (*LV*) longitudinal strain evaluation by 2D speckle-tracking echocardiography in apical four- (**a**), two- (**b**), and long-axis (**c**) views in a dilated cardiomyopathy (DCM) patient. In each view, the LV region of interest in the 2D speckle-tracking analysis is shown (*upper half of each panel*), together with longitudinal strain curves for each segment (*lower half of each panel*). Final results of the strain analysis for each LV segment are displayed in a bulls-eye plot (**d**). Global longitudinal strain is automatically calculated by the software and is importantly reduced (−12 %)

parameters, including longitudinal, circumferential, and radial strain and torsion, are reduced in DCM patients (Fig. 6.2, Clips 6.2a, 6.2b, and 6.2c) [11].

6.3 Left Ventricular Diastolic Function

TDI of the mitral annulus is a relatively novel method for assessing diastolic function. It is performed in apical four-chamber view, placing the pulsed-wave tissue Doppler on the septal or lateral annulus of the mitral valve (MV), showing a Doppler pattern with E' and A' waves. The ratio of transmitral E velocity to mitral annular E' velocity (E/E') is a marker of left atrial (LA) pressure, is related to exercise capacity in DCM, and provides prognostic value [12]. On the other hand, E/E' ratio has a wide grey zone, and its accuracy is questionable, particularly in patients with advanced DCM and severe heart failure (HF). In fact, a study with invasive hemodynamic correlations showed that E/E' ratio had a weak correlation with LV filling pressures in DCM patients, particularly in those with severe LV dilation and after CRT [13].

Other new indices for diastolic function evaluation obtained by speckle-tracking analysis are promising. Circumferential strain and strain rate during late diastolic LV filling, E/circumferential strain rate at early diastolic LV filling, and E/circumferential strain at the time of peak E wave showed greater area under the curve than the E/E' ratio for predicting pulmonary capillary wedge pressure (PCWP) >12 mmHg [14]. Also, LA strain assessment with speckle-tracking technique demonstrated a better correlation than other Doppler indices, such as E/E' ratio, with LV filling pressure as measured by right catheterization, in patients with advanced systolic HF [15]. Specifically, peak atrial longitudinal strain is a parameter for functional assessment of the atrial reservoir phase (which is essential for LV filling), and results progressively reduced with the increase of LV filling pressure. Therefore, peak atrial longitudinal strain demonstrated a strong inverse correlation with PCWP and excellent diagnostic accuracy in predicting elevated filling pressure [15].

6.4 Left Ventricular Dyssynchrony

There is evidence that LV mechanical dyssynchrony is an independent determinant of response to CRT and long-term survival [16]. Advanced indices of intraventricular mechanical dyssynchrony are based on TDI, speckle-tracking imaging, and 3D echocardiography [17].

The rocking motion of the apex (apical rocking) can be quantified by TDI by measuring the transverse motion of the LV apex perpendicular to the LV long axis. This index is clinically feasible, reproducible, and has predictive value for response and long-term survival following CRT [18]. Furthermore, the time from QRS onset to peak systolic velocity can be measured by TDI imaging at the level of different basal and mid-LV segments: the time difference between peak contraction of opposite segments is an index for LV dyssynchrony. Contraction delay between the basal septum and the basal lateral wall in the apical four-chamber view is usually considered, but this index can be measured from multiple apical views in up to 12 segments. Moreover, TDI-derived longitudinal strain and strain-rate imaging allows LV dyssynchrony evaluation by measuring the time delay between peak systolic strain rate [19]. The Predictors of Response to CT (PROSPECT) trial demonstrated a low sensitivity and specificity of echocardiographic TDI markers of LV dyssynchrony for predicting response to CRT [20]. The TDI markers indeed show low feasibility and reproducibility. In particular, in advanced DCM patients with extended areas of akinesis, identifying systolic contraction timing and measurements of TDI parameters are particularly problematic and can be misleading, as it is impossible to discriminate passive from active myocardial movements.

New echocardiographic techniques not included in the PROSPECT trial involve speckle-tracking strain evaluation and 3D echocardiography, even if the temporal resolution of these techniques is relatively low and inferior compared with TDI [21, 22].

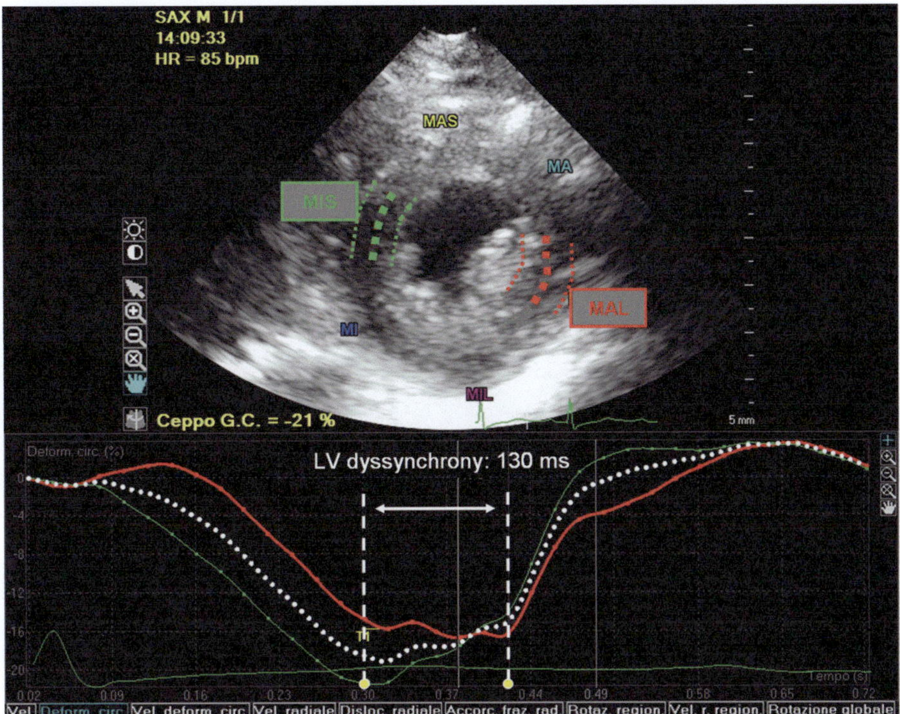

Fig. 6.3 Evaluation of left ventricular (*LV*) dyssynchrony with 2D speckle-tracking strain analysis calculated as the time difference in peak circumferential strain between opposing segments (mid-inferoseptal and mid-anterolateral wall) in the short-axis plane. In this case of advanced dilated cardiomyopathy (DCM), there was significant LV dyssynchrony (130 ms). *MA* mid anterior, *MAL* mid anterolateral, *MAS* mid anteroseptal, *MI* mid inferior, *MIL* mid inferolateral, *MIS* mid inferoseptal

LV dyssynchrony with speckle-tracking strain analysis (Fig. 6.3) is calculated as the time difference in peak strain values (radial and circumferential in the short-axis plane, longitudinal and transverse in the long-axis plane) between opposing segments (most frequently between the anteroseptal and posterolateral wall) [21]. Longitudinal and radial strain parameters appear to be more reproducible and accurate for quantifying LV mechanical dyssynchrony [21, 23]. In the prospective multicenter Speckle Tracking and Resynchronization (STAR) study [24], radial and transverse LV strains were both significantly associated with EF response and long-term outcome (death, heart transplant, LV assist device) after CRT. Lack of baseline radial or transverse LV dyssynchrony (defined as ≥130 ms opposing wall delay) appeared to be a marker of adverse prognosis following CRT [24].

Furthermore, 3D echocardiography has emerged as a novel technique for dyssynchrony quantification based on analysis of volume variations of each segment in the same cardiac cycle: if the contraction is dyssynchronous, there is dispersion in the time each segment takes to reach its minimum volume. The 3D systolic dyssynchrony index is defined as the standard deviation of the time to minimum systolic regional

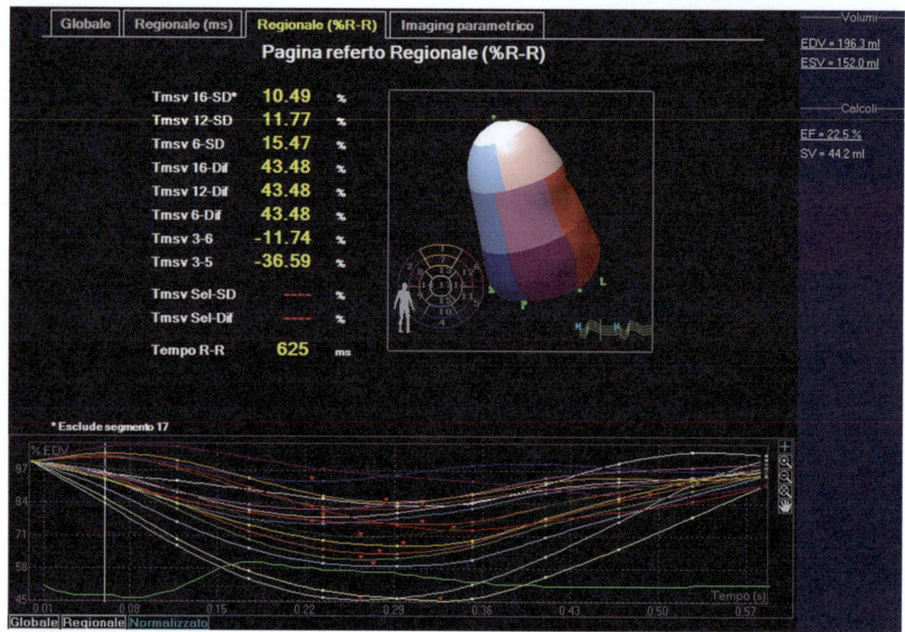

Fig. 6.4 Quantification of left ventricular (LV) dyssynchrony by 3D echocardiography: the systolic dyssynchrony index (defined as the standard deviation of the time to minimum systolic regional volume using a 16-segment model) was 10.49 % in this patient, indicating significant LV dyssynchrony

volume using a 16-segment model (Fig. 6.4). A cutoff value of systolic dyssynchrony index ≥5.6 % has been proposed to predict response to CRT [25]. More recently, 3D speckle-tracking imaging has emerged for calculating LV dyssynchrony by assessing myocardial deformation within the LV 3D full volume [26]. With this technique, the maximal opposing wall delay and the standard deviation of time to peak (radial) strain of 16 LV segments are derived as LV dyssynchrony indices. HF patients show higher 3D dyssynchrony indices compared with normal individuals; moreover, in patients who underwent CRT, 3D imaging demonstrated effective LV resynchronization with considerably improved systolic function [26].

Larger studies are needed to determine the best LV mechanical dyssynchrony echocardiographic parameter for predicting CRT response and long-term survival. Moreover, besides LV mechanical dyssynchrony, it seems important to use advanced imaging to evaluate other aspects to maximize response to CRT, including detecting necrotic tissue, presence of viability, and availability of coronary veins for optimal LV lead position [27]. Echocardiography might play a role in identifying the optimal site for LV pacing, first by detecting the myocardial area of latest mechanical activation (in particular, by 2D and 3D speckle-tracking imaging) [28]; and second, by excluding the presence of scar tissue in the area considered for LV pacing (for instance, by speckle-tracking imaging or dobutamine stress echocardiography). Scarred LV tissue assessed using speckle-tracking global longitudinal strain was a strong determinant of response to CRT in patients with ischemic DCM and was significantly related with total scar burden quantified by CMR [29].

6.5   Functional Mitral Regurgitation

It is well known that the 2D proximal isovelocity surface area (PISA) method for evaluating mitral regurgitation (MR) has several limitations, as it is based on geometric assumptions. There are advantages of 3D over 2D echocardiography in evaluating MR grade due to the direct planimetry of the effective regurgitant orifice area, which is typically elliptical in functional MR (Fig. 6.5, Clip 6.3). Previous studies demonstrated the additional value of 3D echocardiography in patients with functional MR, whereas 2D imaging significantly underestimated the size of the regurgitant orifice [30]. Furthermore, dedicated software permits 3D quantification of MV annulus dimensions, MV leaflet surface, tenting volume, aortomitral angle, and papillary muscle geometry [31].

6.6   Other Features

Echocardiography with integrated backscatter imaging (i.e., a technique that allows assessment of myocardial ultrasound reflectivity) permits identification of myocardial fibrosis, which appears as high-echogenic myocardial areas. Integrated backscattering is an index of myocardial echogenicity that demonstrated a significant correlation with the quantity of fibrosis at biopsy [32]. Other authors [33] demonstrated a reduction of integrated backscattering in patients with DCM and worse prognosis, possibly due to reduced contractility and/or myocardial fibrosis.

Fig. 6.5 Evaluation of mitral regurgitation (MR) grade with 3D transthoracic echocardiography from a 3D full volume with color Doppler acquisition of the regurgitant jet (*mid right panel*): the software permits measurement of the vena contracta in two perpendicular planes (as shown in the *upper panels*); furthermore, it is possible to trace the direct planimetry of the effective regurgitant orifice area, which is typically elliptical in functional MR (*mid left and lower panels*). In this case of severe functional MR, the effective regurgitant orifice area was 0.5 cmq

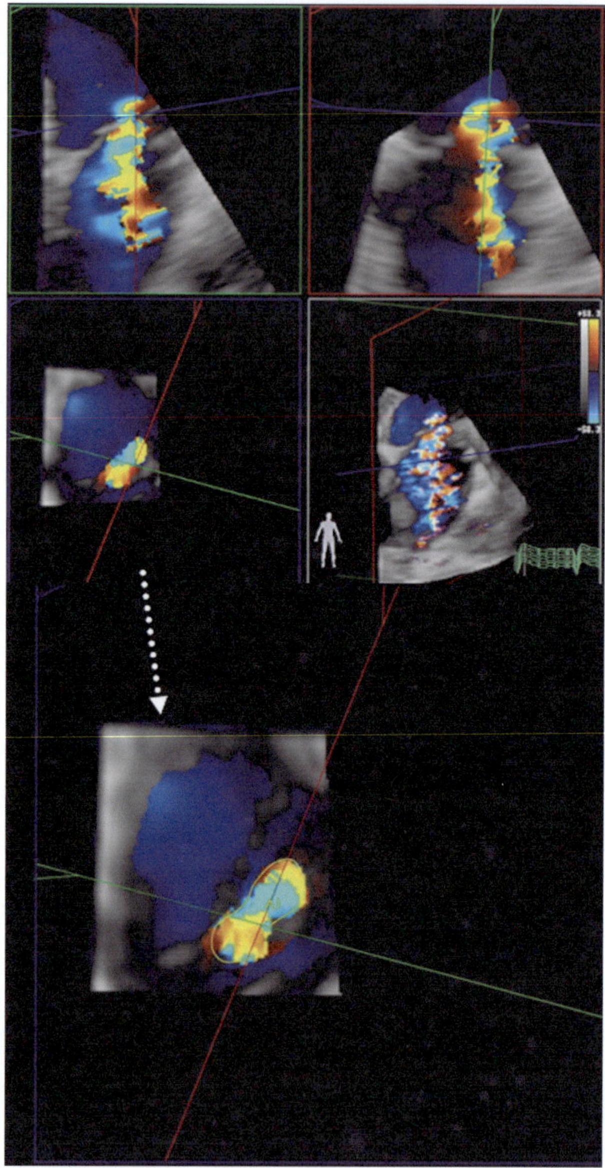

References

1. Otterstad JE, Froeland G, St John Sutton M et al (1997) Accuracy and reproducibility of biplane two-dimensional echocardiographic measurements of left ventricular dimensions and function. Eur Heart J 18:507–513
2. Gutierrez-Chico JL, Zamorano JL, Perez de Isla L et al (2005) Comparison of left ventricular volumes and ejection fractions measured by three-dimensional echocardiography versus by two-dimensional echocardiography and cardiac magnetic resonance in patients with various cardiomyopathies. Am J Cardiol 95:809–813
3. Shiota T, McCarthy PM, White RD et al (1999) Initial clinical experience of real-time three-dimensional echocardiography in patients with ischemic and idiopathic dilated cardiomyopathy. Am J Cardiol 84:1068–1073
4. Lang RM, Badano LP, Tsang W et al (2012) EAE/ASE recommendations for image acquisition and display using three-dimensional echocardiography. Eur Heart J Cardiovasc Imaging 13:1–46
5. Mu Y, Chen L, Tang Q et al (2010) Real time three-dimensional echocardiographic assessment of left ventricular regional systolic function and dyssynchrony in patients with dilated cardiomyopathy. Echocardiography 27:415–420
6. Corsi C, Lang RM, Veronesi F et al (2005) Volumetric quantification of global and regional left ventricular function from real-time three-dimensional echocardiographic images. Circulation 112:1161–1170
7. Gopal AS, Schnellbaecher MJ, Shen Z et al (1997) Freehand three-dimensional echocardiography for determination of left ventricular volume and mass in patients with abnormal ventricles: comparison with magnetic resonance imaging. J Am Soc Echocardiogr 10:853–861
8. Mor-Avi V, Sugeng L, Weinert L et al (2004) Fast measurement of left ventricular mass with real-time three-dimensional echocardiography: comparison with magnetic resonance imaging. Circulation 110:1814–1818
9. Shan K, Bick RJ, Poindexter BJ et al (2000) Relation of tissue Doppler derived myocardial velocities to myocardial structure and beta-adrenergic receptor density in humans. J Am Coll Cardiol 36:891–896
10. Mor-Avi V, Lang RM, Badano LP et al (2011) Current and evolving echocardiographic techniques for the quantitative evaluation of cardiac mechanics: ASE/EAE consensus statement on methodology and indications endorsed by the Japanese Society of Echocardiography. Eur J Echocardiogr 12:167–205
11. Meluzin J, Spinarova L, Hude P et al (2009) Left ventricular mechanics in idiopathic dilated cardiomyopathy: systolic-diastolic coupling and torsion. J Am Soc Echocardiogr 22:486–493
12. Oki T, Tabata T, Yamada H et al (1997) Clinical application of pulsed Doppler tissue imaging for assessing abnormal left ventricular relaxation. Am J Cardiol 79:921–928
13. Mullens W, Borowski AG, Curtin RJ et al (2009) Tissue Doppler imaging in the estimation of intracardiac filling pressure in decompensated patients with advanced systolic heart failure. Circulation 119:62–70
14. Meluzin J, Spinarova L, Hude P et al (2011) Estimation of left ventricular filling pressures by speckle tracking echocardiography in patients with idiopathic dilated cardiomyopathy. Eur J Echocardiogr 12:11–18
15. Cameli M, Lisi M, Mondillo S et al (2010) Left atrial longitudinal strain by speckle tracking echocardiography correlates well with left ventricular filling pressures in patients with heart failure. Cardiovasc Ultrasound 8:14
16. Delgado V, Bax JJ (2011) Assessment of systolic dyssynchrony for cardiac resynchronization therapy is clinically useful. Circulation 123:640–655
17. Gorcsan J 3rd, Abraham T, Agler DA et al (2008) Echocardiography for cardiac resynchronization therapy: recommendations for performance and reporting–a report from the American Society of Echocardiography Dyssynchrony Writing Group endorsed by the Heart Rhythm Society. J Am Soc Echocardiogr 21:191–213

18. Szulik M, Tillekaerts M, Vangeel V et al (2010) Assessment of apical rocking: a new, integrative approach for selection of candidates for cardiac resynchronization therapy. Eur J Echocardiogr 11:863–869
19. Bax JJ, Bleeker GB, Marwick TH et al (2004) Left ventricular dyssynchrony predicts response and prognosis after cardiac resynchronization therapy. J Am Coll Cardiol 44:1834–1840
20. Chung ES, Leon AR, Tavazzi L et al (2008) Results of the Predictors of Response to CRT (PROSPECT) trial. Circulation 117:2608–2616
21. Delgado V, Ypenburg C, van Bommel RJ et al (2008) Assessment of left ventricular dyssynchrony by speckle tracking strain imaging comparison between longitudinal, circumferential, and radial strain in cardiac resynchronization therapy. J Am Coll Cardiol 51:1944–1952
22. Mele D, Agricola E, Galderisi M et al (2009) Real-time three-dimensional echocardiography: current applications, advantages and limits for the evaluation of the left ventricle. G Ital Cardiol (Rome) 10:516–532
23. Faletra FF, Conca C, Klersy C et al (2009) Comparison of eight echocardiographic methods for determining the prevalence of mechanical dyssynchrony and site of latest mechanical contraction in patients scheduled for cardiac resynchronization therapy. Am J Cardiol 103:1746–1752
24. Tanaka H, Nesser HJ, Buck T et al (2010) Dyssynchrony by speckle-tracking echocardiography and response to cardiac resynchronization therapy: results of the Speckle Tracking and Resynchronization (STAR) study. Eur Heart J 31:1690–1700
25. Marsan NA, Bleeker GB, Ypenburg C et al (2008) Real-time three-dimensional echocardiography permits quantification of left ventricular mechanical dyssynchrony and predicts acute response to cardiac resynchronization therapy. J Cardiovasc Electrophysiol 19:392–399
26. Tanaka H, Hara H, Saba S et al (2010) Usefulness of three-dimensional speckle tracking strain to quantify dyssynchrony and the site of latest mechanical activation. Am J Cardiol 105:235–242
27. Ypenburg C, van Bommel RJ, Delgado V et al (2008) Optimal left ventricular lead position predicts reverse remodeling and survival after cardiac resynchronization therapy. J Am Coll Cardiol 52:1402–1409
28. Van de Veire NR, Yu CM, Ajmone-Marsan N et al (2008) Triplane tissue Doppler imaging: a novel three-dimensional imaging modality that predicts reverse left ventricular remodelling after cardiac resynchronisation therapy. Heart 94:e9
29. D'Andrea A, Caso P, Scarafile R et al (2009) Effects of global longitudinal strain and total scar burden on response to cardiac resynchronization therapy in patients with ischaemic dilated cardiomyopathy. Eur J Heart Fail 11:58–67
30. Iwakura K, Ito H, Kawano S et al (2006) Comparison of orifice area by transthoracic three-dimensional Doppler echocardiography versus proximal isovelocity surface area (PISA) method for assessment of mitral regurgitation. Am J Cardiol 97:1630–1637
31. Sugeng L, Spencer KT, Mor-Avi V et al (2003) Dynamic three-dimensional color flow Doppler: an improved technique for the assessment of mitral regurgitation. Echocardiography 20:265–273
32. Fujimoto S, Mizuno R, Nakagawa Y et al (1999) Ultrasonic tissue characterization in patients with dilated cardiomyopathy: comparison with findings from right ventricular endomyocardial biopsy. Int J Card Imaging 15:391–396
33. Dagdeviren B, Akdemir O, Eren M et al (2002) Prognostic implication of myocardial texture analysis in idiopathic dilated cardiomyopathy. Eur J Heart Fail 4:41–48

Other Imaging Techniques in Dilated Cardiomyopathy

7

Giancarlo Vitrella, Marco Bobbo, Manuel Belgrano, Andrea Perkan, and Giorgio Faganello

7.1 Introduction

Cardiac magnetic resonance (CMR) can be used to explore multiple aspects of dilated cardiomyopathy (DCM). In particular, it is useful for differential diagnosis of left ventricular (LV) dysfunction, prognostic stratification, assessment of LV dyssynchrony, prediction of outcome after cardiac resynchronization therapy (CRT) implantation, and assessment of LV thrombosis.

7.2 Differential Diagnosis

Etiologic characterization of DCM may be achieved by evaluating the presence and distribution of macroscopic myocardial fibrosis with late-gadolinium-enhancement (LGE) sequences (Fig. 7.1). In particular, subendocardial or transmural LGE is always found in patients with LV dysfunction secondary to coronary artery disease distributed in coronary perfusion territories. Conversely, LGE is frequently absent in patients with LV dysfunction of nonischemic origin. When LGE is found, the pattern of distribution is often a patchy midwall without coronary distribution. A minority of patients with DCM exhibit a pseudoischemic pattern despite absence

G. Vitrella (✉) • M. Bobbo • A. Perkan
Department of Cardiology, University Hospital of Trieste,
Via P. Valdoni 7, Trieste 34139, Italy
e-mail: giancarlo.vitrella@gmail.com

M. Belgrano, MD
Radiology Unit, University Hospital of Trieste, Via P. Valdoni 7, Trieste 34139, Italy
e-mail: belgranom@gmail.com

G. Faganello, MD
Cardiovascular Center, Azienda per i Servizi Sanitari n° 1, via Slataper, 9, Trieste 34125, Italy
e-mail: giorgio.faganello@libero.it

B. Pinamonti, G. Sinagra (eds.), *Clinical Echocardiography and Other Imaging Techniques in Cardiomyopathies*, DOI 10.1007/978-3-319-06019-4_7,
© Springer International Publishing Switzerland 2014

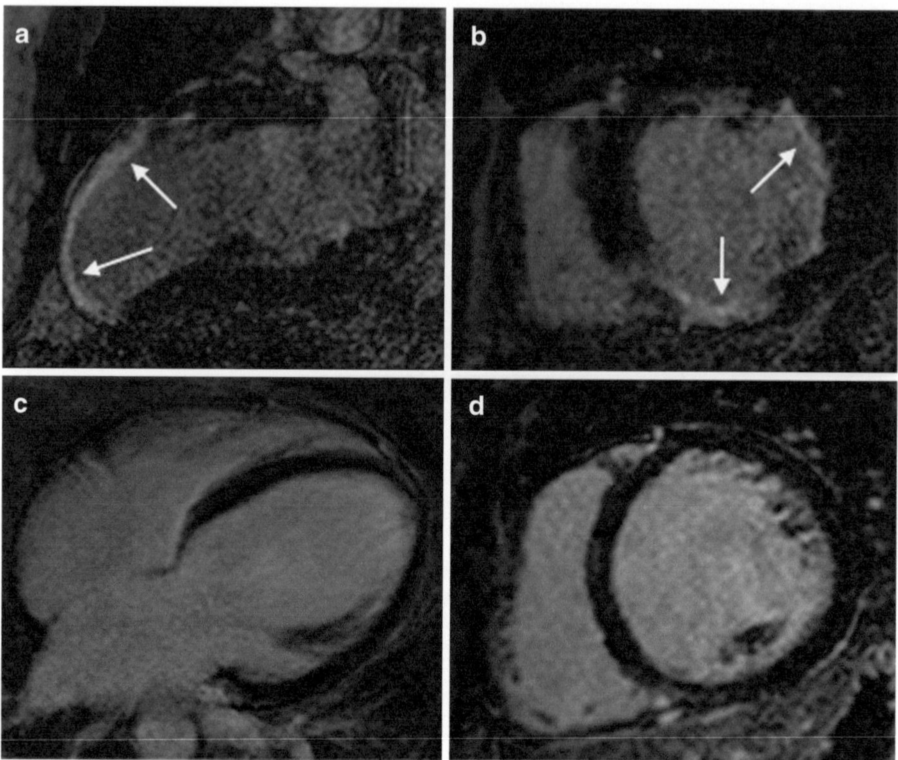

Fig. 7.1 Late gadolinium enhancement (LGE) cardiac magnetic resonance (CMR) images in patients with ischemic (**a, b**) and nonischemic (**c, d**) dilated cardiomyopathy (DCM). Note the absence of LGE in patients with nonischemic DCM and the presence of subendocardial LGE distributed along coronary segments in ischemic DCM images (*arrows*)

of coronary artery disease [1, 2]. LGE with a subepicardial distribution may be suggestive of DCM secondary to myocarditis [3].

7.3 Macroscopic vs Diffuse Fibrosis

LGE sequences are not able to identify diffuse interstitial fibrosis [4] (Fig. 7.2). T1 mapping sequences are able to evaluate interstitial fibrosis and are shown to correlate well with histologically detected fibrosis [5–8], although they require some postprocessing and are time consuming.

7.4 Left Ventricular Dyssynchrony

CMR is able to assess LV dyssynchrony [9] by assessing segmental radial wall motion in short-axis steady-state free precession (SSFP) views. Patients with heart failure (HF) display increased dyssynchrony despite normal QRS duration. Increasing degrees of dyssynchrony are predictive of poor outcomes in patients who

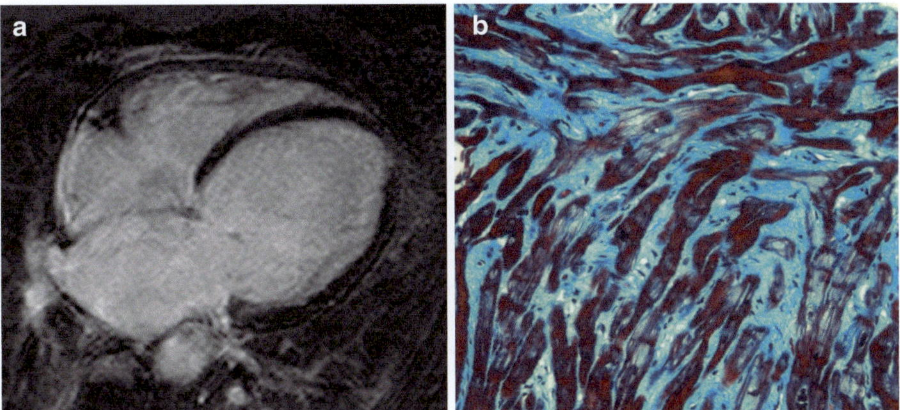

Fig. 7.2 Absence of late gadolinium enhancement (LGE) at cardiac magnetic resonance (CMR) in a patient with dilated cardiomyopathy (DCM) (**a**). Histologic specimen (Masson trichrome stain) from endomyocardial biopsy of the same patient showing diffuse interstitial fibrosis (**b**)

undergo CRT and patients who do not [10, 11]. LV dyssynchrony may also be evaluated with velocity-encoded sequences, with results similar to tissue Doppler imaging [12]. This may be useful in patients with poor acoustic window.

7.5 Assessment of Left Ventricular Thrombosis

Contrast-enhanced CMR is more sensitive and specific in detecting intraventricular thrombus compared with standard 2D echocardiography [13], particularly through SSFP sequences and especially through inversion recovery (IR) sequences with a very long inversion time early after gadolinium administration (Fig. 7.3).

7.6 Single Photon Emission Computed Tomography

Single-photon-emission computed tomography (SPECT) was evaluated to assess ventricular volumes and function [14], myocardial stress, rest perfusion, and sympathetic nervous activity. The presence and extent of perfusion abnormalities, possibly reflecting fibrosis, correlate with poor prognosis [15–17]. The pattern of occurrence may be helpful to differentiate ischemic from nonischemic forms of DCM [18–20]. SPECT imaging may be an alternative to CMR—although it is less reliable—in identifying patients with areas of LV scarring responsible for poor response to CRT [21, 22]. Iodine 123-metaiodobenzylguanidine (MIBG), a norepinephrine analog, is used as a tracer to investigate cardiac sympathetic nervous function [23]. In some studies, altered cardiac sympathetic nervous activity, assessed by MIBG imaging, is predictive of ventricular arrhythmias, appropriate implantable cardioverter defibrillator (ICD) therapy [24], and adverse prognosis in DCM [25–27].

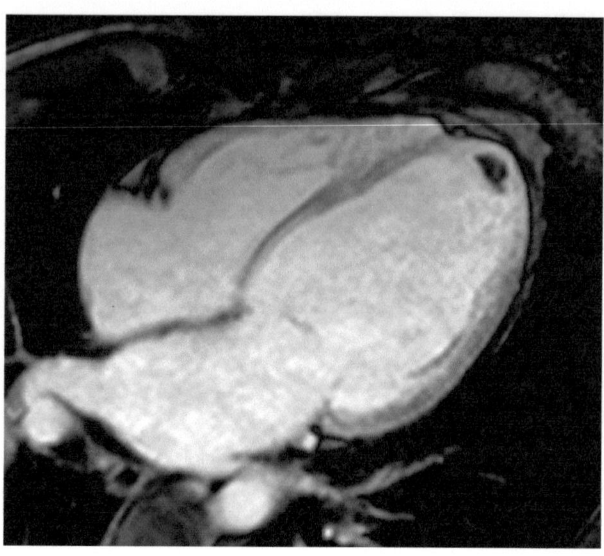

Fig. 7.3 Advanced dilated cardiomyopathy (DCM). Cardiac magnetic resonance (CMR) image acquired early after contrast administration, with long inversion time, showing a small intraventricular thrombus as hypointense (*dark*) area at left ventricular (LV) apex

7.7 Positron Emission Tomography

Myocardial metabolic activity may be assessed with [^{18}F]-fluorodeoxyglucose positron emission tomography (PET). In patients with DCM, finding heterogeneous regional myocardial metabolic activity is predictive of a poor outcome, whereas a homogeneous pattern is predictive of functional improvement [28]. Absolute myocardial blood flow measured by dynamic PET and [^{13}N]-ammonia or ^{15}O-labeled water (^{15}O-H$_2$O) [29] is impaired both at rest and in response to vasodilating stimuli in DCM patients [30, 31]. The degree of impairment is independently associated with disease progression and adverse outcome [31, 32]. Conversely, patients on beta-blockers who experience improved LV ejection fraction (EF) also show improved myocardial blood flow assessed by PET [33, 34].

7.8 Computed Tomography

Computed tomography (CT) is a noninvasive cardiac imaging technique that is mainly used to test for the presence of coronary artery disease. Multidetector CT is thus accurate in identifying patients with idiopathic versus ischemic forms of DCM and may represent a valid alternative to coronary angiography [35, 36]. Data acquisition in CT is continuous throughout the cardiac cycle. Therefore, end-diastolic and end-systolic images may be used to analyze ventricular volumes and function, with good correlation with CMR and contrast-enhanced echocardiography [37, 38].

7.9   Dystrophinopathy-Associated Cardiomyopathy

CMR studies in patients with dystrophinopathy-associated CMP show abnormalities of myocardial strain through SSFP and tagging sequences [39–41], midwall/subepicardial fibrosis by LGE imaging [42–44], diffuse fibrosis identified by T1 mapping techniques [45], fatty replacement [46, 47], and inflammation through T2 and early gadolinium enhancement sequences [48]. The latter sign is a harbinger of rapid LV function deterioration [48]. Subclinical CMP is also reported at CMR (SSFP and LGE) in mother-carriers of Duchenne and Becker muscular dystrophy [49]. Myocardial perfusion with ^{201}Tl imaging shows distinct perfusion defects in the LV free wall in patients with Duchenne muscular dystrophy [50–52]. Large perfusion defects have adverse prognostic significance [50, 53]. PET identifies areas of myocardial perfusion/metabolism mismatch (increased [^{18}F]-FDG activity and decreased [^{13}N]-ammonia activity) in the LV free wall in patients with Duchenne and Becker dystrophy [54, 55].

References

1. McCrohon JA, Moon JC, Prasad SK et al (2003) Differentiation of heart failure related to dilated cardiomyopathy and coronary artery disease using gadolinium-enhanced cardiovascular magnetic resonance. Circulation 108:54–59
2. Bello D, Shah DJ, Farah GM et al (2003) Gadolinium cardiovascular magnetic resonance predicts reversible myocardial dysfunction and remodeling in patients with heart failure undergoing beta-blocker therapy. Circulation 108:1945–1953
3. Voigt A, Elgeti T, Durmus T et al (2011) Cardiac magnetic resonance imaging in dilated cardiomyopathy in adults–towards identification of myocardial inflammation. Eur Radiol 21:925–935
4. Schalla S, Bekkers SC, Dennert R et al (2010) Replacement and reactive myocardial fibrosis in idiopathic dilated cardiomyopathy: comparison of magnetic resonance imaging with right ventricular biopsy. Eur J Heart Fail 12:227–231
5. Sibley CT, Noureldin RA, Gai N et al (2012) T1 Mapping in cardiomyopathy at cardiac MR: comparison with endomyocardial biopsy. Radiology 265:724–732
6. Iles L, Pfluger H, Phrommintikul A et al (2008) Evaluation of diffuse myocardial fibrosis in heart failure with cardiac magnetic resonance contrast-enhanced T1 mapping. J Am Coll Cardiol 52:1574–1580
7. Messroghli DR, Greiser A, Frohlich M et al (2007) Optimization and validation of a fully-integrated pulse sequence for modified look-locker inversion-recovery (MOLLI) T1 mapping of the heart. J Magn Reson Imaging 26:1081–1086
8. Piechnik SK, Ferreira VM, Dall'Armellina E et al (2010) Shortened Modified Look-Locker Inversion recovery (ShMOLLI) for clinical myocardial T1-mapping at 1.5 and 3 T within a 9 heartbeat breathhold. J Cardiovasc Magn Reson 12:69
9. Chalil S, Stegemann B, Muhyaldeen S et al (2007) Intraventricular dyssynchrony predicts mortality and morbidity after cardiac resynchronization therapy: a study using cardiovascular magnetic resonance tissue synchronization imaging. J Am Coll Cardiol 50:243–252
10. Foley PW, Khadjooi K, Ward JA et al (2009) Radial dyssynchrony assessed by cardiovascular magnetic resonance in relation to left ventricular function, myocardial scarring and QRS duration in patients with heart failure. J Cardiovasc Magn Reson 11:50

11. Leyva F, Foley PW, Stegemann B et al (2009) Development and validation of a clinical index to predict survival after cardiac resynchronisation therapy. Heart 95:1619–1625

12. Westenberg JJ, Lamb HJ, van der Geest RJ et al (2006) Assessment of left ventricular dyssynchrony in patients with conduction delay and idiopathic dilated cardiomyopathy: head-to-head comparison between tissue doppler imaging and velocity-encoded magnetic resonance imaging. J Am Coll Cardiol 47:2042–2048

13. Mollet NR, Dymarkowski S, Volders W et al (2002) Visualization of ventricular thrombi with contrast-enhanced magnetic resonance imaging in patients with ischemic heart disease. Circulation 106:2873–2876

14. Wang F, Zhang J, Fang W et al (2009) Evaluation of left ventricular volumes and ejection fraction by gated SPECT and cardiac MRI in patients with dilated cardiomyopathy. Eur J Nucl Med Mol Imaging 36:1611–1621

15. Doi YL, Chikamori T, Tukata J et al (1991) Prognostic value of thallium-201 perfusion defects in idiopathic dilated cardiomyopathy. Am J Cardiol 67:188–193

16. Li LX, Nohara R, Okuda K et al (1996) Comparative study of 201Tl-scintigraphic image and myocardial pathologic findings in patients with dilated cardiomyopathy. Ann Nucl Med 10:307–314

17. Watanabe M, Gotoh K, Nagashima K et al (2001) Relationship between thallium-201 myocardial SPECT and findings of endomyocardial biopsy specimens in dilated cardiomyopathy. Ann Nucl Med 15:13–19

18. Danias PG, Papaioannou GI, Ahlberg AW et al (2004) Usefulness of electrocardiographic-gated stress technetium-99 m sestamibi single-photon emission computed tomography to differentiate ischemic from nonischemic cardiomyopathy. Am J Cardiol 94:14–19

19. Juilliere Y, Marie PY, Danchin N et al (1993) Radionuclide assessment of regional differences in left ventricular wall motion and myocardial perfusion in idiopathic dilated cardiomyopathy. Eur Heart J 14:1163–1169

20. Chikamori T, Doi YL, Yonezawa Y et al (1992) Value of dipyridamole thallium-201 imaging in noninvasive differentiation of idiopathic dilated cardiomyopathy from coronary artery disease with left ventricular dysfunction. Am J Cardiol 69:650–653

21. Sciagra R, Giaccardi M, Porciani MC et al (2004) Myocardial perfusion imaging using gated SPECT in heart failure patients undergoing cardiac resynchronization therapy. J Nucl Med 45:164–168

22. Yokokawa M, Tada H, Toyama T et al (2009) Magnetic resonance imaging is superior to cardiac scintigraphy to identify nonresponders to cardiac resynchronization therapy. Pacing Clin Electrophysiol 32(Suppl 1):S57–S62

23. Henderson EB, Kahn JK, Corbett JR et al (1988) Abnormal I-123 metaiodobenzylguanidine myocardial washout and distribution may reflect myocardial adrenergic derangement in patients with congestive cardiomyopathy. Circulation 78:1192–1199

24. Boogers MJ, Borleffs CJ, Henneman MM et al (2010) Cardiac sympathetic denervation assessed with 123-iodine metaiodobenzylguanidine imaging predicts ventricular arrhythmias in implantable cardioverter-defibrillator patients. J Am Coll Cardiol 55:2769–2777

25. Merlet P, Benvenuti C, Moyse D et al (1999) Prognostic value of MIBG imaging in idiopathic dilated cardiomyopathy. J Nucl Med 40:917–923

26. Verberne HJ, Brewster LM, Somsen GA et al (2008) Prognostic value of myocardial 123I-metaiodobenzylguanidine (MIBG) parameters in patients with heart failure: a systematic review. Eur Heart J 29:1147–1159

27. Jacobson AF, Senior R, Cerqueira MD et al (2010) Myocardial iodine-123 meta-iodobenzylguanidine imaging and cardiac events in heart failure. Results of the prospective ADMIRE-HF (AdreView Myocardial Imaging for Risk Evaluation in Heart Failure) study. J Am Coll Cardiol 55:2212–2221

28. Yokoyama I, Momomura S, Ohtake T et al (1998) Role of positron emission tomography using fluorine-18 fluoro-2-deoxyglucose in predicting improvement in left ventricular function in patients with idiopathic dilated cardiomyopathy. Eur J Nucl Med 25:736–743

29. Kaufmann PA, Camici PG (2005) Myocardial blood flow measurement by PET: technical aspects and clinical applications. J Nucl Med 46:75–88

30. Canetti M, Akhter MW, Lerman A et al (2003) Evaluation of myocardial blood flow reserve in patients with chronic congestive heart failure due to idiopathic dilated cardiomyopathy. Am J Cardiol 92:1246–1249
31. Neglia D, Parodi O, Gallopin M et al (1995) Myocardial blood flow response to pacing tachycardia and to dipyridamole infusion in patients with dilated cardiomyopathy without overt heart failure. A quantitative assessment by positron emission tomography. Circulation 92:796–804
32. Neglia D, Michelassi C, Trivieri MG et al (2002) Prognostic role of myocardial blood flow impairment in idiopathic left ventricular dysfunction. Circulation 105:186–193
33. Slart RH, Tio RA, van der Vleuten PA et al (2010) Myocardial perfusion reserve and contractile pattern after beta-blocker therapy in patients with idiopathic dilated cardiomyopathy. J Nucl Cardiol 17:479–485
34. Neglia D, De Maria R, Masi S et al (2007) Effects of long-term treatment with carvedilol on myocardial blood flow in idiopathic dilated cardiomyopathy. Heart 93:808–813
35. Andreini D, Pontone G, Pepi M et al (2007) Diagnostic accuracy of multidetector computed tomography coronary angiography in patients with dilated cardiomyopathy. J Am Coll Cardiol 49:2044–2050
36. Ghostine S, Caussin C, Habis M et al (2008) Non-invasive diagnosis of ischaemic heart failure using 64-slice computed tomography. Eur Heart J 29:2133–2140
37. Juergens KU, Grude M, Maintz D et al (2004) Multi-detector row CT of left ventricular function with dedicated analysis software versus MR imaging: initial experience. Radiology 230:403–410
38. Burianova L, Riedlbauchova L, Lefflerova K et al (2009) Assessment of left ventricular function in non-dilated and dilated hearts: comparison of contrast-enhanced 2-dimensional echocardiography with multi-detector row CT angiography. Acta Cardiol 64:787–794
39. Ashford MW Jr, Liu W, Lin SJ et al (2005) Occult cardiac contractile dysfunction in dystrophin-deficient children revealed by cardiac magnetic resonance strain imaging. Circulation 112:2462–2467
40. Hor KN, Wansapura J, Markham LW et al (2009) Circumferential strain analysis identifies strata of cardiomyopathy in Duchenne muscular dystrophy: a cardiac magnetic resonance tagging study. J Am Coll Cardiol 53:1204–1210
41. Smith GC, Kinali M, Prasad SK et al (2006) Primary myocardial dysfunction in autosomal dominant EDMD. A tissue doppler and cardiovascular magnetic resonance study. J Cardiovasc Magn Reson 8:723–730
42. Silva MC, Meira ZM, Gurgel Giannetti J et al (2007) Myocardial delayed enhancement by magnetic resonance imaging in patients with muscular dystrophy. J Am Coll Cardiol 49:1874–1879
43. Yilmaz A, Gdynia HJ, Baccouche H et al (2008) Cardiac involvement in patients with Becker muscular dystrophy: new diagnostic and pathophysiological insights by a CMR approach. J Cardiovasc Magn Reson 10:50
44. Puchalski MD, Williams RV, Askovich B et al (2009) Late gadolinium enhancement: precursor to cardiomyopathy in Duchenne muscular dystrophy? Int J Cardiovasc Imaging 25:57–63
45. Turkbey EB, Gai N, Lima JA et al (2012) Assessment of cardiac involvement in myotonic muscular dystrophy by T1 mapping on magnetic resonance imaging. Heart Rhythm 9:1691–1697
46. Wahbi K, Meune C, el Hamouda H et al (2008) Cardiac assessment of limb-girdle muscular dystrophy 2I patients: an echography, Holter ECG and magnetic resonance imaging study. Neuromuscul Disord 18:650–655
47. Rosales XQ, Moser SJ, Tran T et al (2011) Cardiovascular magnetic resonance of cardiomyopathy in limb girdle muscular dystrophy 2B and 2I. J Cardiovasc Magn Reson 13:39
48. Mavrogeni S, Papavasiliou A, Spargias K et al (2010) Myocardial inflammation in Duchenne Muscular Dystrophy as a precipitating factor for heart failure: a prospective study. BMC Neurol 10:33
49. Mavrogeni S, Bratis K, Papavasiliou A et al (2013) CMR detects subclinical cardiomyopathy in mother-carriers of Duchenne and Becker muscular dystrophy. JACC Cardiovasc Imaging 6:526–528

50. Kawai N, Sotobata I, Okada M et al (1985) Evaluation of myocardial involvement in Duchenne's progressive muscular dystrophy with thallium-201 myocardial perfusion imaging. Jpn Heart J 26:767–775
51. Yamamoto S, Matsushima H, Suzuki A et al (1988) A comparative study of thallium-201 single-photon emission computed tomography and electrocardiography in Duchenne and other types of muscular dystrophy. Am J Cardiol 61:836–843
52. Nagamachi S, Jinnouchi S, Ono S et al (1989) Tl-201 myocardial SPECT in patients with Duchenne's muscular dystrophy: a long-term follow-up. Clin Nucl Med 14:827–830
53. Miyoshi K, Fujikawa K (1995) Comparison of thallium-201 myocardial single-photon emission computed tomography and cine magnetic resonance imaging in Duchenne's muscular dystrophy. Am J Cardiol 75:1284–1286
54. Perloff JK, Henze E, Schelbert HR (1984) Alterations in regional myocardial metabolism, perfusion, and wall motion in Duchenne muscular dystrophy studied by radionuclide imaging. Circulation 69:33–42
55. Quinlivan RM, Lewis P, Marsden P et al (1996) Cardiac function, metabolism and perfusion in Duchenne and Becker muscular dystrophy. Neuromuscul Disord 6:237–246

Dilated Cardiomyopathy: Usefulness of Imaging in Prognostic Stratification and Choice of Treatment

8

Marco Merlo, Francesco Negri, Davide Stolfo, Anita Iorio, Bruno Pinamonti, Massimo Zecchin, Laura Vitali Serdoz, and Andrea Di Lenarda

8.1   Introduction

The role of imaging in prognostic stratification of idiopathic dilated cardiomyopathy (DCM), due to the rarity of this pathology, has some problems. In particular, difficult therapeutic choices in clinical practice, (i.e., heart transplantation or implantable device therapy), which mainly depend on prognostic stratification, are often based on clinical trials assessing patients with heart failure (HF), due to multiple etiologies (mostly ischemic) or retrospective studies on small populations, which have subsequent limitations. Nevertheless, idiopathic DCM patient profiles are somehow different from those in patients who present with secondary forms of DCM (i.e. ischemic, hypertensive, or valvular heart disease), because idiopathic DCM is usually found in younger people with fewer comorbidities. Echocardiography and cardiac magnetic resonance (CMR) represent useful imaging techniques for prognostic assessment of DCM.

Besides imaging tools, it must be noted that some functional tests, such as cardiopulmonary exercise test, or other nonimaging tests, such as T-wave alternans, QT dynamicity, as well as genetic characterization, can be prognostically helpful in selected scenarios, such as arrhythmic risk stratification, especially in the early

M. Merlo (✉) • F. Negri • D. Stolfo • A. Iorio •B. Pinamonti • M. Zecchin • L.V. Serdoz
Department of Cardiology, University Hospital of Trieste,
via P. Valdoni 7, Trieste 34139, Italy
e-mail: supermerloo@libero.it; francesco_negri@yahoo.it; davide.stolfo@gmail.com;
anita.iorio@hotmail.it; bruno.pinamonti@gmail.it; massimo.zecchin@alice.it;
lavise@gmail.com

A. Di Lenarda
Cardiovascular Center, Azienda per i Servizi Sanitari n°1 di Trieste,
Via Slataper 9, Trieste 34100, Italy
e-mail: andrea.dilenarda@aots.sanita.fvg.it

B. Pinamonti, G. Sinagra (eds.), *Clinical Echocardiography and Other Imaging Techniques in Cardiomyopathies*, DOI 10.1007/978-3-319-06019-4_8,
© Springer International Publishing Switzerland 2014

phases of DCM, which remains a critical issue for the cardiologic community, as sudden death (SD) accounts for 30–40 % of all idiopathic DCM deaths. However, these variables are not yet validated in randomized prospective clinical trials. Considerations such as these, connected to the generally young age of patients and to their family history, make this issue very important and difficult for cardiologists. That is why it is often better to refer patients to tertiary care centers for diagnostic–therapeutic assessment and prognostic stratification of cardiomyopathies (CMP).

8.2 Echocardiography and Prognosis

8.2.1 Left Ventricular Dimensions and Systolic Dysfunction

Quantitative assessment of left ventricular (LV) dimensions and systolic function has a particular relevance in the long-term follow-up of DCM patients for assessing disease progression or response to treatment. LV ejection fraction (EF) emerged as the only instrumental baseline parameter that could predict SD in the long term, which confirms its known role in this specific field [1]. The presence of markedly dilated LV (end-diastolic LV diameter $\geq$38 mm/m^2) associated with severely depressed EF is a predictor for SD if evaluated within 1 year before the event. These two parameters probably identify a subgroup of patients with a very advanced and severe disease characterized by predicting a higher risk of SD [2].

Notably, implanted cardiac defibrillator (ICD) implantation emerged as the only therapy with an independent protective role against SD [1]. Since publication of the Sudden Cardiac Death in Heart Failure (SCD-HeFT) and Defibrillators in Non-Ischemic Cardiomyopathy Treatment Evaluation (DEFINITE) trials [3, 4] ICD indication for primary prevention of SD has been extended to patients affected by DCM presenting LVEF $\leq$0.35 and New York Heart Association (NYHA) functional classes II or III (class I indication, level of evidence B) [5], despite $\geq$3 months of optimal pharmacological therapy. However, it is not clear whether a longer interval could modify the proportion of patients who are candidates for ICD. In clinical practice, timing of ICD implantation for primary prevention remains a critical and very common issue [6], particularly in idiopathic DCM [5].

In this sense, the Canadian Cardiovascular Society recommended a different timing in ICD therapy, depending on the etiology of heart failure (HF). Patients with nonischemic DCM with EF $\leq$0.35 and NYHA functional classes II or III are recommended for an ICD after at least 9 months of optimal medical therapy (strong recommendation, high-quality evidence), whereas in patients with ischemic DCM, ICD therapy is recommended after only $\geq$3 months of optimal medical therapy [7]. However, the risk of waiting before implanting an ICD is not specified. In clinical practice, there is often the attitude not to delay implantation for too long, especially when cardiac resynchronization is required. In patients with a high probability of improvement, ICD implantation could be safely delayed [8].

This issue remains a challenge for the cardiologist community; in fact, according to recent evidence, even in patients considered at very high risk (i.e., those presenting with important enlargement of LV dimensions and very severe LV systolic dysfunction), the probability of maintaining ICD indications after optimization of medical treatment, or SD in the meantime, was only 40 %, even in more impaired patients (unpublished data). Therefore, early ICD implantation should not be generally recommended in the majority of cases but should at least be considered a closer follow-up (i.e., 3 or 4 weeks) in patients who will less likely improve after baseline evaluation. The need of further parameters, useful in arrhythmic stratification, clearly emerges regardless of LVEF. In this sense, only a few reports provided by retrospective studies are available, such as those assessing the presence of nonsustained ventricular tachycardia (VT) during Holter monitoring in patients with moderate systolic dysfunction [9] or T-wave alternans [10].

8.2.2 Left Ventricular Reverse Remodeling

Several studies have demonstrated the importance of echocardiography for re-evaluating patients after an appropriate follow-up under optimal medical treatment. A study by our group [11] (361 patients consecutively enrolled in a cohort of idiopathic DCM) emphasizes the importance of considering both clinical and laboratory data at baseline and during follow-up to improve prognostic stratification of idiopathic DCM patients. In that study, LV reverse remodeling characterized about one third of the entire cohort alive at midterm follow-up. Those patients received tailored pharmacological treatment, and the condition emerged as an independent predictor of long-term prognosis. Therefore, evolution to LV reverse remodeling suggests less structural cardiac damage at diagnosis and a higher probability of better response to treatment [11].

8.2.3 Diastolic Dysfunction

Conventional echo Doppler assessment of LV diastolic dysfunction (transmitral filling pattern) provides important diagnostic and prognostic information in patients with idiopathic DCM. To fully define the category of diastolic dysfunction, it is important to include methods such as tissue Doppler analysis (TDI) of the mitral annulus (E' velocity), pulsed-wave Doppler of pulmonary venous inflow, and left atrial (LA) size.

LV restrictive filling pattern (RFP), frequent in idiopathic DCM, is associated with more severe disease and is as a powerful long-term indicator of increased mortality risk and need for heart transplantation [12, 13]. Furthermore in patients with idiopathic DCM, the persistence of RFP despite optimized treatment is associated with high mortality and transplantation rates, provides additional prognostic information with respect to the baseline study, and might be used in conjunction with the clinical assessment to select patients for a more strict follow-up or for cardiac transplantation [14]. No data exist at present regarding the role of diastolic function calculated by TDI regarding the prognosis of idiopathic DCM. E/E' could represent an easy tool that can be used earlier to assess early diastolic dysfunction compared with RFP.

8.2.4 Right Ventricular Dysfunction

Right ventricular (RV) dysfunction may be present in idiopathic DCM and is an important adverse prognostic marker associated with significantly worse functional class and outcome [15]. However, there is a lack of studies and data on large populations of such patients due to the relative rarity of the disease and difficulty in assessing RV function. RV dysfunction can be related to LV dysfunction severity and subsequently secondary to high LV filling pressures and pulmonary hypertension; however, biventricular involvement in the disease process may be present. The tricuspid annular proximal systolic excursion (TAPSE), a well-validated and simple measurement of RV longitudinal function, provides a prognostic factor in patients with advanced HF [15]. Nevertheless, there is a lack of exhaustive data regarding RV dysfunction impact specifically on the outcome in idiopathic DCM.

8.2.5 Functional Mitral Regurgitation

Functional mitral regurgitation (MR), a common finding in ischemic and nonischemic LV dysfunction, is independently associated with a worse prognosis [11, 16], and increasing functional MR severity correlates with adverse clinical conditions and reduced survival [17]. The adverse hemodynamic consequence of MR are particularly relevant in idiopathic DCM, in which it increases volume overload of a failing ventricle, which, in turn, stimulates modifications at several levels (molecular, cellular, tissue, and cardiac chamber level), further promoting adverse LV remodeling [16]. In patients where it is difficult to find out whether MR is primary or secondary, a detailed assessment of valve morphology is required, often employing the transesophageal approach (TEE). This assessment has important management implications because medical therapy and cardiac resynchronization therapy (CRT) improve secondary MR but are not helpful in the setting of significant leaflet disease [18]. Moreover, interventional approaches, both, surgical and percutaneous, can be considered to correct functional MR. MitraClip is emerging as a new percutaneous technique. However, to date, selection of patients as candidates for MitraClip intervention is an open and important issue.

8.2.6 Mechanical Dyssynchrony

Newer echocardiographic techniques to evaluate LV dyssynchrony involving real-time 3D echo, TDI-derived strain imaging, and 2D-derived speckle-tracking strain analysis have all been described and potentially offer solutions to some of the problems encountered with tissue velocity imaging. To date, however, NYHA class, LV ejection fraction, and electrocardiography (ECG) are the only validated parameters for determining the appropriateness of CRT implantation. Furthermore, biventricular pacing seems to have more effect in idiopathic DCM patients than in patients with ischemic heart disease [19].

8.2.7 Ventricular Thrombosis

The presence of spontaneous echo contrast is often seen in severely impaired ventricles and should prompt a careful assessment for thrombus. Again, LV contrast agents can be used where resolution of the LV apex and differentiation of thrombus from artefacts is difficult.

8.2.8 Prognostic Significance of Stress Echocardiography with Dobutamine

The prognostic role of dobutamine stress test has been used to evaluate the contractile reserve [20, 21]. The presence of viability is related to better prognosis and higher probability for improved LV function at follow-up [22]. In our experience, positive dobutamine response is frequent in idiopathic DCM (43 % of cases), with improvement in systolic and diastolic LV function, RV function, and MR; it is also associated with a better prognosis. Moreover, patients who respond to dobutamine are less symptomatic and show less severe ventricular dilation and dysfunction and lower LV filling pressure [20]. Finally, assessment of LV contractile reserve by 3D speckle-tracking global circumferential strain during dobutamine stress test demonstrates a predictive value for cardiovascular events in patients with idiopathic DCM [23]. However, in clinical practice, the dobutamine test, due to its only moderate accuracy, is not commonly employed for prognostic stratification of idiopathic DCM patients and in selecting patients for heart transplantation.

8.3 Cardiac Magnetic Resonance

CMR provides additional prognostic information in patients with DCM because it is the gold-standard technique for both biventricular morphologic and functional quantitative assessment and tissue characterization. However, few studies are available that specifically assess patients with idiopathic DCM. Nazarian et al. reported on 26 patients with nonischemic DCM who had predominant scar localization and distribution characterized by the transmural extent of late gadolinium enhancement (LGE) of 26–75 % of wall thickness, which was significantly predictive of inducible ventricular tachycardia (VT) on electrophysiological stimulation and remained predictive after adjustment for LVEF. Thus, scar distribution may identify the substrate for inducible VT and may identify high-risk patients for SD [24]. Assomull et al. found midwall fibrosis using LGE-CMR in 35 % of 101 consecutive patients with nonischemic DCM and HF. This finding was associated with a higher rate of all-cause deaths and hospitalizations for a cardiovascular event and for predicting SD and/or sustained VT [25]. Finally, Hombach et al. demonstrated that in addition to cardiac index and RV end-diastolic volume index derived from CMR imaging, a QRS duration >110 ms and presence of diabetes mellitus provided prognostic impact in a large cohort of patients with idiopathic DCM over a 4-year period [26].

However, it is important to emphasize that CMR has some limitations: it always involves accessibility problems and requires expert cardiology and radiology personnel. Additionally, it is not usually permitted for heart-device carriers and so frequently it turns out to be complementary to echocardiography, mainly limited to the initial phase of the disease and ceased during the follow-up period, when a device could be implanted.

References

1. Merlo MPA, Pinamonti B, Zecchin M et al (2013) Long-term prognostic impact of therapeutic strategies in patients with idiopathic dilated cardiomyopathy: changing mortality over the last 30 years. Eur J Heart Fail 16(3):317–324
2. Zecchin M, Lenarda AD, Bonin M et al (2001) Incidence and predictors of sudden cardiac death during long-term follow-up in patients with dilated cardiomyopathy on optimal medical therapy. Ital Heart J 2:213–221
3. Bardy GH, Lee KL, Mark DB et al (2005) Amiodarone or an implantable cardioverter-defibrillator for congestive heart failure. N Engl J Med 352:225–237
4. Kadish A, Dyer A, Daubert JP, et al. (2004) Defibrillators in non-ischemic cardiomyopathy treatment evaluation (DEFINITE) investigators. Prophylactic defibrillator implantation in patients with nonischemic dilated cardiomyopathy. N Engl J Med 350(21):2151–2158
5. Epstein AE, DiMarco JP, Ellenbogen KA et al (2008) ACC/AHA/HRS 2008 Guidelines for Device-Based Therapy of Cardiac Rhythm Abnormalities: a report of the American College of Cardiology/American Heart Association Task Force on Practice Guidelines (Writing Committee to Revise the ACC/AHA/NASPE 2002 Guideline Update for Implantation of Cardiac Pacemakers and Antiarrhythmia Devices) developed in collaboration with the American Association for Thoracic Surgery and Society of Thoracic Surgeons. J Am Coll Cardiol 51:e1–e62
6. Al-Khatib SM, Hellkamp A, Curtis J et al (2011) Non-evidence-based ICD implantations in the United States. JAMA 305:43–49
7. McKelvie RS, Moe GW, Ezekowitz JA et al (2013) The 2012 Canadian Cardiovascular Society heart failure management guidelines update: focus on acute and chronic heart failure. Can J Cardiol 29:168–181
8. Metra M, Nodari S, Parrinello G et al (2003) Marked improvement in left ventricular ejection fraction during long-term beta-blockade in patients with chronic heart failure: clinical correlates and prognostic significance. Am Heart J 145:292–299
9. Zecchin M, Di Lenarda A, Gregori D et al (2008) Are nonsustained ventricular tachycardias predictive of major arrhythmias in patients with dilated cardiomyopathy on optimal medical treatment? Pacing Clin Electrophysiol 31:290–299
10. Klingenheben T, Zabel M, D'Agostino RB et al (2000) Predictive value of T-wave alternans for arrhythmic events in patients with congestive heart failure. Lancet 356:651–652
11. Merlo M, Pyxaras SA, Pinamonti B et al (2011) Prevalence and prognostic significance of left ventricular reverse remodeling in dilated cardiomyopathy receiving tailored medical treatment. J Am Coll Cardiol 57:1468–1476
12. Vanoverschelde JL, Raphael DA, Robert AR et al (1990) Left ventricular filling in dilated cardiomyopathy: relation to functional class and hemodynamics. J Am Coll Cardiol 15:1288–1295
13. Pinamonti B, Di Lenarda A, Sinagra G et al (1993) Restrictive left ventricular filling pattern in dilated cardiomyopathy assessed by Doppler echocardiography: clinical, echocardiographic and hemodynamic correlations and prognostic implications. Heart Muscle Disease Study Group. J Am Coll Cardiol 22:808–815

14. Pinamonti B, Zecchin M, Di Lenarda A et al (1997) Persistence of restrictive left ventricular filling pattern in dilated cardiomyopathy: an ominous prognostic sign. J Am Coll Cardiol 29: 604–612
15. Ghio S, Recusani F, Klersy C et al (2000) Prognostic usefulness of the tricuspid annular plane systolic excursion in patients with congestive heart failure secondary to idiopathic or ischemic dilated cardiomyopathy. Am J Cardiol 85:837–842
16. Rossi A, Dini FL, Faggiano P et al (2011) Independent prognostic value of functional mitral regurgitation in patients with heart failure. A quantitative analysis of 1256 patients with ischaemic and non-ischaemic dilated cardiomyopathy. Heart 97:1675–1680
17. Karaca O, Avci A, Guler GB et al (2011) Tenting area reflects disease severity and prognosis in patients with non-ischaemic dilated cardiomyopathy and functional mitral regurgitation. Eur J Heart Fail 13:284–291
18. Whitlow PL, Feldman T, Pedersen WR et al (2012) Acute and 12-month results with catheter-based mitral valve leaflet repair: the EVEREST II (Endovascular Valve Edge-to-Edge Repair) High Risk Study. J Am Coll Cardiol 59:130–139
19. Molhoek SG, Bax JJ, van Erven L et al (2004) Comparison of benefits from cardiac resynchronization therapy in patients with ischemic cardiomyopathy versus idiopathic dilated cardiomyopathy. Am J Cardiol 93:860–863
20. Pinamonti B, Perkan A, Di Lenarda A et al (2002) Dobutamine echocardiography in idiopathic dilated cardiomyopathy: clinical and prognostic implications. Eur J Heart Fail 4:49–61
21. Pratali L, Picano E, Otasevic P et al (2001) Prognostic significance of the dobutamine echocardiography test in idiopathic dilated cardiomyopathy. Am J Cardiol 88:1374–1378
22. Naqvi TZ, Goel RK, Forrester JS et al (1999) Myocardial contractile reserve on dobutamine echocardiography predicts late spontaneous improvement in cardiac function in patients with recent onset idiopathic dilated cardiomyopathy. J Am Coll Cardiol 34:1537–1544
23. Matsumoto K, Tanaka H, Kaneko A et al (2012) Contractile reserve assessed by three-dimensional global circumferential strain as a predictor of cardiovascular events in patients with idiopathic dilated cardiomyopathy. J Am Soc Echocardiogr 25:1299–1308
24. Nazarian S, Bluemke DA, Lardo AC et al (2005) Magnetic resonance assessment of the substrate for inducible ventricular tachycardia in nonischemic cardiomyopathy. Circulation 112:2821–2825
25. Assomull RG, Prasad SK, Lyne J et al (2006) Cardiovascular magnetic resonance, fibrosis, and prognosis in dilated cardiomyopathy. J Am Coll Cardiol 48:1977–1985
26. Hombach V, Merkle N, Torzewski J et al (2009) Electrocardiographic and cardiac magnetic resonance imaging parameters as predictors of a worse outcome in patients with idiopathic dilated cardiomyopathy. Eur Heart J 30:2011–2018

Part III
Hypertrophic Cardiomyopathy

Hypertrophic Cardiomyopathy: Clinical Assessment and Differential Diagnosis

9

Marco Merlo, Andrea Cocciolo, Francesca Brun, and Gianfranco Sinagra

9.1 Introduction

Hypertrophic cardiomyopathy (HCM) is a common genetic disorder characterized by unexplained left ventricular (LV) hypertrophy associated with a nondilated ventricular chamber in the absence of any other cardiac or systemic cause of LV pressure overload (such as hypertension, aortic stenosis, congenital heart disease, etc). Conventionally, in adulthood, HCM is diagnosed in the presence of at least one segment with a maximal LV wall thickness >15 mm. In childhood, any degree of unexplained LV hypertrophy could be compatible with such a diagnosis, even if it is usually recognized that a wall thickness >2 standard deviations above the mean for age, sex, and body surface area (BSA) is the universally accepted criteria [1]. Histologically characterized by myocyte and fiber disarray (Fig. 9.1), interstitial fibrosis and small-vessel disease, this cardiomyopathy (CMP) is diagnosed through clinical (including familial history) and instrumental features, principally echocardiographic; however, cardiac magnetic resonance (CMR) is increasingly used as an essential diagnostic tool.

9.2 Epidemiology

HCM is a disease widespread worldwide, with similar prevalence reported in different countries: 1:500 individuals [2]. It can be diagnosed throughout life, from childhood to old age, but it is most commonly seen for the first time among young adults. The disease shows rapid, sometimes exponential, phenotypic onset and expression

M. Merlo (✉) • A. Cocciolo • F. Brun • G. Sinagra, MD, FESC
Department of Cardiology, University Hospital of Trieste,
via P. Valdoni 7, Trieste, 34139, Italy
e-mail: supermerloo@libero.it; coccioloandrea@gmail.com; frabrun77@gmail.com;
gianfranco.sinagra@aots.sanita.fvg.it

B. Pinamonti, G. Sinagra (eds.), *Clinical Echocardiography and Other Imaging Techniques in Cardiomyopathies*, DOI 10.1007/978-3-319-06019-4_9,
© Springer International Publishing Switzerland 2014

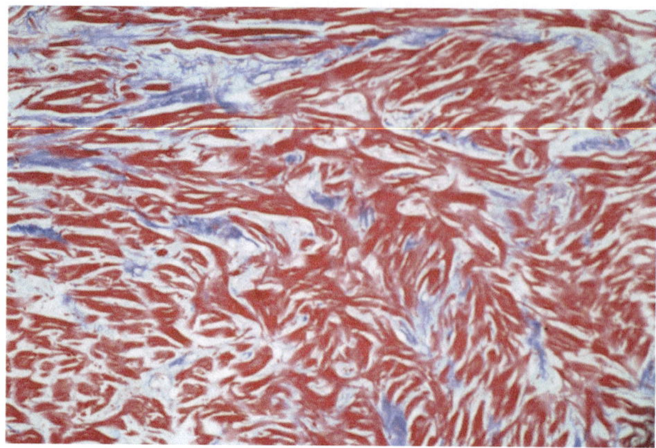

Fig. 9.1 Histologic specimen (Azan-Mallory, ×25) of a patient with hypertrophic cardiomyopathy (HCM) showing myocardial fiber disarray and interstitial fibrosis

throughout adolescence, in parallel with growth, indicating close noninvasive clinical and echocardiographic screening during this period. This applies above all to individuals with a family history or known to be carriers of a sarcomeric-causing disease mutation (genotype-positive/phenotype-negative individuals). Probably, many cases of HCM remain undiagnosed because of its asymptomatic course and normal life expectancy.

9.3 Genetics, Pathogenesis, and Pathophysiology

HCM is considered a genetic disease and is generally transmitted with an autosomal dominant pattern, shows a variable penetrance, and has great variability in phenotypic expression. Familial HCM accounts for 50 % of cases, with the remaining sporadic cases assumed to be de novo mutations [3]. The disease is caused by a singular mutated allele in one of more than 11 genes encoding for sarcomeric contractile myofilament proteins or components of the Z-disc. Mutations in two genes, the β-myosin heavy chain (*MYH7*) and myosin-binding protein C (*MYBPC3*), account for ~70 % of cases, >1,400 mutations have been identified thus far, mostly missense mutations [2].

Great phenotypic heterogeneity can be seen between and within families in terms of age at onset, degree and segmental distribution of hypertrophy, clinical manifestation, and outcome, suggesting a possible role for gene modifiers and environmental factors [2, 4]. The main four pathophysiological features and clinical manifestations of this CMP are LV diastolic dysfunction, LV outflow tract (OT) obstruction, heart failure (HF) symptoms, and sudden death (SD). The marked LV hypertrophy associated with increased ventricular wall stiffness due to interstitial fibrosis are responsible for LV diastolic dysfunction characterized by reduced compliance and abnormal relaxation, leading to diastolic HF. LV systolic function is usually preserved or is supernormal in the majority of patients, with a small subset (5–10 %) developing systolic dysfunction [e.g., LV ejection fraction (EF) <50 %) in the advanced stage (the so called end-stage evolution). This is a result of marked LV fibrosis, which is frequently associated with wall thinning and cavity dilatation. This unfavorable evolution, sometimes morphologically indistinguishable from a dilated cardiomyopathy, is associated with increased mortality (up to 11 % annual risk) and morbidity for HF and increased risk of SD [5, 6].

Dynamic LV OT obstruction can be appreciated in the resting condition in ~30 % of HCM patients (obstructive HCM), with a consequent dynamic LV OT pressure gradient at rest ≥30 mmHg. One third of patients show no LV OT obstruction at rest but only during exercise or other provocative maneuvers, such as Valsalva (labile LV OT obstruction). This peculiar feature of the disease is the consequence of vigorous systolic contraction, with an accelerated systolic ejection trough and narrowed LV OT due to systolic anterior motion (SAM) of the anterior mitral leaflet during mid systole, thus generating dynamic obstruction that assumes the aspect of a dynamic LV OT pressure gradient. The SAM of the mitral valve (MV), in association with abnormalities of the valve apparatus, leading to incomplete leaflet coaptation in mid systole, can also be responsible for a certain degree of mitral regurgitation (MR) that is often observed. SD in HCM seems to be less frequent than it was once thought. Recent data [2] indicate a prevalence of ~5 % in a hospital-based population. Nevertheless, HCM is the most common cause of SD in young athletes participating in competitive activity, without significant difference between genders [7]; SD may be the first clinical manifestation of the disease.

9.4 Clinical Diagnosis

As a result of its variability in phenotypic expression, the spectrum of clinical manifestations ranges from asymptomatic patients with normal life expectancy to severely symptomatic individuals. Dyspnea, angina pectoris under stress, palpitations, and occasionally syncope are the most common subjective manifestations, the most dramatic of which can be SD. SD most frequently occurs during or after strenuous physical exercise and is generally consequence of malignant arrhythmias.

Even if physical examination can often be silent, some affected patients manifest signs of systemic or pulmonary congestion, especially in the end stage of the disease. Irregular cardiac rhythm due to atrial fibrillation (AF) or presence of a fourth heart sound in patients in sinus rhythm can be detected on auscultation as a systolic murmur due to dynamic LV OT obstruction—the auscultatory stigmata of the disease—often associated with MR murmur. Every maneuver capable of reducing the preload or afterload (such as Valsalva or inhalation of amyl nitrite) or increasing contractility may result in an increase in intensity of this characteristic systolic heart murmur. Presence of particular syndromic findings (dysmorphic facies in patients with Noonan syndrome or typical maculopapular skin lesions in those with Anderson-Fabry disease) may suggest systemic disease presenting with an hypertrophied LV, which can be considered phenocopies of HCM [3, 8].

Electrocardiogram (ECG) is rarely normal in HCM patients, with about 6–10 % showing normal ECG at presentation [9]. More frequently, patients present with ECG signs of LV hypertrophy (Fig. 9.2), pathological Q waves, negative T waves,

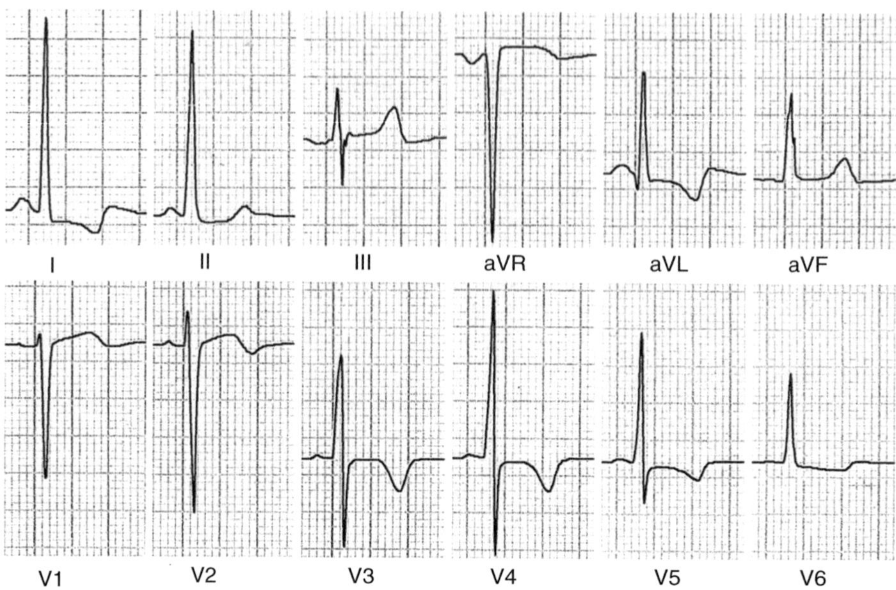

Fig. 9.2 Electrocardiograph (ECG) in a patient with hypertrophic cardiomyopathy (HCM) showing left ventricular (LV) hypertrophy and T-wave inversion

left-atrial (LA) enlargement, and intraventricular conduction abnormalities. Patients with a normal ECG at presentation seem to have a less advanced stage of the disease and a better prognosis [9].

9.5 Other Diagnostic Tools

Ambulatory Holter ECG recording is part of the primary diagnostic and follow-up approach in detecting nonsustained ventricular tachycardia (e.g., an important risk factor for SD) and is therefore essential for risk stratification. Invasive electrophysiological examination has become less important in recent years [3]. The exercise test can be useful for risk stratification in selected patients for monitoring stress-induced ventricular arrhythmias and blood pressure response to physical exercise (systolic pressure fall) (*see* Chap. 13). Cardiac catheterization and endomyocardial biopsy are rarely employed in clinical practice.

9.6 Genetic Testing

Genetic testing is used to identify affected relatives in families known to have HCM. Because familial HCM is a dominant disorder, the risk that an affected patient will transmit the disease is 50 %. When a pathogenic mutation is identified in an index

Table 9.1 Incidence of major cardiovascular events in HCM patients in the Heart Muscle Disease Registry of Trieste (1983–2013)

	Events per 100 patients per year
All-cause death/heart transplant	2.97
Heart-failure death/heart transplant	1.8
Sudden cardiac death/major ventricular arrhythmias	1.21

patient, genetic testing may be extended to each family member. Genetic counseling must be performed before genetic testing to improve patient and family understanding of implications of test results, potential risks, and benefits. Genetic counseling should be performed even if genetic testing is not undertaken. Genetic screening of first-degree relatives can identify family members carrying a mutation (genotype positive) but without overt cardiac hypertrophy (phenotype negative). In such cases, noninvasive clinical screening with physical examination, ECG, and 2D echocardiography or CMR is recommended due to the possibility of an age-related expression of the disease phenotype [1].

9.7 Natural History

HCM heterogeneity is manifested even in clinical presentation, symptoms severity, and clinical course (Table 9.1). Many affected patients (with the hypertrophic phenotype) present with no symptoms or major disability and experience a normal life expectancy without complications. On the other hand, symptomatic disease may present with different, not mutually exclusive, clinical settings. Some patients may experience SD, which can be the first and last manifestation of the disease, especially in individuals <35 years of age. Some other patients develop signs and symptoms of HF due to diastolic dysfunction (diastolic HF) with a well-preserved LV systolic function. A minority of those patients (~5–10 %) manifests progression toward end-stage disease, with impaired contractility and systolic dysfunction due to massive myocardial fibrosis. Those patients are at very high risk both for refractory HF and malignant arrhythmias. Finally, some affected individuals developed AF as a consequence of increased filling pressure and atrial dilatation, which can contribute to HF symptoms and brings with it major or minor systemic thromboembolic complications (e.g., cardioembolic stroke) [1, 10].

9.8 Differential Diagnosis

HCM enters into differential diagnosis with several other clinical or physiological conditions characterized by LV hypertrophy, such as hypertensive heart disease, athlete's heart, mitochondrial diseases, cardiac amyloidosis (CA), and other infiltrative/storage CMP. Although sometimes problematic, only a comprehensive assessment considering familial and clinical history, physical signs, and integrated instrumental evaluation help to achieve a correct diagnosis [5, 8]. In this sense, clinical cardiologists must pay attention to some small, but sometimes fundamental, clinical–instrumental signs—red flags—capable of orienting differential diagnosis.

The most common, important, and challenging differential diagnosis with HCM is hypertensive heart disease, as the two conditions may coexist and they widely overlap, particularly in individuals in whom severe LV hypertrophy is out of proportion compared with systemic blood pressure levels. In the presence of overlap cases, the term hypertensive HCM is sometimes used [11]. Distinguishing HCM from positive physiologic response to intense physical activity seen in athlete's heart is very important, considering the overlapping age of presentation of the two conditions and the implications derived from a diagnosis of HCM on participation in competitive activity. Family history of HCM or SD and presence of symptoms, particularly syncope during exertion, suggest a diagnosis of HCM. The LV hypertrophy seen in athletes manifests with a symmetric distribution without reaching the magnitude seen in HCM ($\leq$16 mm) [7]. Differential diagnosis may be particularly difficult in African American athletes in whom LV hypertrophy tends to be very marked and the ECG is often abnormal. Nevertheless, an adequate detraining period will show hypertrophy regression and reduced LV cavity dimension in healthy young athletes, which is different from patients affected with HCM.

Many characteristic features help differentiate CA from HCM, including familial and individual history, physical examination, and evidence of signs and symptoms of systemic involvement of other organs and apparatus (kidney, nervous system, liver, etc). Vitreous opacities, paraesthesia, and bilateral carpal tunnel syndrome are characteristic of transthyretin (TTR)-related amyloidosis. Some biochemical laboratory tests, such as serum immunoglobulin-free light-chains assay, serum and urine immunofixation, and urine electrophoresis, can be used to detect the abnormal clonal immunoglobulin light-chain production associated with plasma-cell dyscrasias in the most common form of CA: AL-related amyloidosis. In CA, the ECG may show atrioventricular blocks, and low QRS voltage, in contrast to the degree of hypertrophy visible at echocardiographic evaluation, even if this feature manifests low sensitivity. Much more important is the relation of the arithmetic sum of positive and negative QRS deflections in the limb or in the 12 leads to the LV mass. A low ratio suggests a diagnosis of CA (especially AL and TTR amyloidosis), in contrast to a high value often seen in HCM. Moreover, LV hypertrophy in CA manifests a symmetric, homogenous distribution, with a characteristic, although not always seen, granular-sparkling myocardial echogenicity [8].

Another important diagnostic possibility is Anderson-Fabry disease, a genetically transmitted storage disease thought to account for 6–10 % of cases of phenotypic nonobstructive HCM. It is difficult to distinguish Fabry disease from HCM with echocardiography alone, and the diagnosis is often the result of familiar and personal history (in this sense, an X-linked pathway of inheritance may suggest the diagnosis), clinical examination, and evidence of signs and symptoms of systemic involvement, such as cutaneous angiokeratomata, anhidrosis, Raynaud-like symptoms, neuropathy, ocular manifestations, tinnitus, diarrhea, and proteinuria. ECG may show atrioventricular blocks. It is interesting to note that storage diseases rarely manifest in adults, but Fabry disease represents an exception, with a mean age of presentation between the fourth and fifth decade of life [8]. Differential diagnosis is relevant for patients because treatment with human α-galactosidase A produced with genetic technology can improve most Fabry disease manifestations.

Danon disease (also known as glycogen storage disease type IIb) due to *LAMP2* gene mutation, and Pompe disease (or glycogen storage disease type II) caused by mutations in the gene encoding for alpha-glucosidase lysosomal enzyme, are metabolic storage disorders that also enter into differential diagnosis with HCM because of their hypertrophic phenotype. What may help differentiating these conditions from sarcomeric HCM are the pathways of inheritance (X-linked for Danon and autosomal recessive for Pompe disease); expression in a child or adolescent with massive and concentric ventricular hypertrophy, often with coexistent systolic dysfunction; presence of neuromuscular symptoms (e.g., skeletal muscle weakness, progressive exercise intolerance, cognitive impairment, and retinitis pigmentosa in Danon disease); atrioventricular blocks; ventricular pre-excitation and high QRS voltage on ECG; and raised levels of serum creatine phosphokinase [8].

PRKAG2 cardiac syndrome is a rare autosomal dominant disorder, the consequence of mutation in the protein kinase, adenosine monophosphate (AMP)-activated, noncatalytic, gamma-2 (*PRKAG2*) gene, commonly characterized by LV hypertrophy, ventricular pre-excitation for the presence of an accessory pathway, and conduction disorders, often leading to pacemaker implantation [12].

Even if rare, mitochondrial diseases [e.g., mitochondrial encephalomyopathy, lactic acidosis, and stroke-like episodes (MELAS), myoclonic epilepsy with ragged red fibers (MERRF), Barth syndrome] caused by mutations in mitochondrial DNA, deserve a mention in the differential diagnostic process in HCM. They are inherited with a matrilinear transmission, a unique feature that helps distinguish these disorders form HCM. Clinical manifestations appear early in life, with a characteristic multisystemic involvement of organs with high-energy requests. Cardiac involvement is almost always present and is characterized by concentric hypertrophy, often with associated systolic impairment. Signs and symptoms frequently seen are hypoacousia, palpebral ptosis, myopathy with ragged red fibers, ophthalmoplegia, encephalopathy, and retinitis pigmentosa, with a phenotypic heterogeneity at the organ level. ECG shows atrioventricular blocks and ventricular pre-excitation, whereas laboratory studies may evidence increased creatine phosphokinase and transaminase serum levels, lactic acidosis, myoglobinuria, and leukocytopenia [8].

HCM phenotype may be a feature of rare congenital autosomal dominant dysmorphic syndromes—such as Noonan syndrome—characterized by short stature, variable developmental delay, cutaneous abnormalities, hypertelorism, ptosis, low-set and posteriorly rotated ears, and a webbed neck, as well as LEOPARD syndrome (lentigines, ECG abnormalities, ocular hypertelorism, pulmonary stenosis, abnormal genitalia, retardation of growth, and sensory–neural deafness). In these cases, differential diagnosis is usually simple due to evident morphological abnormalities, but somatic features may sometimes be subtle [8].

9.9   Implantable Cardioverter Defibrillator Implantation and Therapeutic Options

HCM is the most common cause of SD in young people, including trained athletes. Implantable cardioverter defibrillator (ICD) therapy represents the only strategy for prolonging life expectancy in HCM patients. ICDs are effective in preventing this life-threatening complication, with appropriate intervention rates of 11 % for secondary and 4 % for primary prevention. On the other hand, antiarrhythmic pharmacologic therapy (such as beta-blockers and amiodarone) does not provide adequate protection from SD [13].

Pharmacological treatments are indicated only in symptomatic patients [1]. Beta-blockers are considered the first-line drugs for treating angina or exertional dyspnea. When beta-blockers are contraindicated or not well tolerated, verapamil can be used. In patients not responding to single-drug therapy, the association between beta-blockers and verapamil or diltiazem may be an alternative. In patients not responding to these drugs, disopyramide may be given, exploiting its negative inotropic effect. This drug should always be used in association with verapamil or diltiazem or with a beta-blocker, particularly in patients with AF, due to the risk of increasing ventricular rate.

In patients presenting with symptoms or signs of HF, evidence-based therapy for HF should be used. Vasodilators, such as angiotensin-converting enzyme (ACE) inhibitors or dihydropyridinic calcium-channel blockers, in symptomatic patients showing significant LV OT obstruction are generally contraindicated because of the risk of increasing the dynamic gradient. In patients with either paroxysmal, persistent, or chronic AF, anticoagulation with vitamin K antagonists to an International Normalized Ratio (INR) of 2.0–3.0 is indicated. In this setting, controlling ventricular rate may require high doses of beta-blockers and nondihydropyridine calcium-channel blockers, whereas disopyramide (with ventricular-rate-controlling agents) and amiodarone are useful in a rhythm control strategy. Sotalol, dofetilide, and dronedarone might be used, but clinical evidence with these drugs is limited. Patients with refractory symptoms or who are unable to take antiarrhythmic drugs should be considered for AF radiofrequency ablation or, in highly select cases, surgical Maze procedure with closure of the LA appendage [1].

Invasive septal-reduction strategies are indicated only in patients with obstructive HCM who remain severely symptomatic [New York Heart Association (NYHA) functional class 3–4] despite optimal medical therapy [1]. Surgical septal myectomy (with or without MV repair or replacement) represents the most effective treatment, particularly in patients who are candidates for cardiac surgery for other reasons (coronary artery disease, etc.) [1]. The alternative of catheter alcohol septal ablation may be considered in patients with severe comorbidities or contraindication to cardiac surgery, thus representing a second choice. It is unadvisable in children and in patients with massive septal hypertrophy, in whom it will probably be unsuccessful. Alcohol septal ablation may also be a therapeutic option for patients who are candidates for surgery and who reject this therapeutic option; careful and complete discussion with the patient is essential [1].

In symptomatic patients with LV OT obstruction in whom an ICD has already been implanted for high-risk status and who are suboptimal candidates for septal reduction therapies because of severe comorbidities, dual-chamber atrioventricular pacing (DDD pacing) may be considered. Pacing the right ventricular apex and maintaining atrioventricular synchrony may result in decreased LV OT gradient and improved symptoms, even if a real, long-term benefit is seen in a minority of patients only, probably largely due to a placebo effect [14].

In patients in sinus rhythm and end-stage disease, severe LV dysfunction (e.g., LVEF ≤35 %), highly symptomatic for HF despite optimal medical therapy and left bundle branch block (LBBB) on ECG, cardiac resynchronization therapy (CRT) with biventricular pacing should be considered as a therapeutic option. Nevertheless, due to paucity of published data on CRT in HCM patients, the real benefit of this strategy it is still unclear [15].

The very last therapeutic option for patients with end-stage disease and severe HF symptoms (NYHA functional class III–IV) who are unresponsive to all other interventions is represented by heart transplantation and, in some selected cases, often a bridge to transplantation using a mechanical ventricular-assist device. Rarely, heart transplantation can be considered, even in the absence of significant LV dysfunction, for patients with refractory angina or arrhythmias [1].

References

1. Gersh BJ, Maron BJ, Bonow RO et al (2011) 2011 ACCF/AHA guideline for the diagnosis and treatment of hypertrophic cardiomyopathy: a report of the American College of Cardiology Foundation/American Heart Association Task Force on Practice Guidelines. Circulation 124:783–831
2. Maron BJ, Maron MS (2013) Hypertrophic cardiomyopathy. Lancet 381:242–255
3. Prinz C, Farr M, Hering D et al (2011) The diagnosis and treatment of hypertrophic cardiomyopathy. Dtsch Arztebl Int 108:209–215
4. Alcalai R, Seidman JG, Seidman CE (2008) Genetic basis of hypertrophic cardiomyopathy: from bench to the clinics. J Cardiovasc Electrophysiol 19:104–110
5. Williams LK, Frenneaux MP, Steeds RP (2009) Echocardiography in hypertrophic cardiomyopathy diagnosis, prognosis, and role in management. Eur J Echocardiogr 10:9–14
6. Harris KM, Spirito P, Maron MS et al (2006) Prevalence, clinical profile, and significance of left ventricular remodeling in the end-stage phase of hypertrophic cardiomyopathy. Circulation 114:216–225
7. Dilsizian V, Bonow RO, Epstein SE et al (1993) Myocardial ischemia detected by thallium scintigraphy is frequently related to cardiac arrest and syncope in young patients with hypertrophic cardiomyopathy. J Am Coll Cardiol 22:796–804
8. Rapezzi C, Arbustini E, Caforio AL et al (2013) Diagnostic work-up in cardiomyopathies: bridging the gap between clinical phenotypes and final diagnosis. A position statement from the ESC Working Group on Myocardial and Pericardial Diseases. Eur Heart J 34:1448–1458
9. McLeod CJ, Ackerman MJ, Nishimura RA et al (2009) Outcome of patients with hypertrophic cardiomyopathy and a normal electrocardiogram. J Am Coll Cardiol 54:229–233
10. Melacini P, Basso C, Angelini A et al (2010) Clinicopathological profiles of progressive heart failure in hypertrophic cardiomyopathy. Eur Heart J 31:2111–2123
11. Topol EJ, Traill TA, Fortuin NJ (1985) Hypertensive hypertrophic cardiomyopathy of the elderly. N Engl J Med 312:277–283

12. Fabris E, Brun F, Porto AG et al (2013) Cardiac hypertrophy, accessory pathway, and conduction system disease in an adolescent: the PRKAG2 cardiac syndrome. J Am Coll Cardiol 62:e17
13. Maron BJ, Rowin EJ, Casey SA et al (2013) Risk stratification and outcome of patients with hypertrophic cardiomyopathy >=60 years of age. Circulation 127:585–593
14. Fananapazir L, Epstein ND, Curiel RV et al (1994) Long-term results of dual-chamber (DDD) pacing in obstructive hypertrophic cardiomyopathy. Evidence for progressive symptomatic and hemodynamic improvement and reduction of left ventricular hypertrophy. Circulation 90:2731–2742
15. Rogers DP, Marazia S, Chow AW et al (2008) Effect of biventricular pacing on symptoms and cardiac remodelling in patients with end-stage hypertrophic cardiomyopathy. Eur J Heart Fail 10:507–513

Basic Echocardiography in Hypertrophic Cardiomyopathy

10

Gherardo Finocchiaro, Bruno Pinamonti, and Elena Abate

10.1 Introduction

As in the other cardiomyopathies (CMP), echocardiography has a major role in the diagnostic assessment and prognostic stratification of hypertrophic cardiomyopathy (HCM) [1]. The clinical–echocardiographic diagnosis of HCM is based on the demonstration of significant left ventricular (LV) hypertrophy in the absence of another disease process that could reasonably account for the magnitude of hypertrophy present [2].

10.2 Left Ventricular Structural Abnormalities

The echocardiographic hallmark of HCM is a pathologic increase in LV wall thickness, with a corresponding increase in LV mass [3]. In adults, the diagnostic cut-off for end-diastolic LV wall thickness is 15 mm. In the pediatric population, LV hypertrophy is defined considering LV end-diastolic wall thickness indexed for body surface area (BSA) [more than two standard deviations (SD) above the mean value for a normal population of infants, children, and adolescents with similar BSA] [4].

Degree and location of increased LV wall thickness vary significantly. Various morphologic categories have traditionally been used to describe hypertrophic LV appearance. Wigle et al. [5] proposed a points scoring system that takes into account

Electronic supplementary material The online version of this chapter (doi: 10.1007/978-3-319-06019-4_10) contains supplementary material, which is available to authorized users. Videos can also be accessed at http://www.springerimages.com/videos/978-3-319-06018-7.

G. Finocchiaro (✉) • B. Pinamonti, MD • E. Abate
Department of Cardiology, University Hospital of Trieste,
via P. Valdoni 7, Trieste 34139, Italy
e-mail: gherardobis@yahoo.it; bruno.pinamonti@gmail.com; abate.elena@gmail.com

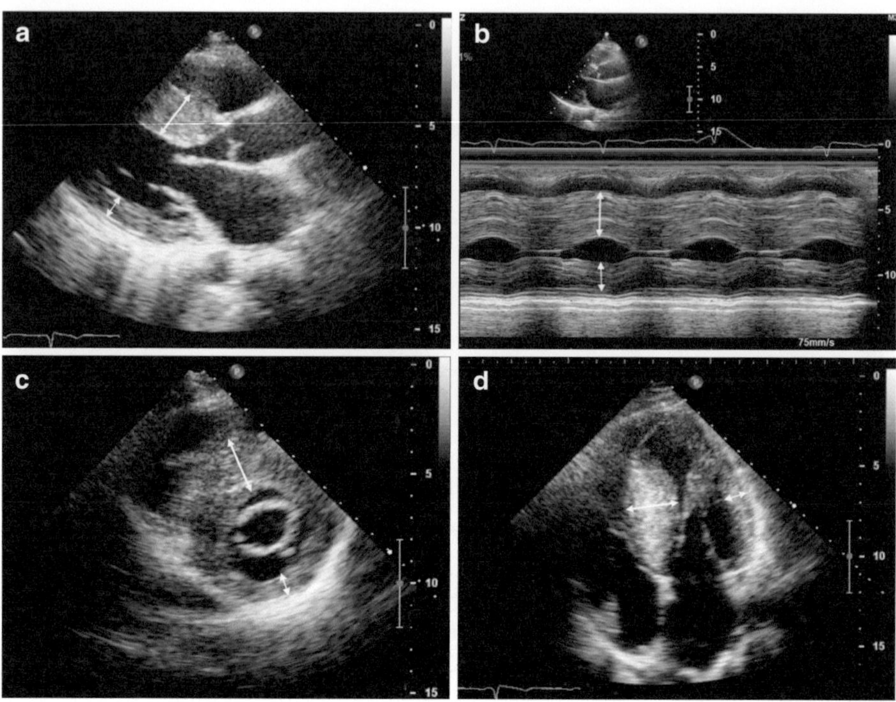

Fig. 10.1 Parasternal long-axis view (**a**), M-mode (**b**), parasternal short-axis view (**c**), apical four-chamber view (**d**), end-diastolic frames, of a 39-year-old woman with hypertrophic cardio-myopathy and asymmetric hypertrophy. There is severe septal hypertrophy (24 mm) and normal thickness of posterior and lateral walls (*arrows*)

the degree of interventricular septum (IVS) thickness, starting from a value of 15 mm, and the extension of hypertrophy from the base to the apex. Spirito et al. [6] developed a method to quantify the magnitude of hypertrophy, comprehensive of the parasternal long- and short-axis and apical views.

In HCM, hypertrophy is most frequently asymmetric (ratio of end-diastolic IVS to posterior wall thicknesses >1.3–1.5) (Fig. 10.1, Clips 10.1a, 10.1b, 10.1c, 10.1d, 10.1e, and 10.1f). In the most recent classification, the morphology and distribution of hypertrophy is classified into four categories according to IVS morphology and curvature: reverse curve, sigmoidal, neutral, apical (Fig. 10.2) [7, 8]. Reverse curvature IVS morphology is generally associated with more severe hypertrophy and more frequent demonstration of abnormal genetics [7, 8]. Apical HCM (Fig. 10.3, Clips 10.2a, 10.2b, 10.2c, 10.2d, and 10.2e) is more frequently seen in the Asian population, especially Japanese, than in the Western population, and could be associated with midventricular obstruction and apical aneurysms [9].

Hypertrophy severity varies, ranging from mild to very severe (wall thickness >30 mm) (Fig. 10.4, Clips 10.3a, 10.3b, 10.3c, 10.3d, and 10.3e). LV mass assessment, which is useful for hypertrophy quantification, is problematic and unreliable

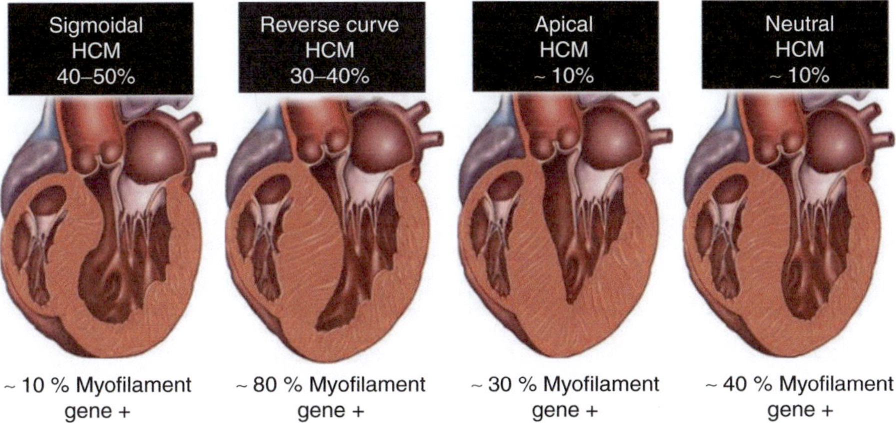

Fig. 10.2 Septal morphologies in hypertrophic cardiomyopathy. Prevalence of septal morphologies (*top*) among a large cohort of patients with hypertrophic cardiomyopathy. Data from genetic testing in each subgroup of patients (*bottom*). *HCM* hypertrophic cardiomyopathy (From [7], with permission)

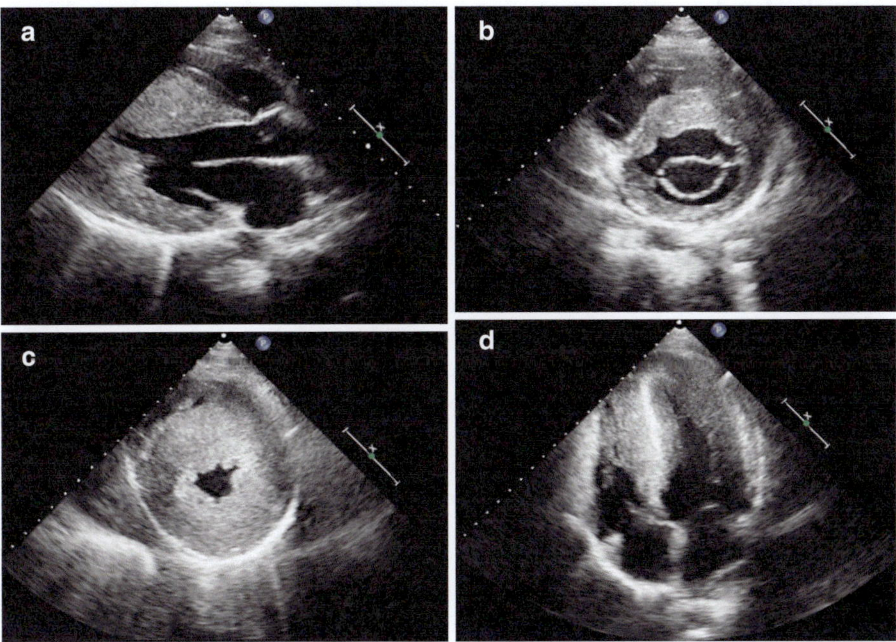

Fig. 10.3 A 16-year-old patient with apical hypertrophic cardiomyopathy. Parasternal long-axis (**a**), short-axis at the mitral valve level (**b**), short-axis at the apical level (**c**), and apical four-chamber view (**d**), end-diastolic frames, demonstrating severe left ventricular hypertrophy at the midapical level (maximal septal thickness 36 mm)

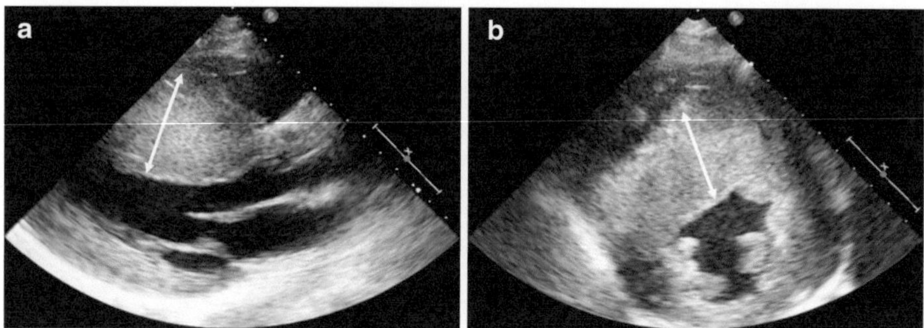

Fig. 10.4 Massive hypertrophy of the left ventricular septum (*arrows*) in an 18-year-old patient with asymmetrical hypertrophic cardiomyopathy. Parasternal long-axis (**a**) and parasternal short-axis (**b**) views, end-diastolic frames. Maximal septal thickness 43 mm

by traditional echocardiographic formulae based on M-mode due to the irregular distribution of hypertrophy [10]. Sometimes, the extent of hypertrophy is difficult to visualize; thus LV cavity opacification by intravenous administration of contrast material [11] or cardiac magnetic resonance (CMR) may be helpful. In particular, apical HCM and apical aneurysms can be missed on transthoracic echocardiography (TTE) [12, 13]. The HCM phenotype could be associated with accentuated trabeculations, sometimes in a continuum with LV noncompaction [14].

10.3 Left Ventricular Systolic Function

In the majority of patients with the classic form of HCM, LV systolic function is described to be normal or supranormal (Clips 10.1a, 10.1c, 10.1d, and 10.1e).

However, although LV ejection fraction (EF) is frequently seen as more than 70 %, significant hypertrophy hesitates in small LV end-diastolic volumes and cavity size, with abnormal filling and these features explain the reduced stroke volume [1]. A minority (5–10 %) of patients develop LV systolic dysfunction (end-stage phase with EF <50 %) (Fig. 10.5, Clips 10.4a and 10.4b) [15]. End-stage HCM seems to have a strong genetic background: Girolami et al. [16] showed that can be associated with multiple genetic mutations.

Overt dysfunction is characterized by severe functional LV deterioration subtended by extreme degrees of fibrosis and remodeling and generally associated with increased dimensions and wall thinning (apparent regression of hypertrophy), thus mimicking dilated cardiomyopathy (DCM). Progressive heart failure (HF) and adverse outcome are common. There are primarily two morphofunctional manifestations of HCM in the advanced stage: the hypokinetic-dilated form, and the hypokinetic-restrictive form. The first is characterized by LV volume increase and spherical remodeling; in the second, the distinctive feature is a small hypertrophic LV with severe diastolic dysfunction and mild systolic impairment [17].

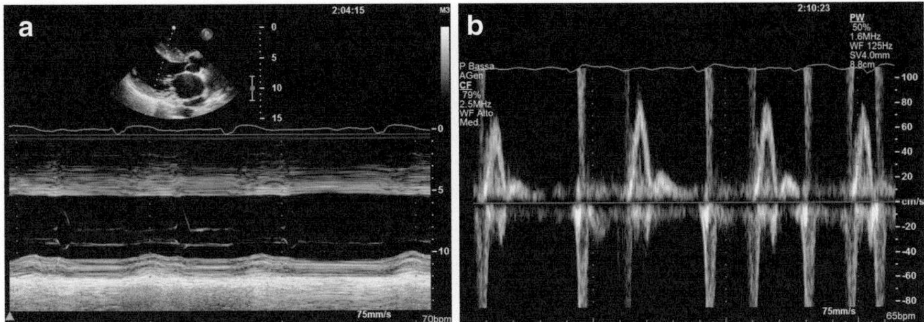

Fig. 10.5 Woman with end-stage hypertrophic cardiomyopathy with a progression to significant left ventricular systolic dysfunction. M-mode echocardiography (**a**) shows severe septal hypertrophy (25 mm) associated with left ventricular dilatation (end-diastolic diameter 59 mm, end-diastolic diameter corrected for body surface area 35 mm/mq), and systolic dysfunction (fractional shortening 16 %, ejection fraction 22 %). Transmitral pulsed Doppler shows severe diastolic dysfunction with restrictive filling pattern (**b**)

10.4 Left Ventricular Diastolic Function

Diastolic dysfunction is the main and most frequent hemodynamic abnormality described in HCM. Its importance led to an extensive search for accurate, noninvasive methods of quantifying its severity. Doppler echocardiography allows assessment of diastolic dysfunction in HCM, even if conventional parameters, such as E-wave deceleration time and E/A ratio on transmitral flow, do not correlate well with LV filling pressure, as it does in other CMP, such as DCM [18]. Conversely, atrial reversal velocity from the pulmonary veins and its duration, recorded at pulsed-wave (PW) Doppler, significantly correlate with LV end-diastolic pressures [19]. A restrictive filling pattern can be present in a minority of patients and corresponds to severe diastolic dysfunction, as in other heart diseases (Fig. 10.5) [20].

Considering tissue Doppler imaging (TDI) assessment of diastolic dysfunction, previous studies noted reasonable correlations between E/E' ratio and LV filling pressures in HCM [19]. However, the E/E' ratio is poorly correlated with capillary wedge pressures measurements at catheterization [12, 13]. Therefore, it must be considered as unreliable as a single parameter for assessing LV diastolic dysfunction in patients with HCM.

Left-atrial (LA) volume can be useful as a surrogate for diastolic dysfunction, particularly in the absence of significant mitral regurgitation (MR) and atrial fibrillation (AF) [21].

In conclusion, as suggested by international guidelines on echo Doppler assessment of diastolic dysfunction [22], a comprehensive echocardiographic approach is recommended when predicting LV filling pressures in patients with HCM, taking into consideration transmitral Doppler and TDI velocities and ratios, as well as pulmonary vein flow pattern, pulmonary artery pressure, and LA volume.

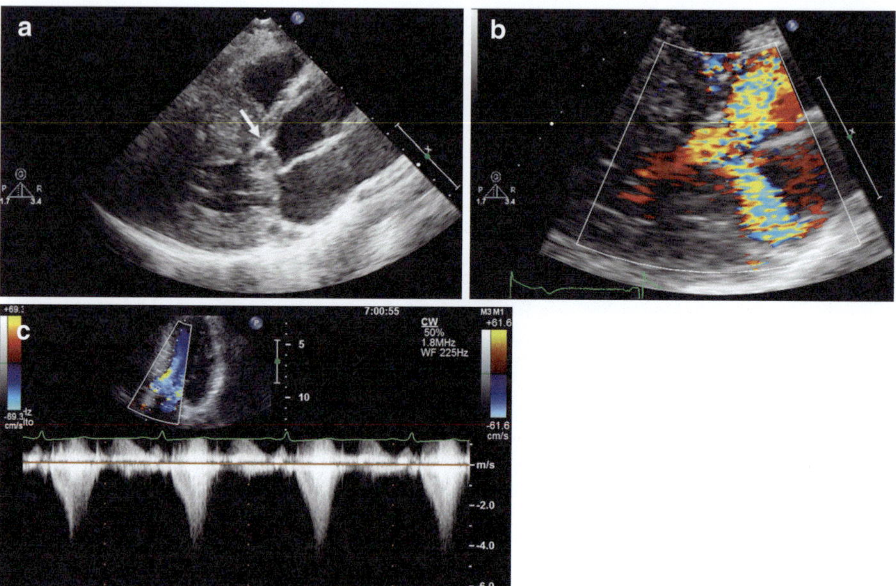

Fig. 10.6 Doppler echocardiography in a patient with obstructive hypertrophic cardiomyopathy. Parasternal long-axis view, systolic frame (**a**), demonstrating systolic anterior motion of the anterior mitral leaflet (*arrow*). Color Doppler examination, systolic frame (**b**), shows marked turbulence in the left ventricular outflow tract and a posteriorly directed jet of mitral regurgitation. The continuous-wave Doppler image recorded through the left ventricular outflow tract (**c**) shows a late-peaking systolic gradient with peak pressure gradient of 64 mmHg at rest

10.5 Mitral Valve

HCM may be associated with a variety of intrinsic abnormalities of the mitral valve (MV), including anomalous mitral papillary muscles or chordae, direct papillary insertion into the mitral leaflets, MV prolapse, and chordal rupture. Furthermore, MV abnormalities may have a major role in generating LV obstruction [23]. Systolic anterior motion (SAM) of the anterior mitral leaflet—with or without a pressure gradient across the LV outflow tract (LVOT)—although not pathognomonic, is highly indicative of HCM (Fig. 10.6, Clips 10.5a and 10.5b) [24].

The first study using cardiac ultrasound (US) to establish MV SAM was published in 1969 [25]. Even if subsequent advances in echocardiography substantially increased our comprehension of the processes underlying LV OT obstruction, the mechanism of SAM in HCM is not yet completely defined. SAM typically involves the anterior—and, less often—the posterior leaflet. Initially it was thought to be related to the Venturi effect and that raised flow velocities in a LVOT anatomically distorted by septal hypertrophy could pull the MV leaflets toward the septum, inducing a significant obstruction. The true mechanism is probably much more complex and involves the subvalvular apparatus and drag forces created by a hyperdynamic

LV, which predispose the leaflets to being swept into the LVOT [26]. Studies using both transesophageal echocardiography (TEE) and CMR show that both mitral leaflets—in particular, the anterior—are longer than those of control individuals, which could be a factor predisposing to SAM [27].

MR and its severity are correlated with the degree of SAM and obstruction [28]. Grigg et al. [29], studying 32 HCM patients with intraoperative TEE during myectomy, found that in 56 %, neither MV leaflet coapted in midsystole secondary to severe SAM, leading to a jet originating from the gap between the two leaflets.

Considering papillary muscles, the currently described abnormalities are papillary muscle hypertrophy, papillary muscle fusion with IVS, anterior apically displaced papillary muscles, papillary muscle insertion directly in the anterior mitral leaflet, papillary muscle fusion with the LV free wall, double-bifid papillary muscles, and accessory papillary muscles [30, 31]. Even if echocardiography plays a major role in identifying these abnormalities, studies in patients undergoing septal myectomy show that they are frequently not identified by TTE and are often identified only during direct inspection at the time of operation [32]. Therefore, TEE and/ or CMR are indicated in patients with HCM and severe MR who are potential candidates for surgery.

In clinical practice, MR jet direction at color Doppler examination is useful to predict its mechanism (posterolateral jet direction in SAM-related MR; anterior MV leaflet prolapse; anteromedial jet direction in MR due to posterior MV leaflet prolapse) (Fig. 10.6, Clip 10.5c).

10.6　Left Ventricular Obstruction

A significant pressure gradient at rest or during exercise affects more than 70 % of the patients with HCM [33]. Doppler echocardiography plays a primary role in assessing patients with obstructive HCM. Using the simplified Bernoulli equation on continuous-wave Doppler signal from the LV—as in valvular heart diseases—it is possible to reliably estimate peak and mean intraventricular systolic pressure gradients. In addition, accurate echocardiographic examination provides important insights about mechanisms that generate LV obstruction, and color and PW Doppler mapping are highly useful for determining the obstruction site [34].

A LV gradient >30 mmHg at rest and >50 mmHg at stress is considered significant (Fig. 10.6) [4]. Midcavitary obstruction can occur with and without LVOT obstruction in ventricles with hyperdynamic function and concentric and/or apical hypertrophy (Fig. 10.7, Clips 10.6a and 10.6b) and is sometimes accompanied by an apical aneurysm [3].

Echocardiography can be useful for tailoring therapeutic approaches to obstructive HCM, especially when a septal reduction (septal myectomy or alcohol septal ablation) is considered [1]. In particular, in the setting of alcohol septal ablation, echocardiographic monitoring enables visualization of the strategic septal area involved in outflow gradient formation, thereby defining the area and extent of future necrosis [35]. Furthermore, TEE with direct intracoronary contrast injection

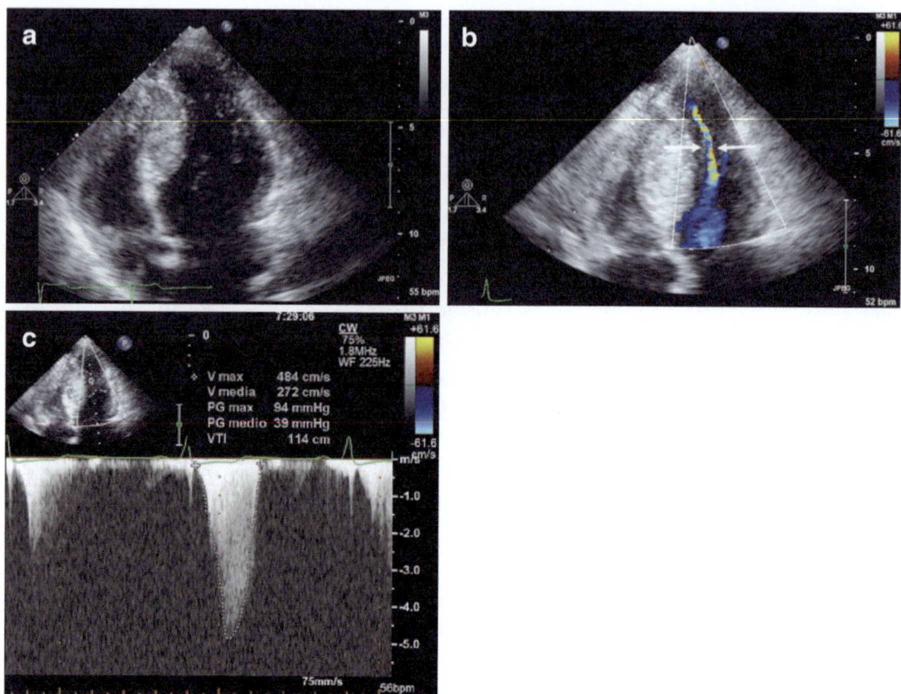

Fig. 10.7 A 20-year-old woman with hypertrophic cardiomyopathy, hyperdynamic left ventricular function, and midcavitary obstruction. Apical four-chamber view, end-diastolic frame, demonstrating severe left ventricular septal hypertrophy at midapical level (septal thickness 29 mm) (**a**). Apical four-chamber view, systolic frame, with color Doppler imaging, showing midcavity obliteration with a very narrow residual left ventricular cavity (*arrows*) (**b**). Continuous-wave Doppler image recorded at midcavity showing a peak systolic pressure gradient of 94 mmHg (**c**)

immediately before septal alcohol ablation, is crucial for assessing the site and extension of the myocardial area to be treated [36]. On the other hand, intraoperative TEE is useful for assessing residual obstruction and/or MR during septal myectomy.

10.7 Right Ventricle

Although HCM is a disease known to affect mainly the LV, studies show involvement of the right ventricle (RV). RV abnormalities range from hypertrophy, systolic and diastolic dysfunction, RV systolic gradient, and consequences of secondary pulmonary hypertension [37].

Severino et al. demonstrated that in HCM, despite the absence of RV systolic dysfunction, the majority of patients show signs of abnormal RV filling patterns [38]. Finocchiaro et al. [39] show how RV dysfunction, based on the RV myocardial performance index, is common in HCM patients (with significantly higher values than a healthy control cohort: 0.51 ± 0.18 vs 0.25 ± 0.06, $p < 0.001$) and is more frequently observed in patients with LV dysfunction and pulmonary hypertension. RV hypertrophy and function can be better assessed by CMR [40] (Chap. 12).

10.8 Differential Diagnosis with Other Causes of Hypertrophy

It is important to remember that LV and/or RV hypertrophy cannot be considered pathognomonic of HCM. Secondary forms—for example, in the context of hypertension, infiltrative and storage CMP such as cardiac amyloidosis (CA) and Anderson-Fabry disease—may be very difficult to distinguish from HCM. This fact has generated some confusion also in terminology [41].

In some case, the degree and the distribution of hypertrophy may help in discriminating HCM from other forms of LV hypertrophy. For example, in CA, wall thickening is usually concentric; in Anderson-Fabry disease, the binary appearance at echocardiography of the LV endocardial border has been questioned as a possible characteristic [42], although not specific [43], feature.

Even if echocardiography could be helpful in the differential diagnosis with other causes of hypertrophy, its role must be considered in the context of the clinical picture and electrocardiography, possibly gathering information from genetics and histopathology. Furthermore, other imaging modalities, particularly CMR (Chap. 12) can be helpful in the differential diagnosis.

10.9 Athlete Heart and Hypertrophic Cardiomyopathy

Because of the potentially adverse consequences of underlying cardiovascular disease in young athletes, considerable attention has focused on discriminating physiologically based athlete's heart from various structural heart diseases. In particular, in athletes, it is important to rule out a disease that can potentially lead to sudden death (SD), such as HCM, and echocardiography plays a primary role in this setting [44].

First, significant hypertrophy may occur only in athletes who undergo very intensive training, and a discrepancy between the intensity of physical activity and the degree of hypertrophy is an important clue in the differential diagnosis. Maximum LV end-diastolic wall thickness of 15 mm in young trained athletes likely represents the upper limit of physiologic LV hypertrophy. However, an important minority of patients with HCM show only mild to moderate wall thickening in a grey zone of 13–15 mm, which overlaps with that found in elite athletes. Therefore, absolute LV wall thickness itself is often not helpful in discriminating the two conditions. Usually, hypertrophy in HCM is asymmetric and the LV cavity is small, whereas athletes show a concentric hypertrophy and enlarged cavity. LV obstruction at rest or during exercise is common (two of three patients) in HCM but is not present in trained athletes [31]. Besides, various degrees of diastolic dysfunction are frequently observed in HCM, whereas athletes have normal filling pattern at transmitral Doppler [45].

TDI and E' velocities should also be evaluated in grey cases. In fact, an E' velocity <9 cm/s provides the best differentiation of pathologic from physiologic hypertrophy, with a sensitivity of 87 % and a specificity of 97 % [46]. LA remodeling can be frequently observed in athletes. In HCM, LA enlargement is often a consequence of diastolic dysfunction and is associated with a small cavity, whereas in athletes, it is dimensionally related to an enlarged LV cavity [47].

10.10 Echocardiography in Preclinical Diagnosis

HCM is caused by known sarcomere gene mutations in ~60 % of patients [48]. One important but challenging point is that phenotypic expression could be highly variable, and some patients do not show LV hypertrophy despite the presence of a gene mutation. Through genetic testing, relatives who have inherited the family's pathogenic sarcomere mutation (G+) can be identified before they exhibit diagnostic clinical features of the disease (LVH−). However, there is evidence that G+/ LVH−mutation carriers have myocardial abnormalities, even when LV wall thickness is normal.

Nagueh et al. [49] demonstrated that subsequent HCM development in patients with initially reduced TDI velocities establishes TDI as a reliable method for early identification of HCM mutation carriers (Chap. 11). Gandjbakhch et al. [50] showed that several parameters are significantly different in LVH−/G+compared with controls, in particular, IVS/posterior wall ratio, relative wall thickness, and septal E/E' ratio. There is a growing evidence that new techniques, such as strain imaging and, in particular, the presence of regional alterations, are indicative of the presence of underlying subclinical disease [51] (Chap. 11).

10.11 Stress Echocardiography

Exercise echocardiography is an important and useful tool for evaluating symptoms and monitoring response to therapy in patients with HCM. One of the main roles of stress echocardiography is the evaluation of latent obstruction. A range of provocative maneuvers—such as standing and Valsalva maneuver—can be used to induce a gradient, but exercise Doppler is considered the best test to unmask and assess the degree of obstruction in HCM (Fig. 10.8) [1].

Maron et al. [33] showed, by a post-treadmill exercise echo Doppler study, that 53 % of symptomatic and asymptomatic HCM patients nonobstructive at rest developed a significant intraventricular pressure gradient after exercise. Provocative medications, such as dobutamine infusion, have also been studied but are considered nonphysiologic and thus are not commonly recommended in this clinical setting [52].

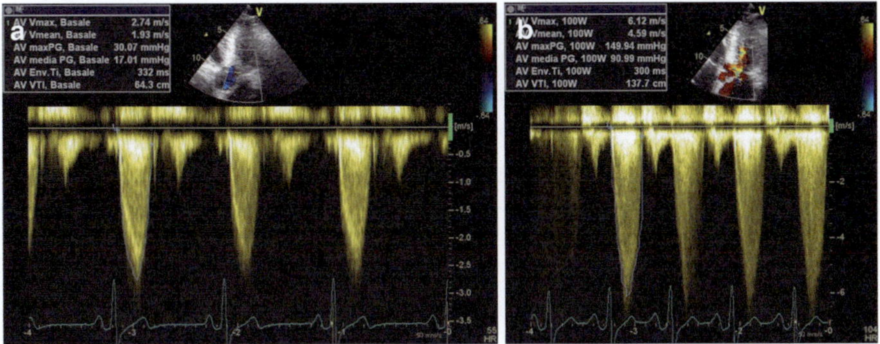

Fig. 10.8 Continuous-wave Doppler imaging recorded through the left ventricular outflow tract at rest (**a**) in a 20-year-old patient with hypertrophic cardiomyopathy. Peak gradient 30 mmHg. During exercise echocardiography, there is an increase in peak gradient to 150 mmHg at 100 W (**b**)

In clinical practice, the best method is employing a dedicated semisitting cycle ergometer, which allows continuous echo Doppler monitoring during a calibrated exercise test. Exercise Doppler echocardiography can also be helpful for better understanding the mechanisms underlying patient symptoms, exercise tolerance limitation, and abnormal blood pressure response to exercise [53, 54]. Patients with HCM can present with a wide and varied spectrum of symptoms, including exertional dyspnea, chest pain, and syncope. The appearance of these symptoms can be related to the development of intraventricular obstruction, wall-motion abnormalities, appearance or worsening of MR, and diastolic dysfunction [55].

References

1. Maron BJ, Maron MS (2013) Hypertrophic cardiomyopathy. Lancet 381:242–255
2. Maron BJ, McKenna WJ, Danielson GK et al (2003) American College of Cardiology/European Society of Cardiology clinical expert consensus document on hypertrophic cardiomyopathy. A report of the American College of Cardiology Foundation Task Force on Clinical Expert Consensus Documents and the European Society of Cardiology Committee for Practice Guidelines. J Am Coll Cardiol 42:1687–1713
3. Maron BJ (2002) Hypertrophic cardiomyopathy: a systematic review. JAMA 287:1308–1320
4. Gersh BJ, Maron BJ, Bonow RO et al (2011) 2011 ACCF/AHA Guideline for the Diagnosis and Treatment of Hypertrophic Cardiomyopathy: a report of the American College of Cardiology Foundation/American Heart Association Task Force on Practice Guidelines. Developed in collaboration with the American Association for Thoracic Surgery, American Society of Echocardiography, American Society of Nuclear Cardiology, Heart Failure Society of America, Heart Rhythm Society, Society for Cardiovascular Angiography and Interventions, and Society of Thoracic Surgeons. J Am Coll Cardiol 58:e212–e260
5. Wigle ED, Sasson Z, Henderson MA et al (1985) Hypertrophic cardiomyopathy. The importance of the site and the extent of hypertrophy. A review. Prog Cardiovasc Dis 28:1–83
6. Spirito P, Watson RM, Maron BJ (1987) Relation between extent of left ventricular hypertrophy and occurrence of ventricular tachycardia in hypertrophic cardiomyopathy. Am J Cardiol 60:1137–1142

7. Bos JM, Towbin JA, Ackerman MJ (2009) Diagnostic, prognostic, and therapeutic implications of genetic testing for hypertrophic cardiomyopathy. J Am Coll Cardiol 54:201–211

8. Binder J, Ommen SR, Gersh BJ et al (2006) Echocardiography-guided genetic testing in hypertrophic cardiomyopathy: septal morphological features predict the presence of myofilament mutations. Mayo Clin Proc 81:459–467

9. Nagueh SF, Bierig SM, Budoff MJ et al (2011) American Society of Echocardiography clinical recommendations for multimodality cardiovascular imaging of patients with hypertrophic cardiomyopathy: Endorsed by the American Society of Nuclear Cardiology, Society for Cardiovascular Magnetic Resonance, and Society of Cardiovascular Computed Tomography. J Am Soc Echocardiogr 24:473–498

10. de Simone G, Verdecchia P, Schillaci G et al (1998) Clinical impact of various geometric models for calculation of echocardiographic left ventricular mass. J Hypertens 16:1207–1214

11. Thanigaraj S, Perez JE (2000) Apical hypertrophic cardiomyopathy: echocardiographic diagnosis with the use of intravenous contrast image enhancement. J Am Soc Echocardiogr 13: 146–149

12. Bravo PE, Zimmerman SL, Luo HC et al (2013) Relationship of delayed enhancement by magnetic resonance to myocardial perfusion by positron emission tomography in hypertrophic cardiomyopathy. Circ Cardiovasc Imaging 6:210–217

13. Moon JC, Fisher NG, McKenna WJ et al (2004) Detection of apical hypertrophic cardiomyopathy by cardiovascular magnetic resonance in patients with non-diagnostic echocardiography. Heart 90:645–649

14. Baker ML MWF, Goldman B (2011) Hypertrophic cardiomyopathy with features of left ventricular non-compaction: how many diseases? Int J Cardiol 148:364–366

15. Harris KM, Spirito P, Maron MS et al (2006) Prevalence, clinical profile, and significance of left ventricular remodeling in the end-stage phase of hypertrophic cardiomyopathy. Circulation 114:216–225

16. Girolami F, Ho CY, Semsarian C et al (2010) Clinical features and outcome of hypertrophic cardiomyopathy associated with triple sarcomere protein gene mutations. J Am Coll Cardiol 55:1444–1453

17. Olivotto I, Cecchi F, Poggesi C et al (2012) Patterns of disease progression in hypertrophic cardiomyopathy: an individualized approach to clinical staging. Circ Heart Fail 5:535–546

18. Nishimura RA, Appleton CP, Redfield MM et al (1996) Noninvasive doppler echocardiographic evaluation of left ventricular filling pressures in patients with cardiomyopathies: a simultaneous Doppler echocardiographic and cardiac catheterization study. J Am Coll Cardiol 28:1226–1233

19. Nagueh SF, Lakkis NM, Middleton KJ et al (1999) Doppler estimation of left ventricular filling pressures in patients with hypertrophic cardiomyopathy. Circulation 99:254–261

20. Pinamonti B, Di Lenarda A, Nucifora G et al (2008) Incremental prognostic value of restrictive filling pattern in hypertrophic cardiomyopathy: a Doppler echocardiographic study. Eur J Echocardiogr 9:466–471

21. Fayssoil A (2010) Left atrial volume index: a predictor of adverse outcome in patients with hypertrophic cardiomyopathy. J Am Soc Echocardiogr 23:456; author reply 456

22. Nagueh SF, Appleton CP, Gillebert TC et al (2009) Recommendations for the evaluation of left ventricular diastolic function by echocardiography. Eur J Echocardiogr 10:165–193

23. Cavalcante JL, Barboza JS, Lever HM (2012) Diversity of mitral valve abnormalities in obstructive hypertrophic cardiomyopathy. Prog Cardiovasc Dis 54:517–522

24. Maron BJ, Gottdiener JS, Perry LW (1981) Specificity of systolic anterior motion of anterior mitral leaflet for hypertrophic cardiomyopathy. Prevalence in large population of patients with other cardiac diseases. Br Heart J 45:206–212

25. Maron BJ, Maron MS, Wigle ED et al (2009) The 50-year history, controversy, and clinical implications of left ventricular outflow tract obstruction in hypertrophic cardiomyopathy from idiopathic hypertrophic subaortic stenosis to hypertrophic cardiomyopathy: from idiopathic hypertrophic subaortic stenosis to hypertrophic cardiomyopathy. J Am Coll Cardiol 54: 191–200

26. Woo A, Jedrzkiewicz S (2011) The mitral valve in hypertrophic cardiomyopathy: it's a long story. Circulation 124:9–12
27. Maron MS, Olivotto I, Harrigan C et al (2011) Mitral valve abnormalities identified by cardiovascular magnetic resonance represent a primary phenotypic expression of hypertrophic cardiomyopathy. Circulation 124:40–47
28. Wigle ED, Adelman AG, Auger P et al (1969) Mitral regurgitation in muscular subaortic stenosis. Am J Cardiol 24:698–706
29. Grigg LE, Wigle ED, Williams WG et al (1992) Transesophageal Doppler echocardiography in obstructive hypertrophic cardiomyopathy: clarification of pathophysiology and importance in intraoperative decision making. J Am Coll Cardiol 20:42–52
30. Kwon DH, Setser RM, Thamilarasan M et al (2008) Abnormal papillary muscle morphology is independently associated with increased left ventricular outflow tract obstruction in hypertrophic cardiomyopathy. Heart 94:1295–1301
31. Klues HG, Schiffers A, Maron BJ (1995) Phenotypic spectrum and patterns of left ventricular hypertrophy in hypertrophic cardiomyopathy: morphologic observations and significance as assessed by two-dimensional echocardiography in 600 patients. J Am Coll Cardiol 26: 1699–1708
32. Sigwart U, Maron BJ, Nishimura RA et al (1999) Pitfalls in clinical recognition and a novel operative approach for hypertrophic cardiomyopathy with severe outflow obstruction due to anomalous papillary muscle. Circulation 100:e99
33. Maron MS, Olivotto I, Zenovich AG et al (2006) Hypertrophic cardiomyopathy is predominantly a disease of left ventricular outflow tract obstruction. Circulation 114:2232–2239
34. Sherrid MV, Wever-Pinzon O, Shah A et al (2009) Reflections of inflections in hypertrophic cardiomyopathy. J Am Coll Cardiol 54:212–219
35. Faber L, Seggewiss H, Welge D et al (2004) Echo-guided percutaneous septal ablation for symptomatic hypertrophic obstructive cardiomyopathy: 7 years of experience. Eur J Echocardiogr 5:347–355
36. Nagueh SF, Lakkis NM, He ZX et al (1998) Role of myocardial contrast echocardiography during nonsurgical septal reduction therapy for hypertrophic obstructive cardiomyopathy. J Am Coll Cardiol 32:225–229
37. Oudiz RJ (2007) Pulmonary hypertension associated with left-sided heart disease. Clin Chest Med 28:233–241
38. Severino S, Caso P, Cicala S et al (2000) Involvement of right ventricle in left ventricular hypertrophic cardiomyopathy: analysis by pulsed Doppler tissue imaging. Eur J Echocardiogr 1:281–288
39. Finocchiaro G, Knowles JW, Pavlovic A et al (2013) Prevalence and clinical correlates of right ventricular dysfunction in patients with hypertrophic cardiomyopathy. Am J Cardiol 113: 361–7
40. Maron MS, Hauser TH, Dubrow E et al (2007) Right ventricular involvement in hypertrophic cardiomyopathy. Am J Cardiol 100:1293–1298
41. Elliott P, Andersson B, Arbustini E et al (2008) Classification of the cardiomyopathies: a position statement from the European Society Of Cardiology Working Group on Myocardial and Pericardial Diseases. Eur Heart J 29:270–276
42. Pieroni M, Chimenti C, De Cobelli F et al (2006) Fabry's disease cardiomyopathy: echocardiographic detection of endomyocardial glycosphingolipid compartmentalization. J Am Coll Cardiol 47:1663–1671
43. Kounas S, Demetrescu C, Pantazis AA et al (2008) The binary endocardial appearance is a poor discriminator of Anderson-Fabry disease from familial hypertrophic cardiomyopathy. J Am Coll Cardiol 51:2058–2061
44. Pelliccia A, Maron MS, Maron BJ (2012) Assessment of left ventricular hypertrophy in a trained athlete: differential diagnosis of physiologic athlete's heart from pathologic hypertrophy. Prog Cardiovasc Dis 54:387–396
45. Lewis JF, Spirito P, Pelliccia A et al (1992) Usefulness of Doppler echocardiographic assessment of diastolic filling in distinguishing "athlete's heart" from hypertrophic cardiomyopathy. Br Heart J 68:296–300

46. Vinereanu D, Florescu N, Sculthorpe N et al (2001) Differentiation between pathologic and physiologic left ventricular hypertrophy by tissue Doppler assessment of long-axis function in patients with hypertrophic cardiomyopathy or systemic hypertension and in athletes. Am J Cardiol 88:53–58
47. Pelliccia A, Maron BJ, Di Paolo FM et al (2005) Prevalence and clinical significance of left atrial remodeling in competitive athletes. J Am Coll Cardiol 46:690–696
48. Maron BJ, Maron MS, Semsarian C (2012) Genetics of hypertrophic cardiomyopathy after 20 years: clinical perspectives. J Am Coll Cardiol 60:705–715
49. Nagueh SF, McFalls J, Meyer D et al (2003) Tissue Doppler imaging predicts the development of hypertrophic cardiomyopathy in subjects with subclinical disease. Circulation 108: 395–398
50. Gandjbakhch E, Gackowski A, Tezenas du Montcel S et al (2010) Early identification of mutation carriers in familial hypertrophic cardiomyopathy by combined echocardiography and tissue Doppler imaging. Eur Heart J 31:1599–1607
51. De S, Borowski AG, Wang H et al (2011) Subclinical echocardiographic abnormalities in phenotype-negative carriers of myosin-binding protein C3 gene mutation for hypertrophic cardiomyopathy. Am Heart J 162:262–267
52. Okeie K, Shimizu M, Yoshio H et al (2000) Left ventricular systolic dysfunction during exercise and dobutamine stress in patients with hypertrophic cardiomyopathy. J Am Coll Cardiol 36:856–863
53. Olivotto I, Maron BJ, Montereggi A et al (1999) Prognostic value of systemic blood pressure response during exercise in a community-based patient population with hypertrophic cardiomyopathy. J Am Coll Cardiol 33:2044–2051
54. Ciampi Q, Betocchi S, Lombardi R et al (2002) Hemodynamic determinants of exercise-induced abnormal blood pressure response in hypertrophic cardiomyopathy. J Am Coll Cardiol 40:278–284
55. Argulian E, Chaudhry FA (2012) Stress testing in patients with hypertrophic cardiomyopathy. Prog Cardiovasc Dis 54:477–482

Advanced Echocardiographic Technologies in Hypertrophic Cardiomyopathy

11

Gherardo Finocchiaro, Elena Abate, and Bruno Pinamonti

11.1 Introduction

The selective employment of advanced echocardiographic techniques has been recently demonstrated to allow a better understanding of hypertrophic cardiomyopathy (HCM) pathophysiology, thus improving diagnostic assessment of this disease. Specific advanced echocardiographic technologies can be applied to investigate in depth the wide spectrum of complexities encountered in HCM—from left ventricular (LV) architectural and morphological changes, to diastolic dysfunction, intraventricular obstruction, and mitral valve (MV) abnormalities.

11.2 Tissue Doppler Imaging

Tissue Doppler imaging (TDI) is a relatively new echocardiographic modality that allows measurement of myocardial tissue motion and provides real-time quantification of axial or longitudinal myocardial function. Annular displacement toward the apex in systole and away from the apex in diastole represents surrogate measures of longitudinal ventricular contraction and relaxation, respectively (Fig. 11.1) [1, 2].

Early diastolic mitral annular velocity (E'), a relatively pre-load-independent index of LV relaxation, is usually reduced in patients with HCM (Fig. 11.1) compared with age-matched controls and relates to LV hypertrophy magnitude [3]. As shown by Nagueh et al. [1], peak systolic myocardial velocity at TDI (S') and early diastolic velocity (E') are also reduced in patients with subclinical disease (early phenotype) in comparison with normal controls.

G. Finocchiaro (✉) • E. Abate • B. Pinamonti, MD
Department of Cardiology, University Hospital of Trieste,
Via P. Valdoni 7, Trieste 34139, Italy
e-mail: gherardobis@yahoo.it; abate.elena@gmail.com; bruno.pinamonti@gmail.com

B. Pinamonti, G. Sinagra (eds.), *Clinical Echocardiography and Other Imaging Techniques in Cardiomyopathies*, DOI 10.1007/978-3-319-06019-4_11,
© Springer International Publishing Switzerland 2014

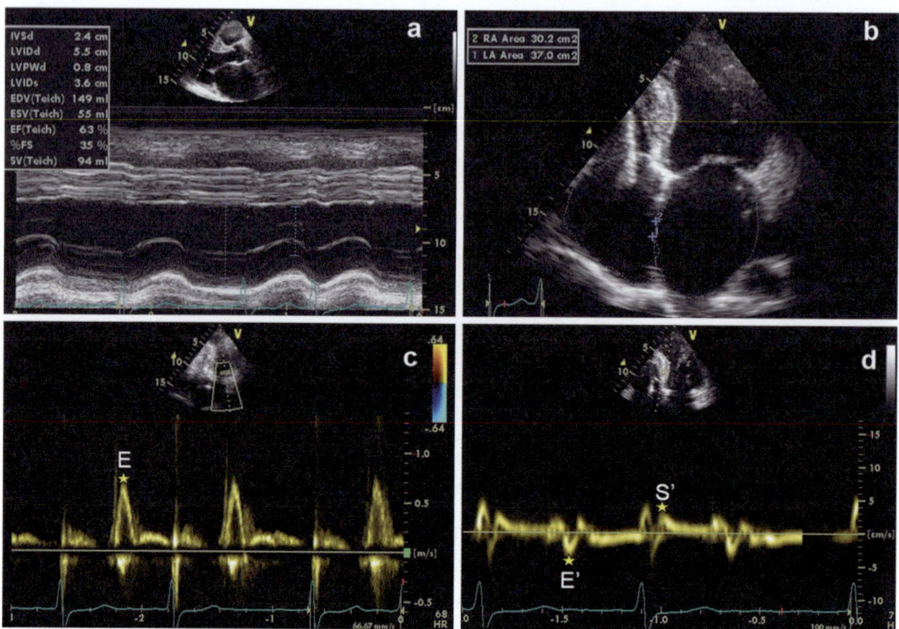

Fig. 11.1 Patient with hypertrophic cardiomyopathy: M-mode echocardiography (**a**) shows a severe left ventricular (LV) septal hypertrophy (24 mm) with preserved systolic function evaluated with conventional echocardiographic indices (fractional shortening 35 %, ejection fraction 63 %). Apical four-chamber view (**b**) demonstrates moderate biatrial dilatation; in the right chambers, the lead of the implantable cardioverter defibrillator (ICD) is visible. Doppler interrogation of the transmitral valve (**c**) shows a restrictive filling pattern (E wave = 80 cm/s, E wave deceleration time = 115 ms). Tissue Doppler imaging curve on the septal mitral valve annulus (**d**) shows low systolic wave velocities (S' = 4 cm/s) and early diastolic wave (E' = 4 cm/s). E/E' = 20

The use of TDI can also assist in differentiating between variants of LV hypertrophy. Vinereanu et al. [4] used TDI to distinguish pathological from physiological LV hypertrophy in a study comprising patients with HCM, patients with systemic hypertension, athletes, and normal individuals. Long-axis systolic and early-diastolic velocities were decreased in patients with pathologic hypertrophy but preserved in athletes. Heterogeneity of annular velocities discriminated between hypertensive patients and HCM.

Evaluation of the E to /E' ratio (E/E') using transmitral Doppler and TDI has allowed noninvasive estimation of LV filling pressures in various cardiac disease patient populations [5]. On the contrary, in symptomatic patients with HCM, Doppler echocardiographic estimates of LV filling pressure using E/E' correlate only modestly with direct measurement of left atrial (LA) pressure [6]. Nevertheless, E/E' has been correlated with exercise tolerance in adults (with an inverse correlation with peak oxygen consumption) [7] and children [8] with HCM. In addition, septal E' velocity appears to be an independent predictor of death and ventricular arrhythmia in children with HCM [8].

TDI assessment of regional myocardial function has some important limitations because of its angle dependence (as with all Doppler techniques) and because it measures absolute tissue velocities and not myocardial deformation, being consequently influenced by cardiac translational motion and tethering. These limitations led to the development of more sophisticated echocardiographic techniques, such as TDI-derived myocardial strain and strain rate and speckle-tracking imaging.

11.2.1 Tissue-Doppler-Imaging-Derived Strain

Longitudinal myocardial strain and strain rate can be estimated by TDI technique and can provide useful information on local myocardial motion or deformation relative to the adjacent myocardium [9]. One of the first studies on strain in HCM was by Yang et al. [10], who reported the assessment of regional myocardial function in 31 adults with HCM diagnosed echocardiographically. Longitudinal strain was evaluated at the basal, mid, and apical segments of septal and lateral walls. It was significantly reduced in the septal segments of patients with HCM compared with control patients. More importantly, within the septum, midseptum longitudinal strain was significantly diminished compared with basal and apical segments. Kato et al. [11] demonstrated a major role of strain rate in differentiating nonobstructive HCM from hypertensive LV hypertrophy. The authors compared an HCM population and hypertensive patients and showed that at multivariate analysis, systolic strain rate and interventricular septum (IVS)/posterior wall thickness ratio were the most powerful predictors for the diagnosis of HCM. However, TDI-derived strain imaging also has technical limitations due to its angle dependence and frequent artifacts.

11.2.2 Speckle-Tracking Imaging

Speckle-tracking echocardiography, relatively a new imaging technique that allows objective and quantitative evaluation of global and regional myocardial deformation independently from the angle of insonation and from cardiac translational movements [12], has been employed in HCM in various settings. Serri et al. [13] applied 2D strain echocardiography to a subset of patients with familial nonobstructive HCM. Despite apparently normal systolic function (with the use of standard criteria), all components of strain (longitudinal, transverse, circumferential, radial) were significantly reduced in HCM in comparison with a healthy control population. Carasso et al. [14] showed that patients compared with controls had higher circumferential strain and lower longitudinal strain. In addition, mid-LV rotation was clockwise (opposite to normal). LV outflow-tract (OT) obstruction and clinical status were related to more circumferentially directed strain and reduced apical biplanar strain.

The ability of predicting the presence of myocardial fibrosis in HCM patients using echocardiography could have important implications, especially when predicting adverse outcomes, such as sudden death (SD). Funabashi et al. [15] used

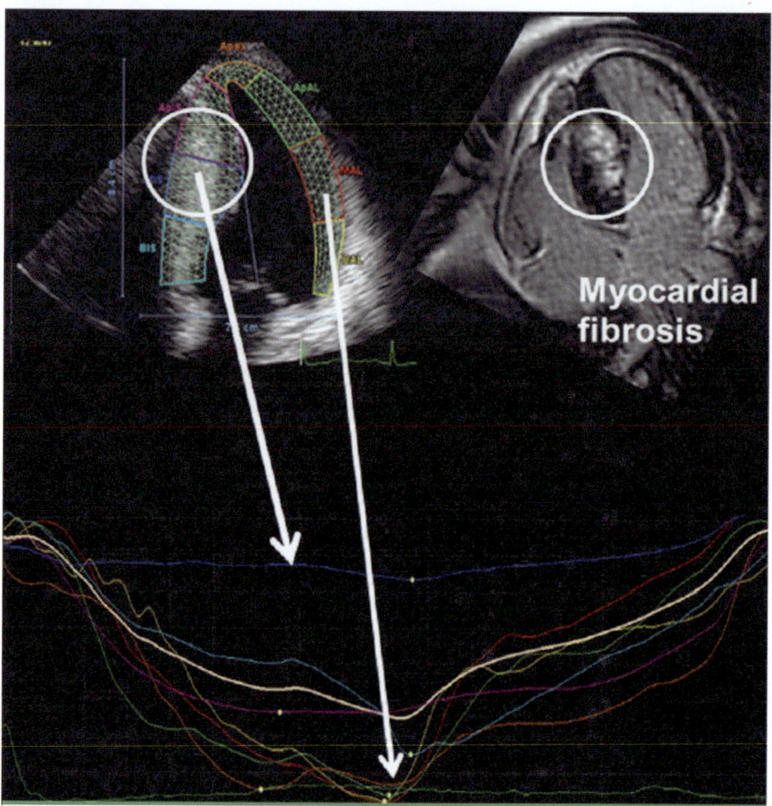

Fig. 11.2 Longitudinal strain measurement in seven left ventricular segments from an apical four-chamber view (*upper left*), regional strain curves (*bottom*), and cardiac magnetic resonance (CMR) (*upper right*) in hypertrophic cardiomyopathy patient with fibrosis in the interventricular septum. The segments with fibrosis at CMR show lower longitudinal strain values (less negative) compared with segments without fibrosis (From [15], with permission)

speckle-tracking echocardiography and cardiac magnetic resonance (CMR) to study 29 HCM patients. The authors showed that absolute peak longitudinal strain values were significantly lower in fibrotic lesions than in nonfibrotic lesions (Fig. 11.2). Moreover, there is an inverse association between various histopathologic findings typical of HCM (myocyte hypertrophy, disarray, small intramural coronary arteriole dysplasia, interstitial fibrosis) and septal strain rate in symptomatic HCM patients who undergo surgical myectomy, as demonstrated by Kobayashi et al. [16]. It is thus possible that myocyte disarray is related to a abnormal ventricular architecture that predisposes to worsening regional LV function. Saito et al. [17] showed that global longitudinal strain might provide useful information regarding myocardial fibrosis [correlating with late gadolinium enhancement (LGE) at CMR] and cardiac events in HCM patients with normal systolic function. Strain imaging of the LA allows for a more direct assessment of LA function. LA longitudinal function, quantified using TDI

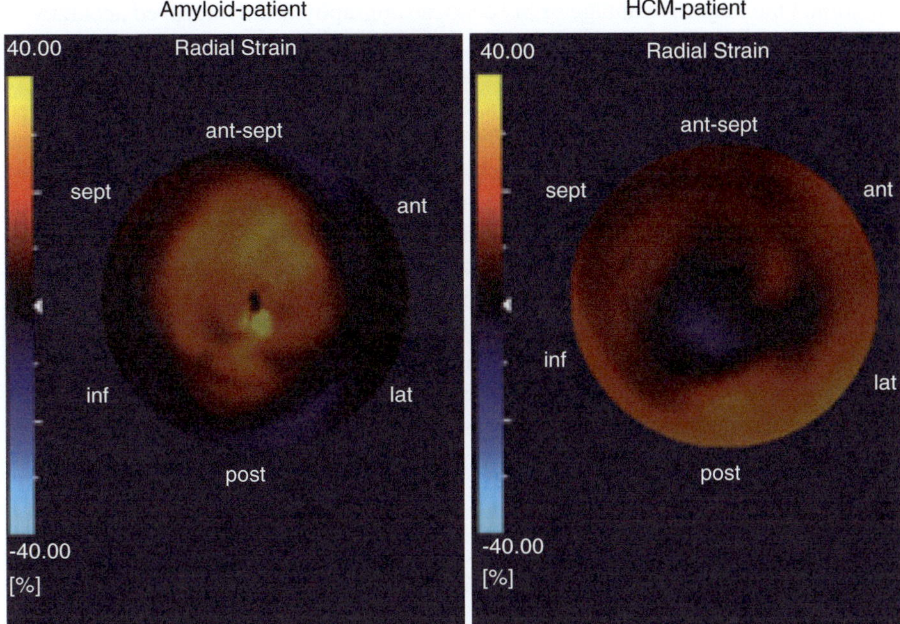

Fig. 11.3 Sixteen-segment polar maps (bull's-eye plot) of 3D speckle-tracking radial strain in a patient with cardiac amyloidosis (*left*) compared with a patient with hypertrophic cardiomyopathy (*right*). The basoapical radial strain gradient displays opposite characteristics in the two diseases: in cardiac amyloidosis, basal radial strain is significantly reduced, with a gradual increase from base to apex; hypertrophic cardiomyopathy shows a physiological gradient of basoapically decreasing radial strain. *ant* anterior, *ant-sept* anteroseptal, *HCM* hypertrophic cardiomyopathy, *inf* inferior, *lat* lateral, *post* posterior, *sept* septal (From [19], with permission)

and 2D strain in HCM patients, was reduced compared with non-HCM patients with LV hypertrophy due to other conditions, as well as with healthy controls [18].

The role of 3D speckle-tracking echocardiography has also been evaluated in HCM. In particular, in the study by Baccouche et al. [19] comparing cardiac amyloidosis (CA) and HCM, basal radial strain was significantly reduced in the former condition (Fig. 11.3). Moreover, in HCM, 3D speckle-tracking parameters showed a remarkably weaker correlation with LGE compared with individuals with CA. This is most likely explained by the focal character of fibrosis, which may be less accessible for 3D strain imaging compared with amyloid changes.

11.3   Three-Dimensional Echocardiography

Another significant advancement in the field of echocardiography is the development and refinement of 3D echocardiography, which can provide insights into mechanics of LV obstruction, LV architecture, and mitral and aortic structure and function. One major advantage of 3D echocardiography is the improved accuracy in evaluating cardiac chamber volumes by eliminating the need for geometric modeling and the errors caused by foreshortened apical views [20].

One of the most common features of HCM is LV obstruction, which is often complex in nature, involving MV leaflets, papillary muscles, and the hypertrophied septum [21]. As demonstrated by Song et al. [22] in 39 patients with obstructive HCM studied with real-time 3D echocardiography, the distance between the IVS and the anterior MV tip in the medial and central plane was significantly smaller than that in the lateral plane; lateral distance was the only independent determinant of LV OT pressure gradient assessed using multiple stepwise regression analysis.

Three-dimensional echocardiography facilitates assessment of the LVOT area after intervention for septal reduction [23], volumetric estimates of LA mechanical function [24], and accurate estimation of LV ejection fraction (EF) and LV mass in hypertrophied hearts [25]. LV mass assessment is limited using conventional 2D echocardiography, considering the asymmetric distribution of hypertrophy typical of the disease [26]. LV mass derived using M-mode American Society of Echocardiography (ASE) formula, the 2D-based truncated ellipsoid method (2D mass), and the real-time 3D technique was assessed in comparison with CMR mass. The closest relationship was with real-time 3D ($r=0.86$, $p<0.001$), emphasizing how this technique is reliable in quantifying LV mass [27]. Moreover, 3D echocardiography can help in the diagnosis of anomalous papillary muscles leading to dynamic LV OT obstruction, which can be challenging with 2D echocardiography [28].

11.4 Contrast Echocardiography

Contrast echocardiography may have a role in HCM diagnosis and assessment, especially when the acoustic window is suboptimal and in the diagnosis of apical HCM [29]. As demonstrated by Nagueh et al. [30], myocardial contrast echocardiography is accurate in determining the perfusion bed of septal perforators and in predicting infarct size after ethanol injection in HCM patients treated with alcohol septal ablation.

References

1. Nagueh SF, McFalls J, Meyer D et al (2003) Tissue Doppler imaging predicts the development of hypertrophic cardiomyopathy in subjects with subclinical disease. Circulation 108: 395–398
2. Michels M, Soliman OI, Kofflard MJ et al (2009) Diastolic abnormalities as the first feature of hypertrophic cardiomyopathy in Dutch myosin-binding protein C founder mutations. JACC Cardiovasc Imaging 2:58–64
3. Yu CM, Sanderson JE, Marwick TH et al (2007) Tissue Doppler imaging a new prognosticator for cardiovascular diseases. J Am Coll Cardiol 49:1903–1914
4. Vinereanu D, Florescu N, Sculthorpe N et al (2001) Differentiation between pathologic and physiologic left ventricular hypertrophy by tissue Doppler assessment of long-axis function in

patients with hypertrophic cardiomyopathy or systemic hypertension and in athletes. Am J Cardiol 88:53–58

5. Ommen SR, Nishimura RA, Appleton CP et al (2000) Clinical utility of Doppler echocardiography and tissue Doppler imaging in the estimation of left ventricular filling pressures: a comparative simultaneous Doppler-catheterization study. Circulation 102:1788–1794

6. Geske JB, Sorajja P, Nishimura RA et al (2007) Evaluation of left ventricular filling pressures by Doppler echocardiography in patients with hypertrophic cardiomyopathy: correlation with direct left atrial pressure measurement at cardiac catheterization. Circulation 116:2702–2708

7. Matsumura Y, Elliott PM, Virdee MS et al (2002) Left ventricular diastolic function assessed using Doppler tissue imaging in patients with hypertrophic cardiomyopathy: relation to symptoms and exercise capacity. Heart 87:247–251

8. McMahon CJ, Nagueh SF, Pignatelli RH et al (2004) Characterization of left ventricular diastolic function by tissue Doppler imaging and clinical status in children with hypertrophic cardiomyopathy. Circulation 109:1756–1762

9. Marwick TH (2006) Measurement of strain and strain rate by echocardiography: ready for prime time? J Am Coll Cardiol 47:1313–1327

10. Yang H, Sun JP, Lever HM et al (2003) Use of strain imaging in detecting segmental dysfunction in patients with hypertrophic cardiomyopathy. J Am Soc Echocardiogr 16:233–239

11. Kato TS, Noda A, Izawa H et al (2004) Discrimination of nonobstructive hypertrophic cardiomyopathy from hypertensive left ventricular hypertrophy on the basis of strain rate imaging by tissue Doppler ultrasonography. Circulation 110:3808–3814

12. Blessberger H, Binder T (2010) NON-invasive imaging: two dimensional speckle tracking echocardiography: basic principles. Heart 96:716–722

13. Serri K, Reant P, Lafitte M et al (2006) Global and regional myocardial function quantification by two-dimensional strain: application in hypertrophic cardiomyopathy. J Am Coll Cardiol 47:1175–1181

14. Carasso S, Yang H, Woo A et al (2008) Systolic myocardial mechanics in hypertrophic cardiomyopathy: novel concepts and implications for clinical status. J Am Soc Echocardiogr 21:675–683

15. Funabashi N, Takaoka H, Horie S et al (2013) Regional peak longitudinal-strain by 2D speckle-tracking TTE provides useful information to distinguish fibrotic from non-fibrotic lesions in LV myocardium on cardiac MR in hypertrophic cardiomyopathy. Int J Cardiol 168:4520–4523

16. Kobayashi T, Popovic Z, Bhonsale A et al (2013) Association between septal strain rate and histopathology in symptomatic hypertrophic cardiomyopathy patients undergoing septal myectomy. Am Heart J 166:503–511

17. Saito M, Okayama H, Yoshii T et al (2012) Clinical significance of global two-dimensional strain as a surrogate parameter of myocardial fibrosis and cardiac events in patients with hypertrophic cardiomyopathy. Eur Heart J Cardiovasc Imaging 13:617–623

18. Paraskevaidis IA, Panou F, Papadopoulos C et al (2009) Evaluation of left atrial longitudinal function in patients with hypertrophic cardiomyopathy: a tissue Doppler imaging and two-dimensional strain study. Heart 95:483–489

19. Baccouche H, Maunz M, Beck T et al (2012) Differentiating cardiac amyloidosis and hypertrophic cardiomyopathy by use of three-dimensional speckle tracking echocardiography. Echocardiography 29:668–677

20. Dorosz JL, Lezotte DC, Weitzenkamp DA et al (2012) Performance of 3-dimensional echocardiography in measuring left ventricular volumes and ejection fraction: a systematic review and meta-analysis. J Am Coll Cardiol 59:1799–1808

21. Maron MS, Olivotto I, Zenovich AG et al (2006) Hypertrophic cardiomyopathy is predominantly a disease of left ventricular outflow tract obstruction. Circulation 114:2232–2239

22. Song JM, Fukuda S, Lever HM et al (2006) Asymmetry of systolic anterior motion of the mitral valve in patients with hypertrophic obstructive cardiomyopathy: a real-time three-dimensional echocardiographic study. J Am Soc Echocardiogr 19:1129–1135

23. Sitges M, Qin JX, Lever HM et al (2005) Evaluation of left ventricular outflow tract area after septal reduction in obstructive hypertrophic cardiomyopathy: a real-time 3-dimensional echocardiographic study. Am Heart J 150:852–858
24. Anwar AM, Soliman OI, Geleijnse ML et al (2007) Assessment of left atrial ejection force in hypertrophic cardiomyopathy using real-time three-dimensional echocardiography. J Am Soc Echocardiogr 20:744–748
25. Oe H, Hozumi T, Arai K et al (2005) Comparison of accurate measurement of left ventricular mass in patients with hypertrophied hearts by real-time three-dimensional echocardiography versus magnetic resonance imaging. Am J Cardiol 95:1263–1267
26. Foppa M, Duncan BB, Rohde LE (2005) Echocardiography-based left ventricular mass estimation. How should we define hypertrophy? Cardiovasc Ultrasound 3:17
27. Chang SA, Kim HK, Lee SC (2013) Assessment of left ventricular mass in hypertrophic cardiomyopathy by real-time three-dimensional echocardiography using single-beat capture image. J Am Soc Echocardiogr 26:436–442
28. Yang HS, Lee KS, Chaliki HP et al (2008) Anomalous insertion of the papillary muscle causing left ventricular outflow obstruction: visualization by real-time three-dimensional echocardiography. Eur J Echocardiogr 9:855–860
29. Soman P, Swinburn J, Callister M et al (2001) Apical hypertrophic cardiomyopathy: bedside diagnosis by intravenous contrast echocardiography. J Am Soc Echocardiogr 14:311–313
30. Nagueh SF, Lakkis NM, He ZX et al (1998) Role of myocardial contrast echocardiography during nonsurgical septal reduction therapy for hypertrophic obstructive cardiomyopathy. J Am Coll Cardiol 32:225–229

Other Imaging Techniques in Hypertrophic Cardiomyopathy

12

Gherardo Finocchiaro, Giancarlo Vitrella, and Bruno Pinamonti

12.1 Introduction

Echocardiography has a primary role in diagnostic assessment of HCM, but other techniques, such as cardiac magnetic resonance (CMR) and positron emission tomography (PET), recently became extremely important and helpful in the general evaluation of the disease and their use is now extremely widespread especially at referral centers.

12.2 Cardiac Magnetic Resonance

If echocardiography has a main role in the diagnosis and prognostic assessment of hypertrophic cardiomyopathy (HCM), in many clinical scenarios, technical limitations and heterogeneous phenotypic expression make such evaluation difficult, and cardiac magnetic resonance (CMR) has emerged as a useful imaging modality to complement routine transthoracic echocardiography [1, 2]. CMR offers not only high spatial resolution and complete 3D coverage of the entire heart but can also allow visualization of myocardial scarring in vivo using late gadolinium enhancement (LGE). Therefore, in many cardiomyopathy (CMP) reference centers, CMR has become a routinely used imaging tool in patients with HCM and it is indicated for establishing the diagnosis in patients with a suspicion of the disease but with no clear diagnostic elements arising from the use of other diagnostic tests [3].

G. Finocchiaro (✉) • G. Vitrella • B. Pinamonti, MD
Department of Cardiology, University Hospital of Trieste,
via P. Valdoni 7, Trieste 34139, Italy
e-mail: gherardobis@yahoo.it; bruno.pinamonti@gmail.com

B. Pinamonti, G. Sinagra (eds.), *Clinical Echocardiography and Other Imaging Techniques in Cardiomyopathies*, DOI 10.1007/978-3-319-06019-4_12,
© Springer International Publishing Switzerland 2014

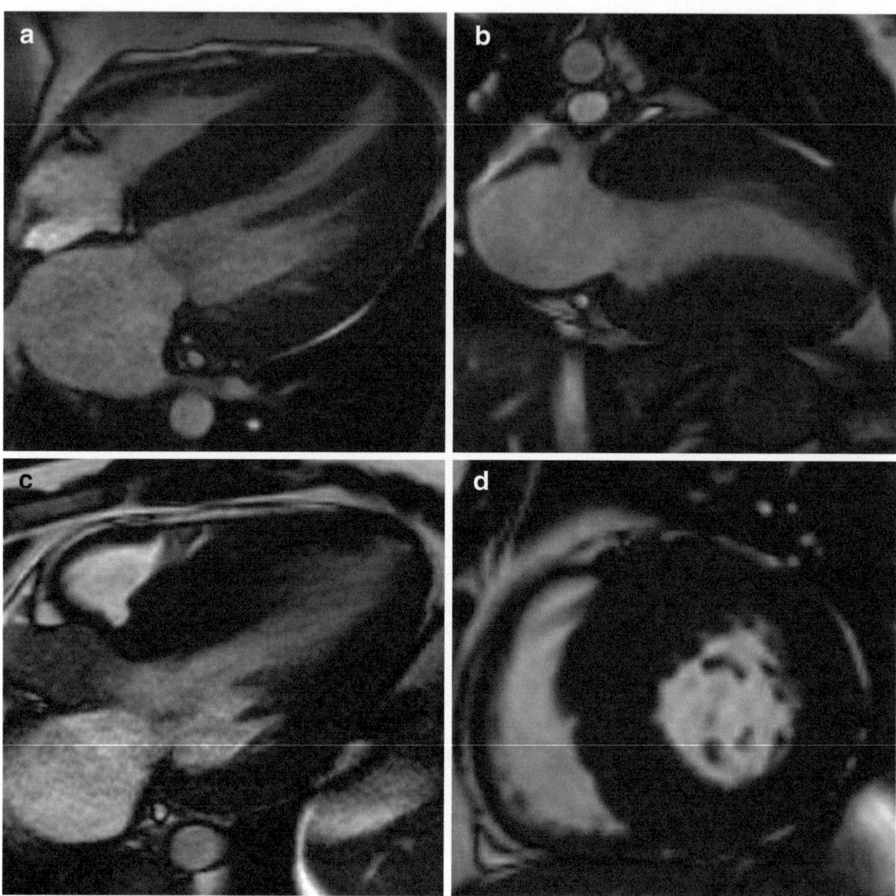

Fig. 12.1 Cardiac magnetic resonance (CMR) of a 35-year-old man with hypertrophic cardiomyopathy (HCM) showing severe asymmetric hypertrophy (maximal wall thickness at the basal septum is 27 mm) and left ventricular outflow tract (LV OT) obstruction. End-diastolic 4 chamber view (a); end-diastolic 2 chamber view (b); end-diastolic 3 chamber view (c); end-diastolic short-axis view

12.2.1 Diagnostic Value

CMR is considered the gold standard for evaluating the complex chamber morphology and function (Fig. 12.1), as well as the heterogeneous distribution of hypertrophy found in HCM patients. In addition, CMR is the best method available to assess the papillary muscle and mitral valve abnormalities, perfusion abnormalities, and fibrosis with LGE [4]. Furthermore, when dealing with left ventricular (LV) obstruction, CMR can characterize the underlying mechanisms, such as MV anatomy, septal systolic anterior motion contact, and subvalvular apparatus [5–7]. Isolated or concomitant midventricular obstruction related to midventricular hypertrophy is also readily demonstrated. CMR is advantageous in identifying the presence and various distribution of LV hypertrophy, particularly when regions of increased wall

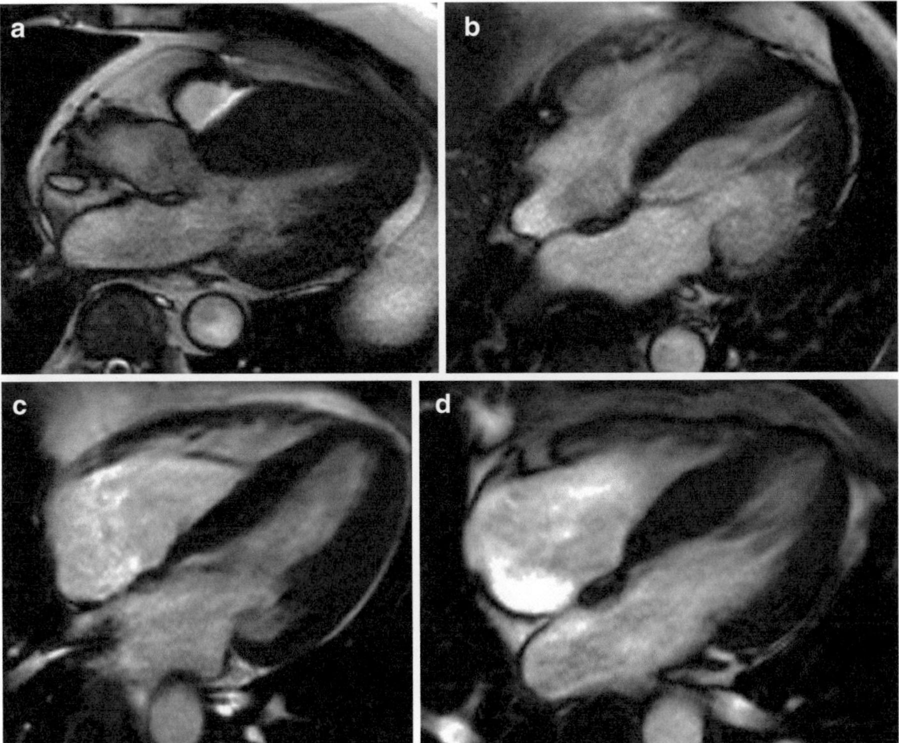

Fig. 12.2 Cardiac magnetic resonance (CMR), four- and three-chamber views, shows different hypertrophic cardiomyopathy (HCM) morphology subtypes. Asymmetric (**a**), apical (**b**), symmetric (**c**), septal bulge (**d**)

thickness are focal, such as the anterior free wall, posterior septum, and apex, and they are not well visualized by echocardiography [8].

The distribution of hypertrophy and distortion of septal anatomy is different among patients with a clinical diagnosis of HCM made later in life compared with younger patients. HCM morphology can be classified into five main subtypes: sigmoid, reverse curve, apical, symmetric, and neutral (Fig. 12.2) [9, 10]. LV apical aneurysms could also be present in HCM and are frequently associated with a mid-ventricular obstruction. They can be a substrate for life-threatening arrhythmias and location of intraventricular thrombi. Echocardiography is not always helpful in their visualization and Contrast-enhanced CMR demonstrates that they are composed predominantly of fibrosis [11].

CMR is also helpful in defining the degree of hypertrophy, which in some cases is massive (Fig. 12.3), and of LV mass, overcoming the limitations of echocardiography [12]. As demonstrated by Olivotto et al. [13], LV mass index in HCM patients significantly exceeds that of control individuals. Interestingly, LV mass index assessed by CMR showed only a modest relationship to maximal LV thickness assessed at echocardiography.

The right ventricle (RV) is often not well visualized by echocardiography, whereas CMR provides optimal assessment of RV volume, systolic function, and

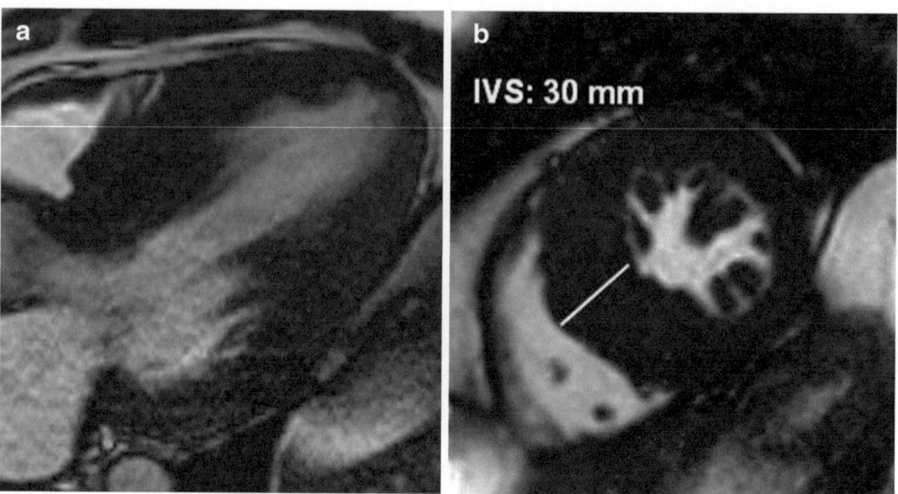

Fig. 12.3 Cardiac magnetic resonance (CMR), three-chamber and short-axis view, of a 40-year-old man with severe hypertrophy. Interventricular septum (IVS) is measured at 30 mm

wall thickness. According to Maron et al. [14], significant RV hypertrophy (end-diastolic RV free wall thickness ≥8 mm) could be demonstrated by CMR in more than one third of HCM patients. In a substantial proportion of patients, RV wall mass is also increased.

Microvascular dysfunction and subsequent ischemia may be present in HCM. As demonstrated by Petersen et al. [15], although resting myocardial blood flow is similar in HCM patients and healthy controls, during hyperemia, it is significantly lower in patients. In addition, this decrease in coronary reserve is related to the extent of LV hypertrophy.

12.2.2 Role in Differential Diagnosis

CMR is helpful in the differential diagnosis between HCM and other pathologic conditions characterized by LV hypertrophy. In particular, hypertrophy pattern and LGE distribution—although heterogeneous in HCM—are often distinctive in other diseases mimicking HCM, such as some infiltrative/storage CMP [15–17] (Chap. 27).

12.2.3 Genotype-Positive/Phenotype-Negative Individuals

CMR plays a role in assessing a particular patient subgroup within the HCM disease spectrum, i.e., genetically affected family members without clinical or morphologic evidence of disease. In this setting, CMR can recognize subtle abnormalities usually not detected by echocardiography [16]. One feature described in this subset of patients is the presence of myocardial crypts, characterized by small invaginations inside the

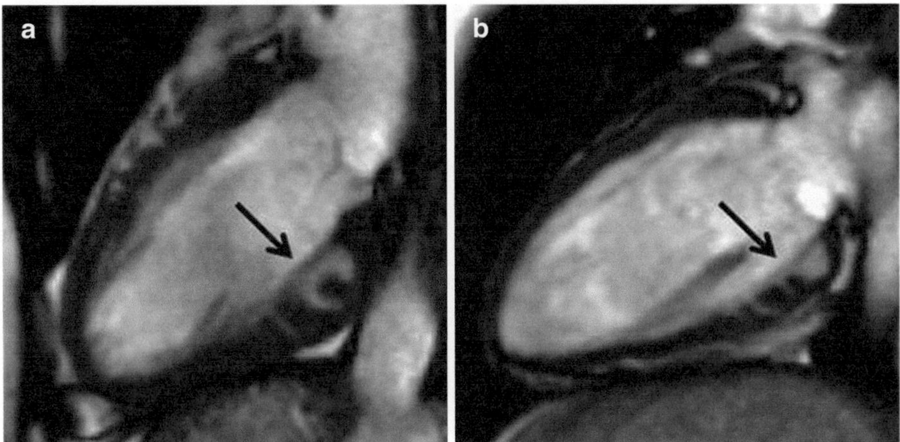

Fig. 12.4 Cardiac magnetic resonance (CMR) two-chamber view of two young carriers—19 (**a**) and 20 (**b**) years—of known disease-causing mutations and overexpression of phenotypes. Note the presence of myocardial crypts at the inferior wall (*black arrows*)

myocardium [17] (Fig. 12.4). Another morphological characteristic observed to be different in comparison with a healthy control population is the presence of longer mitral leaflets [6]. Interestingly, the MV is often abnormal in patients with HCM, and it is possible that abnormalities in its structure could be a primary feature linked to genetic mutation(s) [18]. Valente et al. [19] analyzed 40 genotype-positive/phenotype-negative patients using echocardiography and CMR and found a quite good diagnostic agreement, although CMR measurements of LV wall thickness were 19 % lower than echo, and 10 % of cases had LV hypertrophy appreciated only by CMR.

12.2.4   Assessment of Myocardial Fibrosis

Images acquired following the injection of gadolinium can help in detecting fibrosis in HCM, as in other heart diseases. The presence of myocardial fibrosis can be observed frequently in HCM hearts, and its presence is believed to be a pathological substrate for cardiac arrhythmias (Fig. 12.5).

In the seminal study by Choudhury et al. [20], myocardial scarring visualized by LGE was a common finding in asymptomatic or mildly symptomatic HCM patients (81 %). Also, Moon et al. [21] described a high prevalence of LGE in patients with HCM (79 %). During follow-up, the extent of scar visualized by CMR was associated with progressive ventricular dilation and clinical markers of sudden death (SD). Adabag et al. [22] found that myocardial fibrosis assessed using LGE was associated with greater likelihood and increased frequency of ventricular tachyarrhythmias on ambulatory Holter electrocardiography (ECG). LGE was distributed in different patterns (most commonly within the interventricular septum or in the areas of most extensive hypertrophy) [23]. Extensive LGE was

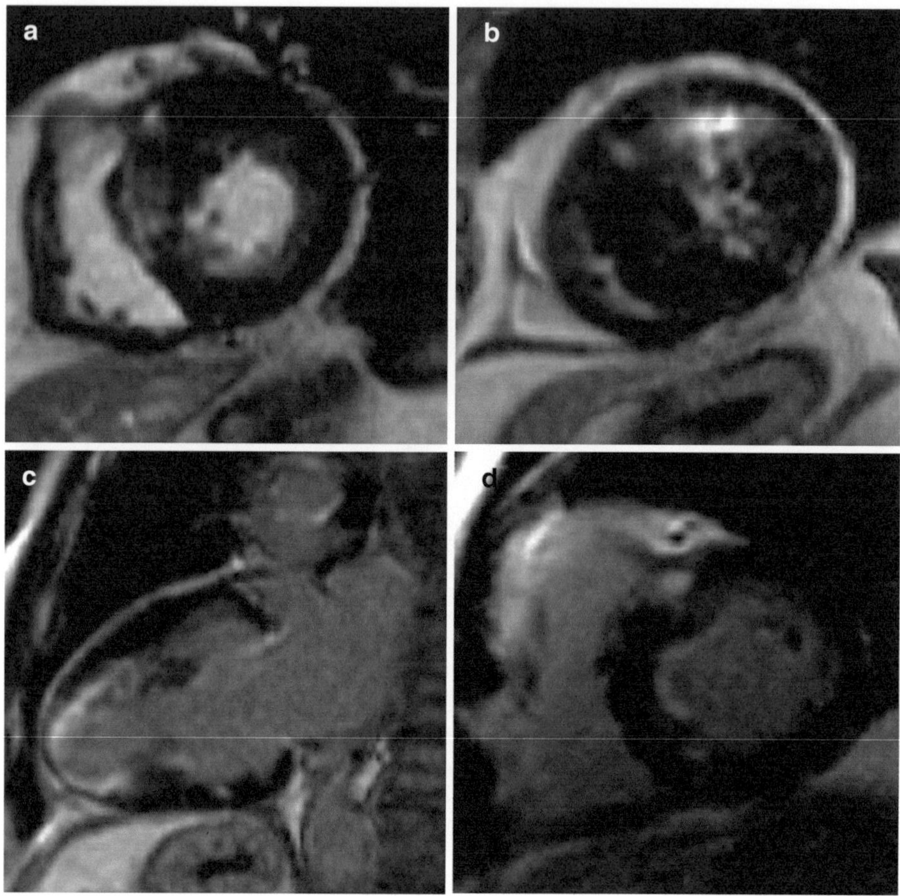

Fig. 12.5 Different late gadolinium enhancement (*LGE*) patterns in hypertrophic cardiomyopathy (*HCM*). Patchy septal LGE (**a**) in a patient with severe asymmetric hypertrophy. Anterior and circumferential LGE in a patient with systolic obliteration (**b**). Apical LGE in apical HCM (**c**). Insertion point LGE (**d**) in a patient with mild hypertrophy

observed in end-stage HCM with significant systolic LV dysfunction. In general, LGE correlates with LV wall thickening and inversely correlates with LV ejection fraction (EF) [24].

Novel techniques for quantifying myocardial extracellular volume, such as T1 mapping, may be promising, particularly for assessing diffuse myocardial interstitial fibrosis in HCM [25]. To date, the roles of these techniques, especially concerning prognostic stratification or relationship with other features such as ventricular arrhythmias, remain undefined.

There is debate around whether genotype-positive/phenotype-negative HCM patients have myocardial fibrosis. Even if some case reports describe the presence of LGE in this condition [26, 27], there is a lack of data on this specific patient population. Moreover, it is possible that these patients may have subtle myocardial fibrosis not detected by LGE. Patients without overt LV hypertrophy and a genetic mutation have a higher myocardial extracellular volume expansion when assessed measuring T1 times pre- and postgadolinium infusion [28].

12.3   Single-Photon-Emission Computed Tomography

Single photon emission computed tomography (SPECT) with thallium-201 radiochemical thallium chloride [^{201}Tl] demonstrates perfusion abnormalities in patients with HCM [29–31]. Abnormal stress myocardial perfusion imaging identifies HCM patients at increased risk of syncope, LV dilatation, reduced exercise capacity, sudden cardiac arrest, and cardiovascular death [31–33]. A possible exception may be found in patients with apical HCM, who seem to maintain a benign prognosis despite the presence of reversible thallium defects [34]. Abnormalities in regional myocardial perfusion, in addition to regional hypertrophy, contribute to early regional diastolic dysfunction in patients with HCM [35].

Fixed ^{201}Tl perfusion defects, possibly representing fibrosis, detected during dipyridamole stress test in patients with HCM are associated with syncope, larger LV cavity dimensions, and reduced exercise capacity [36]. Reduced ^{201}Tl washout was strongly associated with exertional chest pain in HCM patients and was observed in myocardial regions with normal as well as increased thickness [37]. Myocardial perfusion was used to demonstrate the beneficial effects of pharmacologic therapy [29, 30] or surgical or transcatheter septal ablation [38, 39]. Regional fatty acid metabolism abnormalities were demonstrated with ^{201}Tl SPECT and [^{123}] I-beta-methyl-p-iodophenylpentadecanoic acid (^{123}I-BMIPP) mismatch in HCM patients [40–42]. These abnormalities seem to occur before reduction of oxidative metabolism, measured by [^{18}F]-fluorodeoxyglucose (FDG) and ^{11}C-acetate positron emission tomography (PET), in patients with HCM [43]. Studies evaluating the role of regional myocardial sympathetic nerve activity with ^{123}I-metaiodobenzylguanidine (MIBG) suggest sympathetic dysinnervation in patients with HCM [44, 45]. Cardiac sympathetic nervous activity was related to degree of hypertrophy, systolic and diastolic function, and ventricular arrhythmias [46, 47].

12.4   Positron Emission Tomography

The usefulness of PET in patients with HCM was first reported by Grover-McKay et al. [48]. These authors demonstrated that the hypertrophied septum of patients with HCM is viable and not ischemic at rest, as it exhibits normal uptake of the fatty acid tracer ^{11}C-palmitate and normal or only mildly reduced myocardial perfusion. However, it is metabolically different from normal myocardium, as it fails to take up the glucose analog [^{18}F]-FDG despite normal uptake in the rest of the myocardium. Later studies confirmed this finding and demonstrated heterogeneity of [^{18}F]-FDG uptake in hypertrophied segments, possibly reflecting a metabolic abnormality [49]. This heterogeneity was suggested to be related to regional systolic function [50] and was increased in patients with HCM diagnosed at a young age compared with patients diagnosed at middle to old age [51].

Studies using PET with [^{13}N]-ammonia or [^{15}O]-water to assess myocardial blood flow demonstrate that patients with HCM have a blunted response to the vasodilators dipyridamole and adenosine compared with normal controls or patients with secondary hypertrophy, thus suggesting microvascular dysfunction [52–56]. A direct increase in the number of cardiovascular events, including unfavorable LV remodeling, progressive HF, ventricular tachyarrhythmias, and death, was found with increasing coronary reserve impairment [54, 56]. A relationship between LGE CMR and heterogeneous resting myocardial blood flow [57] or microvascular function studied by stress PET were found [58]. Studies with ^{11}C-12177 (CGP) or ^{11}C-hydroxyephedrine (HED) PET demonstrated the presence of cardiac sympathetic dysinnervation: reduced β-adrenergic receptor density with reduced norepinephrine reuptake by presynaptic terminals [59, 60]. These abnormalities seem to be particularly prominent in patients with HF [61].

12.5 Computed Tomography

Cardiac CT has the advantage of clearly delineating the myocardium, thus providing detailed characterization of the HCM phenotype, including accurate wall thickness measurements, and highly reproducible measurements of ventricular volumes, EF, and mass [62, 63]. In addition, it permits simultaneous imaging of coronary arteries, RV and LV volume and mass, and global and regional function [64, 65]. However, this imaging method was not extensively studied in HCM patients and thus is useful only in selected clinical scenarios, following suboptimal echocardiographic images when CMR is contraindicated, or to exclude concomitant coronary disease (Table 12.1).

Table 12.1 Importance of different imaging techniques in assessing hypertrophic cardiomyopathy (HCM) features

	Echocardiography	CMR	PET	CT
Wall thickness evaluation	++	+++	−	++
LV mass	+	+++	−	++
MV abnormalities	++	+++	−	−
MV regurgitation	+++	++	−	−
LV systolic function	++	+++	−	−
LV diastolic function	+++	+	−	−
LV obstruction/quantification of gradient	+++	+	−	−
LA size	++	++	−	+
Apical aneurysm	++	+++	−	+
Perfusion abnormalities	−	++	+++	−
Fibrosis	−	+++	−	−
Screening	+++	++	−	−
Monitoring during septal reduction therapy	+++	−	−	−

LV left ventricular, *MV* mitral valve, *CMR* cardiac magnetic resonance, *PET* positron emission tomography, *CT* computed tomography

Conclusion

Various imaging techniques contribute to the general assessment of HCM. EAch of them has stength and weakness (Table 12.1) and a multiparametric evaluation is pivotal in this setting.

References

1. Lima JA, Desai MY (2004) Cardiovascular magnetic resonance imaging: current and emerging applications. J Am Coll Cardiol 44(6):1164–1171. doi:10.1016/j.jacc.2004.06.033
2. Reichek N, Gupta D (2008) Hypertrophic cardiomyopathy: cardiac magnetic resonance imaging changes the paradigm. J Am Coll Cardiol 52(7):567–568. doi:10.1016/j.jacc.2008.05.014
3. Moon JC, McKenna WJ (2009) The emerging role of cardiovascular magnetic resonance in refining the diagnosis of hypertrophic cardiomyopathy. Nat Clin Pract Cardiovasc Med 6(3):166–167. doi:10.1038/ncpcardio1442
4. Nagueh SF, Bierig SM, Budoff MJ, Desai M, Dilsizian V, Eidem B, Goldstein SA, Hung J, Maron MS, Ommen SR, Woo A (2011) American Society of Echocardiography clinical recommendations for multimodality cardiovascular imaging of patients with hypertrophic cardiomyopathy: Endorsed by the American Society of Nuclear Cardiology, Society for Cardiovascular Magnetic Resonance, and Society of Cardiovascular Computed Tomography. J Am Soc Echocardiogr 24(5):473–498. doi:10.1016/j.echo.2011.03.006
5. Kwon DH, Setser RM, Thamilarasan M, Popovic ZV, Smedira NG, Schoenhagen P, Garcia MJ, Lever HM, Desai MY (2008) Abnormal papillary muscle morphology is independently associated with increased left ventricular outflow tract obstruction in hypertrophic cardiomyopathy. Heart 94(10):1295–1301. doi:10.1136/hrt.2007.118018
6. Maron MS, Olivotto I, Harrigan C, Appelbaum E, Gibson CM, Lesser JR, Haas TS, Udelson JE, Manning WJ, Maron BJ (2011) Mitral valve abnormalities identified by cardiovascular magnetic resonance represent a primary phenotypic expression of hypertrophic cardiomyopathy. Circulation 124(1):40–47. doi:10.1161/CIRCULATIONAHA.110.985812
7. Harrigan CJ, Appelbaum E, Maron BJ, Buros JL, Gibson CM, Lesser JR, Udelson JE, Manning WJ, Maron MS (2008) Significance of papillary muscle abnormalities identified by cardiovascular magnetic resonance in hypertrophic cardiomyopathy. Am J Cardiol 101(5):668–673. doi:10.1016/j.amjcard.2007.10.032
8. Rickers C, Wilke NM, Jerosch-Herold M, Casey SA, Panse P, Panse N, Weil J, Zenovich AG, Maron BJ (2005) Utility of cardiac magnetic resonance imaging in the diagnosis of hypertrophic cardiomyopathy. Circulation 112(6):855–861. doi:10.1161/CIRCULATIONAHA.104.507723
9. Binder J, Ommen SR, Gersh BJ, Van Driest SL, Tajik AJ, Nishimura RA, Ackerman MJ (2006) Echocardiography-guided genetic testing in hypertrophic cardiomyopathy: septal morphological features predict the presence of myofilament mutations. Mayo Clin Proc 81(4):459–467. doi:10.4065/81.4.459
10. Bos JM, Theis JL, Tajik AJ, Gersh BJ, Ommen SR, Ackerman MJ (2008) Relationship between sex, shape, and substrate in hypertrophic cardiomyopathy. Am Heart J 155(6):1128–1134. doi:10.1016/j.ahj.2008.01.005
11. Holloway CJ, Betts TR, Neubauer S, Myerson SG (2010) Hypertrophic cardiomyopathy complicated by large apical aneurysm and thrombus, presenting as ventricular tachycardia. J Am Coll Cardiol 56(23):1961. doi:10.1016/j.jacc.2010.01.078
12. Armstrong AC, Gidding S, Gjesdal O, Wu C, Bluemke DA, Lima JA (2012) LV mass assessed by echocardiography and CMR, cardiovascular outcomes, and medical practice. JACC Cardiovasc Imaging 5(8):837–848. doi:10.1016/j.jcmg.2012.06.003

13. Olivotto I, Maron MS, Autore C, Lesser JR, Rega L, Casolo G, De Santis M, Quarta G, Nistri S, Cecchi F, Salton CJ, Udelson JE, Manning WJ, Maron BJ (2008) Assessment and significance of left ventricular mass by cardiovascular magnetic resonance in hypertrophic cardiomyopathy. J Am Coll Cardiol 52(7):559–566. doi:10.1016/j.jacc.2008.04.047

14. Maron MS, Hauser TH, Dubrow E, Horst TA, Kissinger KV, Udelson JE, Manning WJ (2007) Right ventricular involvement in hypertrophic cardiomyopathy. Am J Cardiol 100(8):1293–1298. doi:10.1016/j.amjcard.2007.05.061

15. Petersen SE, Jerosch-Herold M, Hudsmith LE, Robson MD, Francis JM, Doll HA, Selvanayagam JB, Neubauer S, Watkins H (2007) Evidence for microvascular dysfunction in hypertrophic cardiomyopathy: new insights from multiparametric magnetic resonance imaging. Circulation 115(18):2418–2425. doi:10.1161/CIRCULATIONAHA.106.657023

16. Germans T, Russel IK, Gotte MJ, Spreeuwenberg MD, Doevendans PA, Pinto YM, van der Geest RJ, van der Velden J, Wilde AA, van Rossum AC (2010) How do hypertrophic cardiomyopathy mutations affect myocardial function in carriers with normal wall thickness? Assessment with cardiovascular magnetic resonance. J Cardiovasc Magn Reson 12:13. doi:10.1186/1532-429X-12-13

17. Maron MS, Rowin EJ, Lin D, Appelbaum E, Chan RH, Gibson CM, Lesser JR, Lindberg J, Haas TS, Udelson JE, Manning WJ, Maron BJ (2012) Prevalence and clinical profile of myocardial crypts in hypertrophic cardiomyopathy. Circ Cardiovasc Imaging 5(4):441–447. doi:10.1161/CIRCIMAGING.112.972760

18. Woo A, Jedrzkiewicz S (2011) The mitral valve in hypertrophic cardiomyopathy: it's a long story. Circulation 124(1):9–12. doi:10.1161/CIRCULATIONAHA.111.035568

19. Valente AM, Lakdawala NK, Powell AJ, Evans SP, Cirino AL, Orav EJ, MacRae CA, Colan SD, Ho CY (2013) Comparison of echocardiographic and cardiac magnetic resonance imaging in hypertrophic cardiomyopathy sarcomere mutation carriers without left ventricular hypertrophy. Circ Cardiovasc Genet 6(3):230–237. doi:10.1161/CIRCGENETICS.113.000037

20. Choudhury L, Mahrholdt H, Wagner A, Choi KM, Elliott MD, Klocke FJ, Bonow RO, Judd RM, Kim RJ (2002) Myocardial scarring in asymptomatic or mildly symptomatic patients with hypertrophic cardiomyopathy. J Am Coll Cardiol 40(12):2156–2164

21. Moon JC, McKenna WJ, McCrohon JA, Elliott PM, Smith GC, Pennell DJ (2003) Toward clinical risk assessment in hypertrophic cardiomyopathy with gadolinium cardiovascular magnetic resonance. J Am Coll Cardiol 41(9):1561–1567

22. Adabag AS, Maron BJ, Appelbaum E, Harrigan CJ, Buros JL, Gibson CM, Lesser JR, Hanna CA, Udelson JE, Manning WJ, Maron MS (2008) Occurrence and frequency of arrhythmias in hypertrophic cardiomyopathy in relation to delayed enhancement on cardiovascular magnetic resonance. J Am Coll Cardiol 51(14):1369–1374. doi:10.1016/j.jacc.2007.11.071

23. Maron MS, Appelbaum E, Harrigan CJ, Buros J, Gibson CM, Hanna C, Lesser JR, Udelson JE, Manning WJ, Maron BJ (2008) Clinical profile and significance of delayed enhancement in hypertrophic cardiomyopathy. Circ Heart Fail 1(3):184–191. doi:10.1161/CIRCHEARTFAILURE.108.768119

24. Maron MS (2012) Clinical utility of cardiovascular magnetic resonance in hypertrophic cardiomyopathy. J Cardiovasc Magn Reson 14:13. doi:10.1186/1532-429X-14-13

25. Sado DM, White SK, Piechnik SK, Banypersad SM, Treibel T, Captur G, Fontana M, Maestrini V, Flett AS, Robson MD, Lachmann RH, Murphy E, Mehta A, Hughes D, Neubauer S, Elliott PM, Moon JC (2013) Identification and assessment of Anderson-Fabry disease by cardiovascular magnetic resonance noncontrast myocardial T1 mapping. Circ Cardiovasc Imaging 6(3):392–398. doi:10.1161/CIRCIMAGING.112.000070

26. Rowin EJ, Maron MS, Lesser JR, Maron BJ (2012) CMR with late gadolinium enhancement in genotype positive-phenotype negative hypertrophic cardiomyopathy. JACC Cardiovasc Imaging 5(1):119–122. doi:10.1016/j.jcmg.2011.08.020

27. Strijack B, Ariyarajah V, Soni R, Jassal DS, Greenberg CR, McGregor R, Morris A (2008) Late gadolinium enhancement cardiovascular magnetic resonance in genotyped hypertrophic cardiomyopathy with normal phenotype. J Cardiovasc Magn Reson 10:58. doi:10.1186/1532-429X-10-58

28. Funabashi N, Takaoka H, Horie S, Ozawa K, Daimon M, Takahashi M, Yajima R, Saito M, Fujiwara K, Tani A, Kamata T, Uehara M, Kataoka A, Kobayashi Y (2013) Regional peak longitudinal-strain by 2D speckle-tracking TTE provides useful information to distinguish fibrotic from non-fibrotic lesions in LV myocardium on cardiac MR in hypertrophic cardiomyopathy. Int J Cardiol 168(4):4520–4523. doi:10.1016/j.ijcard.2013.06.105
29. Sugihara H, Taniguchi Y, Ohtsuki K, Umamoto I, Nakazawa T, Shima T, Nakamura T, Azuma A, Kohno Y, Nakagawa M (1993) Assessment of myocardial perfusion abnormalities in patients with apical hypertrophic cardiomyopathy using exercise 201Tl scintigraphy. Kokyu To Junkan 41(11):1089–1093
30. Taniguchi Y, Sugihara H, Ohtsuki K, Umamoto I, Nakagawa T, Shiga K, Nakamura T, Azuma A, Kohno Y, Nakagawa M et al (1994) Effect of verapamil on myocardial ischemia in patients with hypertrophic cardiomyopathy: evaluation by exercise thallium-201 SPECT. J Cardiol 24(1):45–51
31. Dilsizian V, Bonow RO, Epstein SE, Fananapazir L (1993) Myocardial ischemia detected by thallium scintigraphy is frequently related to cardiac arrest and syncope in young patients with hypertrophic cardiomyopathy. J Am Coll Cardiol 22(3):796–804
32. Sorajja P, Chareonthaitawee P, Ommen SR, Miller TD, Hodge DO, Gibbons RJ (2006) Prognostic utility of single-photon emission computed tomography in adult patients with hypertrophic cardiomyopathy. Am Heart J 151(2):426–435. doi:10.1016/j.ahj.2005.02.050
33. Kaimoto S, Kawasaki T, Kuribayashi T, Yamano M, Miki S, Kamitani T, Matsubara H (2012) Myocardial perfusion abnormality in the area of ventricular septum-free wall junction and cardiovascular events in nonobstructive hypertrophic cardiomyopathy. Int J Cardiovasc Imaging 28(7):1829–1839. doi:10.1007/s10554-011-9994-z
34. Lee KH, Jang HJ, Lee SC, Kim YH, Lee EJ, Seo JD, Kim BT (2003) Myocardial thallium defects in apical hypertrophic cardiomyopathy are associated with a benign prognosis. Thallium defects in apical hypertrophy. Int J Cardiovasc Imaging 19(5):381–388
35. Yamanari H, Kakishita M, Fujimoto Y, Hashimoto K, Kiyooka T, Katayama Y, Otsuka F, Emori T, Uchida S, Ohe T (1997) Effect of regional myocardial perfusion abnormalities on regional myocardial early diastolic function in patients with hypertrophic cardiomyopathy. Heart Vessels 12(4):192–198
36. Yamada M, Elliott PM, Kaski JC, Prasad K, Gane JN, Lowe CM, Doi Y, McKenna WJ (1998) Dipyridamole stress thallium-201 perfusion abnormalities in patients with hypertrophic cardiomyopathy. Relationship to clinical presentation and outcome. Eur Heart J 19(3):500–507
37. Takata J, Counihan PJ, Gane JN, Doi Y, Chikamori T, Ozawa T, McKenna WJ (1993) Regional thallium-201 washout and myocardial hypertrophy in hypertrophic cardiomyopathy and its relation to exertional chest pain. Am J Cardiol 72(2):211–217
38. Cannon RO 3rd, Dilsizian V, O'Gara PT, Udelson JE, Tucker E, Panza JA, Fananapazir L, McIntosh CL, Wallace RB, Bonow RO (1992) Impact of surgical relief of outflow obstruction on thallium perfusion abnormalities in hypertrophic cardiomyopathy. Circulation 85(3):1039–1045
39. Lerch H, Schafers M, Gietzen F, Schafers K, Kuwert T, Kuhn H, Schober O (1997) Myocardial perfusion and metabolism after transcoronary ablation of septum hypertrophy (TASH) in hypertrophic obstructive cardiomyopathy. Nuklearmedizin 36(6):218–222
40. Ishida Y, Nagata S, Uehara T, Yasumura Y, Fukuchi K, Miyatake K (2001) Clinical analysis of myocardial perfusion and metabolism in patients with hypertrophic cardiomyopathy by single photon emission tomography and positron emission tomography. J Cardiol 37(Suppl 1):121–128
41. Ito Y, Hasegawa S, Yamaguchi H, Yoshioka J, Uehara T, Nishimura T (2000) Relation between thallium-201/iodine 123-BMIPP subtraction and fluorine 18 deoxyglucose polar maps in patients with hypertrophic cardiomyopathy. J Nucl Cardiol 7(1):16–22. doi:10.1067/mnc.2000.99188
42. Shimonagata T, Nishimura T, Uehara T, Hayashida K, Kumita S, Ohno A, Nagata S, Miyatake K (1993) Discrepancies between myocardial perfusion and free fatty acid metabolism in patients with hypertrophic cardiomyopathy. Nucl Med Commun 14(11):1005–1013

43. Tadamura E, Kudoh T, Hattori N, Inubushi M, Magata Y, Konishi J, Matsumori A, Nohara R, Sasayama S, Yoshibayashi M, Tamaki N (1998) Impairment of BMIPP uptake precedes abnormalities in oxygen and glucose metabolism in hypertrophic cardiomyopathy. J Nucl Med 39(3):390–396

44. Nakajima K, Bunko H, Taki J, Shimizu M, Muramori A, Hisada K (1990) Quantitative analysis of 123I-meta-iodobenzylguanidine (MIBG) uptake in hypertrophic cardiomyopathy. Am Heart J 119(6):1329–1337

45. Shimizu M, Sugihara N, Kita Y, Shimizu K, Horita Y, Nakajima K, Taki J, Takeda R (1992) Long-term course and cardiac sympathetic nerve activity in patients with hypertrophic cardiomyopathy. Br Heart J 67(2):155–160

46. Zhao C, Shuke N, Yamamoto W, Okizaki A, Sato J, Ishikawa Y, Ohta T, Hasebe N, Kikuchi K, Aburano T (2001) Comparison of cardiac sympathetic nervous function with left ventricular function and perfusion in cardiomyopathies by (123)I-MIBG SPECT and (99 m)Tc-tetrofosmin electrocardiographically gated SPECT. J Nucl Med 42(7):1017–1024

47. Terai H, Shimizu M, Ino H, Yamaguchi M, Hayashi K, Sakata K, Kiyama M, Hayashi T, Inoue M, Taki J, Mabuchi H (2003) Cardiac sympathetic nerve activity in patients with hypertrophic cardiomyopathy with malignant ventricular tachyarrhythmias. J Nucl Cardiol 10(3):304–310

48. Grover-McKay M, Schwaiger M, Krivokapich J, Perloff JK, Phelps ME, Schelbert HR (1989) Regional myocardial blood flow and metabolism at rest in mildly symptomatic patients with hypertrophic cardiomyopathy. J Am Coll Cardiol 13(2):317–324

49. Ishiwata S, Maruno H, Senda M, Toyama H, Nishiyama S, Seki A (1997) Myocardial blood flow and metabolism in patients with hypertrophic cardiomyopathy–a study with carbon-11 acetate and positron emission tomography. Jpn Circ J 61(3):201–210

50. Perrone-Filardi P, Bacharach SL, Dilsizian V, Panza JA, Maurea S, Bonow RO (1993) Regional systolic function, myocardial blood flow and glucose uptake at rest in hypertrophic cardiomyopathy. Am J Cardiol 72(2):199–204

51. Kagaya Y, Ishide N, Takeyama D, Kanno Y, Yamane Y, Shirato K, Maruyama Y, Itoh M, Ido T, Matsuzawa T et al (1992) Differences in myocardial fluoro-18 2-deoxyglucose uptake in young versus older patients with hypertrophic cardiomyopathy. Am J Cardiol 69(3):242–246

52. Camici P, Chiriatti G, Lorenzoni R, Bellina RC, Gistri R, Italiani G, Parodi O, Salvadori PA, Nista N, Papi L et al (1991) Coronary vasodilation is impaired in both hypertrophied and non-hypertrophied myocardium of patients with hypertrophic cardiomyopathy: a study with nitrogen-13 ammonia and positron emission tomography. J Am Coll Cardiol 17(4):879–886

53. Lorenzoni R, Gistri R, Cecchi F, Olivotto I, Chiriatti G, Elliott P, McKenna WJ, Camici PG (1998) Coronary vasodilator reserve is impaired in patients with hypertrophic cardiomyopathy and left ventricular dysfunction. Am Heart J 136(6):972–981

54. Cecchi F, Olivotto I, Gistri R, Lorenzoni R, Chiriatti G, Camici PG (2003) Coronary microvascular dysfunction and prognosis in hypertrophic cardiomyopathy. N Engl J Med 349(11):1027–1035. doi:10.1056/NEJMoa025050

55. Choudhury L, Rosen SD, Patel D, Nihoyannopoulos P, Camici PG (1997) Coronary vasodilator reserve in primary and secondary left ventricular hypertrophy. A study with positron emission tomography. Eur Heart J 18(1):108–116

56. Olivotto I, Cecchi F, Gistri R, Lorenzoni R, Chiriatti G, Girolami F, Torricelli F, Camici PG (2006) Relevance of coronary microvascular flow impairment to long-term remodeling and systolic dysfunction in hypertrophic cardiomyopathy. J Am Coll Cardiol 47(5):1043–1048. doi:10.1016/j.jacc.2005.10.050

57. Knaapen P, van Dockum WG, Gotte MJ, Broeze KA, Kuijer JP, Zwanenburg JJ, Marcus JT, Kok WE, van Rossum AC, Lammertsma AA, Visser FC (2006) Regional heterogeneity of resting perfusion in hypertrophic cardiomyopathy is related to delayed contrast enhancement but not to systolic function: a PET and MRI study. J Nucl Cardiol 13(5):660–667. doi:10.1016/j.nuclcard.2006.05.018

58. Bravo PE, Zimmerman SL, Luo HC, Pozios I, Rajaram M, Pinheiro A, Steenbergen C, Kamel IR, Wahl RL, Bluemke DA, Bengel FM, Abraham MR, Abraham TP (2013) Relationship of

delayed enhancement by magnetic resonance to myocardial perfusion by positron emission tomography in hypertrophic cardiomyopathy. Circ Cardiovasc Imaging 6(2):210–217. doi:10.1161/CIRCIMAGING.112.000110

59. Lefroy DC, de Silva R, Choudhury L, Uren NG, Crake T, Rhodes CG, Lammertsma AA, Boyd H, Patsalos PN, Nihoyannopoulos P et al (1993) Diffuse reduction of myocardial beta-adrenoceptors in hypertrophic cardiomyopathy: a study with positron emission tomography. J Am Coll Cardiol 22(6):1653–1660

60. Schafers M, Dutka D, Rhodes CG, Lammertsma AA, Hermansen F, Schober O, Camici PG (1998) Myocardial presynaptic and postsynaptic autonomic dysfunction in hypertrophic cardiomyopathy. Circ Res 82(1):57–62

61. Choudhury L, Guzzetti S, Lefroy DC, Nihoyannopoulos P, McKenna WJ, Oakley CM, Camici PG (1996) Myocardial beta adrenoceptors and left ventricular function in hypertrophic cardiomyopathy. Heart 75(1):50–54

62. Orakzai SH, Orakzai RH, Nasir K, Budoff MJ (2006) Assessment of cardiac function using multidetector row computed tomography. J Comput Assist Tomogr 30(4):555–563

63. Dewey M, Muller M, Eddicks S, Schnapauff D, Teige F, Rutsch W, Borges AC, Hamm B (2006) Evaluation of global and regional left ventricular function with 16-slice computed tomography, biplane cineventriculography, and two-dimensional transthoracic echocardiography: comparison with magnetic resonance imaging. J Am Coll Cardiol 48(10):2034–2044. doi:10.1016/j.jacc.2006.04.104

64. Mangalat D, Kalogeropoulos A, Georgiopoulou V, Stillman A, Butler J (2009) Value of cardiac CT in patients with heart failure. Curr Cardiovasc Imaging Rep 2(6):410–417. doi:10.1007/s12410-009-0052-3

65. Mao S, Budoff MJ, Oudiz RJ, Bakhsheshi H, Wang S, Brundage BH (1999) Effect of exercise on left and right ventricular ejection fraction and wall motion. Int J Cardiol 71(1):23–31

Hypertrophic Cardiomyopathy: Usefulness of Imaging in Prognostic Stratification and Choice of Treatment

13

Gherardo Finocchiaro, Bruno Pinamonti, Elena Abate, Marco Merlo, and Giancarlo Vitrella

13.1 Introduction

In hypertrophic cardiomyopathy (HCM), as in the other cardiomyopathies (CMP), cardiac imaging is not only a main diagnostic tool but offers important prognostic information. It is well known that HCM is a polymorphic disease with a variable natural history. Some patients remain stable over long periods, but a variable number of cases take a progressive evolution toward end-stage disease with refractory heart failure (HF) or sudden death (SD) [1]. A thorough assessment of structural and functional features identifies several risk factors by which the clinician can discriminate severe disease from a more benign condition. O'Mahony et al. [2] described a prognostic model for sudden SD from a large cohort of HCM patients ($n=3,675$). Several factors deriving from imaging assessment [maximal left ventricular (LV) wall thickness, left atrial (LA) diameter, left ventricular (LV) outflow tract (OT) gradient] were predictive of outcome (Table 13.1).

13.2 Left Ventricular Hypertrophy

Being that LV hypertrophy a hallmark of HCM, the degree of LV wall thickness has been tested in several studies as a possible risk factor for adverse outcome. In a large patient population, Spirito et al. [3] demonstrated that the magnitude of hypertrophy is directly related to the risk of SD and is a strong and independent predictor of prognosis. Young patients with extreme hypertrophy (end-diastolic wall thickness $\geq$30 mm) assessed at M-mode and 2D echocardiography, even those with few or no

G. Finocchiaro (✉) • B. Pinamonti, MD • E. Abate • M. Merlo • G. Vitrella
Department of Cardiology, University Hospital of Trieste,
Via P. Valdoni 7, Trieste 34139, Italy
e-mail: gherardobis@yahoo.it; bruno.pinamonti@gmail.com; abate.elena@gmail.com;
supermerloo@libero.it; giancarlo.vitrella@gmail.com

B. Pinamonti, G. Sinagra (eds.), *Clinical Echocardiography and Other Imaging Techniques in Cardiomyopathies*, DOI 10.1007/978-3-319-06019-4_13,
© Springer International Publishing Switzerland 2014

Table 13.1 Risk factors and potential arbitrators for sudden death (SD) in hypertrophic cardio-myopathy (HCM)

Secondary prevention	Primary prevention	Potential arbitrators
Cardiac arrest/sustained VT	Family history of SD	LV apical aneurysms
	Syncope	End-stage phase
	Massive LVH >30 mm	LGE
	NS VT at Holter	LV obstruction
	Abnormal exercise BP response	

VT ventricular tachycardia, *LVH* left ventricular hypertrophy, *NS VT* nonsustained ventricular tachycardia, *LGE* late gadolinium enhancement

symptoms, appeared to be at substantially increased long-term risk, deserving consideration for interventions to prevent SD. Elliott et al. [4] found that patients with LV wall thickness $\geq$30 mm had a higher probability of SD or implanted cardiac defibrillator (ICD) discharge than other HCM patients; however, when considered together, the number of additional risk factors (one to three) was a better predictor of risk than wall thickness alone.

In conclusion, and according to the most recent guidelines [5], severe LV hypertrophy is one of the main factors to be considered for ICD implantation for primary prevention of SD.

13.3 Diastolic Dysfunction

Various degrees of diastolic dysfunction are common in HCM. If severe, it is a marker of adverse outcome. In particular, restrictive filling pattern (RFP) is quite uncommon in HCM, but its evaluation adds prognostic power to the stratification of the patients, as demonstrated by our group [6]. Furthermore, Biagini et al. [7] demonstrated that RFP is a hallmark of severe phenotype, being a strong predictor of SD and progression to end-stage hypokinetic evolution of the disease. In this setting, tissue Doppler imaging (TDI) plays a role—especially in asymptomatic or mildly symptomatic patients—in predicting cardiovascular events. In particular, E wave to E' ratio (E/E') was demonstrated as an independent predictor of adverse outcome [8].

The prognostic role of right ventricular (RV) diastolic function was analyzed in patients with HCM by Pagourelias et al. [9]. Patients presenting with increased RV E/E' ratio (ratio of tricuspid in flow E wave to E' wave obtained by TDI at the lateral tricuspid annulus) had a 1.6-times greater risk for HF mortality, whereas patients with shortened tricuspid E wave deceleration time had a 1.1 greater risk for SD.

13.4 Left Atrial Size

LA size is associated with an adverse prognosis in various cardiovascular diseases [10]. In HCM, LA enlargement is common, is associated with several adverse pathophysiologic consequences such as LV OT obstruction, and is predictive of atrial fibrillation (AF), which is a major predictor of adverse outcome [11]. Nistri et al., using data from an Italian multicentric registry, demonstrated on a large population of patients with HCM ($n = 1{,}491$) that LA dimension is an independent marker of prognosis, particularly relevant in identifying patients at risk for HF-related death [12]. These results were confirmed by studies that considered the independent role of LA diameter in predicting death in the very-long-term follow-up [13].

13.5 Left Ventricular Obstruction

Another feature that frequently affects HCM patients is LV obstruction [14]. As demonstrated by Maron et al. [15] in a population of 1,101 HCM patients, LV OT obstruction is a major risk factor for death related to HCM, stroke, or HF and progression to New York Heart Association (NYHA) class III or IV. The role of LV obstruction in predicting SD is more heatedly debated. Elliott and coworkers [16] reported that it was associated with an increased risk of SD/ICD discharge that was related to obstruction severity and the presence of other recognized risk factors. Conversely, Efthimiadis et al. [17] found that LV OT obstruction did not emerge as an independent predictor of SD. Obstacles to outflow obstruction as a primary risk factor include its dynamic nature, and the high frequency of obstruction encountered in the HCM patient population [15].

13.6 Evolution During Follow-up

HCM can have a highly variable course. Whereas the majority of patients remain stable during the follow-up, some experience adverse LV remodeling with progressive reduction of systolic function (end-stage disease) [18]. In this setting cardiac imaging is pivotal for monitoring during follow-up. As shown by our group [19], of 101 patients affected by HCM and with long-term follow-up, the number of patients who evolve toward systolic or diastolic dysfunction is not negligible (28 and 16 %, respectively). Taking follow-up evaluation into consideration adds accuracy to the general prognostic assessment of the disease.

The outcome of HCM patients in end-stage disease is particularly severe, not only due to high rates of HF-related complications and mortality but because of a considerable incidence of SD [20]. Consequently, accurate and prompt diagnosis of this condition is important and can affect the general therapeutic management (possible indications to ICD, cardiac resynchronization therapy (CRT), heart transplantation).

13.7 Late Gadolinium Enhancement

Cardiac magnetic resonance (CMR) may add important information to the prognostic assessment of HCM patients. In particular, fibrosis, as assessed by late gadolinium enhancement (LGE), is hypothesized to be related to SD. Recent cross-sectional studies demonstrated a strong association between LGE and ventricular tachyarrhythmias on ambulatory Holter electrocardiography (ECG) [21–23]. Adabag et al. [24] found that LGE was an independent risk factor for ventricular arrhythmias and conferred a 7.3-fold [95 % confidence interval (CI) 2.6–20.4; $p < 0.0001$] increased relative risk (RR) of nonsustained ventricular tachycardia (VT), a potential risk factor for SD in HCM. O'Hanlon et al. [21] examined the significance of fibrosis detected by LGE-CMR for predicting major clinical events. Cox proportional hazards modeling revealed the amount of fibrosis to be a significant independent predictor of the primary composite endpoint (cardiovascular death, unplanned cardiovascular hospitalization, sustained VT, ventricular fibrillation, appropriate ICD discharge). Todiere et al. [25] analyzed a cohort of 55 HCM patients with two CMR at an interval of 719 ± 410 days, focusing on LGE progression rate during follow-up. The majority of patients showed a progressive increase in LGE over time, and patients with worsened NYHA functional class presented higher a LGE increase.

Whereas LGE has been identified as a marker of adverse prognosis [22], to date, there is a lack of robust evidence about its role as a predictor of SD in HCM. As a result, recommendations for primary prevention ICDs should not be based solely on the presence of LGE in individual patients. In the most recent HCM guidelines, LGE is classified as an arbitrator, useful in SD prognostic stratification in cases in which the indication for ICD implantation is not clear from conventional risk factors. Another point of discussion regards the extent and site of LGE and the relationship with clinical outcome. In fact, the majority of follow-up studies considered only the presence of LGE rather than its characteristics.

13.8   Microvascular Dysfunction

Microvascular dysfunction is a common feature of HCM, and positron emission tomography (PET) is a reliable method by which to assess it [26]. Cecchi et al. [27], in a PET study of 51 HCM patients, demonstrated that the degree of microvascular dysfunction, assessed using myocardial blood flow values after dipyridamole infusion, is a strong, independent predictor of clinical deterioration and death. Moreover, Olivotto et al. [28] reported severe microvascular dysfunction as being a potent long-term predictor of adverse LV remodeling and systolic dysfunction in HCM, which is thus is a potential target for preventing disease progression and HF in HCM.

References

1. Maron BJ, Maron MS (2013) Hypertrophic cardiomyopathy. Lancet 381(9862):242–255. doi:10.1016/S0140-6736(12)60397-3
2. O'Mahony C, Jichi F, Pavlou M, Monserrat L, Anastasakis A, Rapezzi C, Biagini E, Gimeno JR, Limongelli G, McKenna WJ, Omar RZ, Elliott PM (2013) A novel clinical risk prediction

model for sudden cardiac death in hypertrophic cardiomyopathy (HCM Risk-SCD). Eur Heart J. doi:10.1093/eurheartj/eht439

3. Spirito P, Bellone P, Harris KM, Bernabo P, Bruzzi P, Maron BJ (2000) Magnitude of left ventricular hypertrophy and risk of sudden death in hypertrophic cardiomyopathy. N Engl J Med 342(24):1778–1785. doi:10.1056/NEJM200006153422403

4. Elliott PM, Gimeno Blanes JR, Mahon NG, Poloniecki JD, McKenna WJ (2001) Relation between severity of left-ventricular hypertrophy and prognosis in patients with hypertrophic cardiomyopathy. Lancet 357(9254):420–424. doi:10.1016/S0140-6736(00)04005-8

5. Gersh BJ, Maron BJ, Bonow RO, Dearani JA, Fifer MA, Link MS, Naidu SS, Nishimura RA, Ommen SR, Rakowski H, Seidman CE, Towbin JA, Udelson JE, Yancy CW (2011) 2011 ACCF/AHA Guideline for the Diagnosis and Treatment of Hypertrophic Cardiomyopathy: a report of the American College of Cardiology Foundation/American Heart Association Task Force on Practice Guidelines. Developed in collaboration with the American Association for Thoracic Surgery, American Society of Echocardiography, American Society of Nuclear Cardiology, Heart Failure Society of America, Heart Rhythm Society, Society for Cardiovascular Angiography and Interventions, and Society of Thoracic Surgeons. J Am Coll Cardiol 58(25):e212–e260. doi:10.1016/j.jacc.2011.06.011

6. Pinamonti B, Di Lenarda A, Nucifora G, Gregori D, Perkan A, Sinagra G (2008) Incremental prognostic value of restrictive filling pattern in hypertrophic cardiomyopathy: a Doppler echocardiographic study. Eur J Echocardiogr 9(4):466–471. doi:10.1016/j.euje.2007.06.008

7. Biagini E, Spirito P, Rocchi G, Ferlito M, Rosmini S, Lai F, Lorenzini M, Terzi F, Bacchi-Reggiani L, Boriani G, Branzi A, Boni L, Rapezzi C (2009) Prognostic implications of the Doppler restrictive filling pattern in hypertrophic cardiomyopathy. Am J Cardiol 104(12):1727–1731. doi:10.1016/j.amjcard.2009.07.057

8. Kitaoka H, Kubo T, Hayashi K, Yamasaki N, Matsumura Y, Furuno T, Doi YL (2013) Tissue Doppler imaging and prognosis in asymptomatic or mildly symptomatic patients with hypertrophic cardiomyopathy. Eur Heart J Cardiovasc Imaging 14(6):544–549. doi:10.1093/ehjci/jes200

9. Pagourelias ED, Efthimiadis GK, Parcharidou DG, Gossios TD, Kamperidis V, Karoulas T, Karvounis H, Styliadis IH (2011) Prognostic value of right ventricular diastolic function indices in hypertrophic cardiomyopathy. Eur J Echocardiogr 12(11):809–817. doi:10.1093/ejechocard/jer126

10. Lonborg JT, Engstrom T, Moller JE, Ahtarovski KA, Kelbaek H, Holmvang L, Jorgensen E, Helqvist S, Saunamaki K, Soholm H, Andersen M, Mathiasen AB, Kuhl JT, Clemmensen P, Kober L, Vejlstrup N (2013) Left atrial volume and function in patients following ST elevation myocardial infarction and the association with clinical outcome: a cardiovascular magnetic resonance study. Eur Heart J Cardiovasc Imaging 14(2):118–127. doi:10.1093/ehjci/jes118

11. Olivotto I, Cecchi F, Casey SA, Dolara A, Traverse JH, Maron BJ (2001) Impact of atrial fibrillation on the clinical course of hypertrophic cardiomyopathy. Circulation 104(21):2517–2524

12. Nistri S, Olivotto I, Betocchi S, Losi MA, Valsecchi G, Pinamonti B, Conte MR, Casazza F, Galderisi M, Maron BJ, Cecchi F (2006) Prognostic significance of left atrial size in patients with hypertrophic cardiomyopathy (from the Italian Registry for Hypertrophic Cardiomyopathy). Am J Cardiol 98(7):960–965. doi:10.1016/j.amjcard.2006.05.013

13. Finocchiaro G, Pinamonti B, Merlo M, Brun F, Barbati G, Sinagra G (2012) Prognostic role of clinical presentation in symptomatic patients with hypertrophic cardiomyopathy. J Cardiovasc Med (Hagerstown) 13(12):810–818. doi:10.2459/JCM.0b013e328356a231

14. Maron MS, Olivotto I, Zenovich AG, Link MS, Pandian NG, Kuvin JT, Nistri S, Cecchi F, Udelson JE, Maron BJ (2006) Hypertrophic cardiomyopathy is predominantly a disease of left ventricular outflow tract obstruction. Circulation 114(21):2232–2239. doi:10.1161/CIRCULATIONAHA.106.644682

15. Maron MS, Olivotto I, Betocchi S, Casey SA, Lesser JR, Losi MA, Cecchi F, Maron BJ (2003) Effect of left ventricular outflow tract obstruction on clinical outcome in hypertrophic cardiomyopathy. N Engl J Med 348(4):295–303. doi:10.1056/NEJMoa021332

16. Elliott PM, Gimeno JR, Tome MT, Shah J, Ward D, Thaman R, Mogensen J, McKenna WJ (2006) Left ventricular outflow tract obstruction and sudden death risk in patients with hypertrophic cardiomyopathy. Eur Heart J 27(16):1933–1941. doi:10.1093/eurheartj/ehl041

17. Efthimiadis GK, Parcharidou DG, Giannakoulas G, Pagourelias ED, Charalampidis P, Savvopoulos G, Ziakas A, Karvounis H, Styliadis IH, Parcharidis GE (2009) Left ventricular outflow tract obstruction as a risk factor for sudden cardiac death in hypertrophic cardiomyopathy. Am J Cardiol 104(5):695–699. doi:10.1016/j.amjcard.2009.04.039

18. Olivotto I, Cecchi F, Poggesi C, Yacoub MH (2012) Patterns of disease progression in hypertrophic cardiomyopathy: an individualized approach to clinical staging. Circ Heart Fail 5(4):535–546. doi:10.1161/CIRCHEARTFAILURE.112.967026

19. Pinamonti B, Merlo M, Nangah R, Korcova R, Di Lenarda A, Barbati G, Sinagra G (2010) The progression of left ventricular systolic and diastolic dysfunctions in hypertrophic cardiomyopathy: clinical and prognostic significance. J Cardiovasc Med (Hagerstown) 11(9):669–677. doi:10.2459/JCM.0b013e3283383355

20. Yacoub MH, Olivotto I, Cecchi F (2007) 'End-stage' hypertrophic cardiomyopathy: from mystery to model. Nat Clin Pract Cardiovasc Med 4(5):232–233. doi:10.1038/ncpcardio0859

21. O'Hanlon R, Grasso A, Roughton M, Moon JC, Clark S, Wage R, Webb J, Kulkarni M, Dawson D, Sulaibeekh L, Chandrasekaran B, Bucciarelli-Ducci C, Pasquale F, Cowie MR, McKenna WJ, Sheppard MN, Elliott PM, Pennell DJ, Prasad SK (2010) Prognostic significance of myocardial fibrosis in hypertrophic cardiomyopathy. J Am Coll Cardiol 56(11):867–874. doi:10.1016/j.jacc.2010.05.010

22. Green JJ, Berger JS, Kramer CM, Salerno M (2012) Prognostic value of late gadolinium enhancement in clinical outcomes for hypertrophic cardiomyopathy. JACC Cardiovasc Imaging 5(4):370–377. doi:10.1016/j.jcmg.2011.11.021

23. Alla VM, Koneru S, Hunter C, Mooss A (2012) LGE and the risk of sudden death in HCM. JACC Cardiovasc Imaging 5(7):761–762; author reply 762–763. doi:10.1016/j.jcmg.2012.05.004

24. Adabag AS, Maron BJ, Appelbaum E, Harrigan CJ, Buros JL, Gibson CM, Lesser JR, Hanna CA, Udelson JE, Manning WJ, Maron MS (2008) Occurrence and frequency of arrhythmias in hypertrophic cardiomyopathy in relation to delayed enhancement on cardiovascular magnetic resonance. J Am Coll Cardiol 51(14):1369–1374. doi:10.1016/j.jacc.2007.11.071

25. Todiere G, Aquaro GD, Piaggi P, Formisano F, Barison A, Masci PG, Strata E, Bacigalupo L, Marzilli M, Pingitore A, Lombardi M (2012) Progression of myocardial fibrosis assessed with cardiac magnetic resonance in hypertrophic cardiomyopathy. J Am Coll Cardiol 60(10):922–929. doi:10.1016/j.jacc.2012.03.076

26. Olivotto I, Girolami F, Sciagra R, Ackerman MJ, Sotgia B, Bos JM, Nistri S, Sgalambro A, Grifoni C, Torricelli F, Camici PG, Cecchi F (2011) Microvascular function is selectively impaired in patients with hypertrophic cardiomyopathy and sarcomere myofilament gene mutations. J Am Coll Cardiol 58(8):839–848. doi:10.1016/j.jacc.2011.05.018

27. Camici P, Chiriatti G, Lorenzoni R, Bellina RC, Gistri R, Italiani G, Parodi O, Salvadori PA, Nista N, Papi L et al (1991) Coronary vasodilation is impaired in both hypertrophied and non-hypertrophied myocardium of patients with hypertrophic cardiomyopathy: a study with nitrogen-13 ammonia and positron emission tomography. J Am Coll Cardiol 17(4):879–886

28. Olivotto I, Cecchi F, Gistri R, Lorenzoni R, Chiriatti G, Girolami F, Torricelli F, Camici PG (2006) Relevance of coronary microvascular flow impairment to long-term remodeling and systolic dysfunction in hypertrophic cardiomyopathy. J Am Coll Cardiol 47(5):1043–1048. doi:10.1016/j.jacc.2005.10.050

Part IV

Arrhythmogenic Right Ventricular Cardiomyopathy

Arrhythmogenic Right Ventricular Cardiomyopathy: Clinical Assessment and Differential Diagnosis

14

Francesca Brun, Concetta Di Nora, Marco Merlo, Alberto Pivetta, Luisa Mestroni, and Gianfranco Sinagra

14.1 Introduction

Arrhythmogenic right ventricular cardiomyopathy (ARVC) is an inherited cardiovascular disorder characterized by myocyte loss and fibrofatty tissue replacement leading to life-threatening ventricular arrhythmias, progressive ventricular dysfunction of the right (RV) and left ventricle (LV), and heart failure (HF) [1, 2]. The estimated prevalence of ARVC in the general population ranges from 1:2,000 to 1:5,000 individuals; men are more frequently affected than women, with an approximate ratio of 3:1 [3]. A familial history of ARVC is present in 30–50 % of cases, and the disease is usually inherited in an autosomal dominant pattern, with variable penetrance and expressivity, although autosomal recessive forms are also reported (Naxos disease and Carvajal syndrome). ARVC is considered to be a disease of myocyte adhesion caused by defects at the intercellular junctions. Cardiac myocyte-to-myocyte adhesion is maintained by desmosomes, adherens junctions, and gap junctions, which together comprise the intercalated disc.

Electronic supplementary material The online version of this chapter (doi: 10.1007/978-3-319-06019-4_14) contains supplementary material, which is available to authorized users. Videos can also be accessed at http://www.springerimages.com/videos/978-3-319-06018-7.

F. Brun (✉) • C. Di Nora • M. Merlo • A. Pivetta • G. Sinagra, MD, FESC
Department of Cardiology, University Hospital of Trieste,
via P. Valdoni 7, Trieste 34139, Italy
e-mail: frabrun77@gmail.com; concetta.dinora@gmail.com; supermerloo@libero.it; pivetta.alberto@gmail.com; gianfranco.sinagra@aots.sanita.fvg.it

L. Mestroni, MD, FACC, FESC
Department of Molecular Genetics, Cardiovascular Institute, University of Colorado Denver Anschutz Medical Campus, 12700 E. 19th Ave, F442, Aurora, Colorado 80045-2507, USA
e-mail: luisa.mestroni@ucdenver.edu

B. Pinamonti, G. Sinagra (eds.), *Clinical Echocardiography and Other Imaging Techniques in Cardiomyopathies*, DOI 10.1007/978-3-319-06019-4_14,
© Springer International Publishing Switzerland 2014

A genetic defect can be confirmed in approximately 40 % of cases, and 12 different ARVC loci have been reported, among which five genes (*DSP, PKP2, DSG2, DSC2,* and *JUP*) encode proteins of cell–cell junctions at the intercalated disc. The role of the other three nondesmosomal genes is well established: transforming growth factor beta-3 (*TGF-β3*), the ion-channel subunit *RYR2*, and the transmembrane protein 43 (*TMEM43*) [4]. Novel variants in the giant sarcomeric protein titin (*TTN*) are also associated with ARVC [5]. Structural impairment of titin, which probably leads to proteolysis and apoptosis, constitutes to be a novel mechanism underlying myocardial remodeling and sudden death (SD).

14.2 Clinical Features

ARVC onset usually occurs after childhood, with palpitations and/or syncope. In some cases, severe ventricular arrhythmias are the first presentation of the disease and lead to SD. Since 1995, a recessive form of ARVC has been recognized with a distinct phenotypic expression and cardiocutaneous aspects characterized by palmoplantar keratoderma and woolly hair, well known as Naxos disease. Furthermore, ARVC is the second most frequent cause of SD in young adults and athletes, and cardiac arrest may occur in up to 50 % of index cases [6]. According to Dalal et al. [7], the median age at onset is 29 years. It is rare to manifest clinical signs or symptoms of ARVC before the age of 12 years or after the age of 60 years.

According to the Padua group [8], the natural history of ARVC may be separated into four distinct phases, with progressive development of symptoms and structural abnormalities:

1. Concealed phase: This phase is characterized by minor arrhythmias that usually go unnoticed and subtle or absent structural RV abnormalities. The diagnosis is usually made during family screening in asymptomatic individuals. SD may be the first and unique manifestation of the disease at this initial stage.
2. Overt electrical disorder with palpitations, syncope, and ventricular arrhythmias of RV origin: This manifestation is usually triggered by effort. Arrhythmias range from isolated premature ventricular beats to nonsustained ventricular tachycardia with left bundle-branch block (LBBB) morphology up to ventricular fibrillation leading to cardiac arrest.
3. RV failure due to progressive myocardial fibrofatty replacement: This manifestation leads to RV enlargement and systolic dysfunction with consequent HF.
4. Biventricular failure, which usually develops late in the natural history of the disease: Progressive structural abnormalities involve the LV, with symptoms of overt congestive HF. In such conditions, contractile dysfunction may be so severe as to require cardiac transplantation. Endocavitary mural thrombosis may occur, especially within RV aneurysms or in the atria in the presence of atrial fibrillation (AF). The ultimate phenotype may resemble features of dilated cardiomyopathy (DCM) with biventricular involvement, making differential diagnosis difficult.

The diagnosis of ARVC is often challenging due to heterogeneous clinical presentation, highly variable intra- and interfamily expressivity, and incomplete penetrance. This genotype–phenotype plasticity is as yet largely unexplained.

14.3 Diagnosis

There is no single gold-standard diagnostic test for ARVC. Therefore, diagnosis relies on a scoring system, with major and minor criteria based on demonstration of a combination of abnormalities in RV morphology and function, typical depolarization/repolarization electrocardiographic (ECG) changes (Fig. 14.1), peculiar histological findings, ventricular arrhythmias, family history, and results of genetic testing. Definitive diagnosis, based on the Revised 2010 Task Force Criteria [9] (Table 14.1), requires two major criteria, one major plus two minor criteria, or four minor criteria from different categories. Therefore, initial evaluation of all patients suspected of having ARVC should include physical examination; clinical history; family history of ARVC or arrhythmias or SD; ECG; signal-averaged ECG; 24-h Holter monitoring; and comprehensive nonechocardiography focused on both ventricles. This imaging technique can reveal RV structural abnormalities such as RV dilation, aneurysm formation, and functional abnormalities, including hypo-a-dyskinetic RV regions, RV systolic dysfunction, paradoxical septal motion, and tricuspid regurgitation [10]. In the late stages, LV involvement with biventricular failure is observed. New tools for improving diagnostic accuracy are now available in clinical practice. Among noninvasive investigations, cardiac magnetic resonance (CMR) with late gadolinium enhancement (LGE) can detect myocardial fibrosis

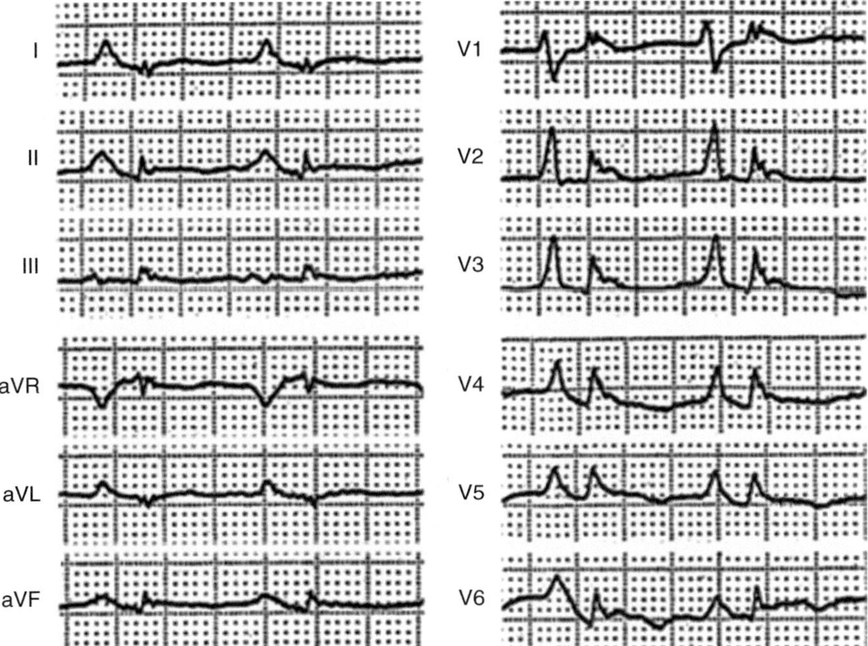

Fig. 14.1 Typical electrocardiogram (ECG) in advanced arrhythmogenic right ventricular cardiomyopathy (ARVC). Right atrial enlargement, low QRS voltages, epsilon waves, and negative T waves in anterior precordial leads are present

Table 14.1 Revised Task Force Criteria 2010

	Major criteria	Minor criteria
RV systolic function and structure	By 2D echo: Regional RV akinesia, dyskinesia, or aneurysm and one of the following (end diastole): PLAX RVOT $\geq$32 mm, PSAX RVOT $\geq$36 mm, or fractional area change $\leq$33 % By MRI: Regional RV akinesia, dyskinesia or aneurysm or dyssynchronous RV contraction and one of following: Ratio of RV end-diastolic volume to BSA $\geq$110 ml/m^2 or $\geq$100 ml/m^2 (or RVEF $\leq$40 %) By RV angiography: Regional RV akinesia, dyskinesia, or aneurysm	By 2D echo: Regional RV akinesia, dyskinesia, or aneurysm and 1 of the following (end diastole): PLAX RVOT $\geq$29 to <32 mm, PSAX RVOT $\geq$32 to <36 mm, or fractional area change >33 to $\leq$40 % By MRI: Regional RV akinesia, dyskinesia or aneurysm or dyssynchronous RV contraction and 1 of the following: Ratio of RV end-diastolic volume to BSA $\geq$100 to <110 ml/m^2 (male) or $\geq$90 to <100 ml/m^2 (female) or RV >40 to $\leq$45 % By RV angiography: Regional RV akinesia, dyskinesia, or aneurysm
Tissue characterization	Residual myocytes <60 % by morphometric analysis, with fibrous replacement of the RV free wall myocardium in $\geq$1 sample, with or without fatty replacement of tissue on EMB	Residual myocytes 60–75 % (or 50–65 % if estimated), with fibrous replacement of RV free wall myocardium in $\geq$1 sample, with or without fatty replacement of tissue on EMB
Repolarization abnormality	Inverted T waves in right precordial leads (V1–3) or beyond in individuals >14 years of age (in the absence of complete RBBB QRS $\geq$120 ms	Inverted T waves in leads V1 and 2 in individuals >14 years (in absence of complete RBBB) or in V4–6 or inverted T waves in leads V1–4 in individuals >14 years (in presence of complete RBBB)
Depolarization abnormality	Epsilon waves in the right precordial leads (V1–3)	Late potential by SAECG in $\geq$1 of 3 parameters in absence of QRS duration $\geq$110 ms on standard ECG; filtered QRS duration $\geq$114 ms; terminal QRS duration <40 μV or $\geq$38 ms; root-mean-square voltage of terminal 40 ms $\leq$20 μV; QRS terminal activation duration $\geq$55 ms measured from S-wave nadir to end of QRS
Arrhythmias	Nonsustained or sustained ventricular tachycardia of LBB morphology with superior axis Frequent ventricular extrasystoles (>1,000 per 24 h) (Holter)	Nonsustained or sustained ventricular tachycardia of RV outflow configuration, LBB morphology with inferior axis, or >500 ventricular extrasystoles per 24 h (Holter)
Familial history	ARVC confirmed pathologically in the first degree or identification of a pathogenic mutation categorized as associated or probably associated with ARVC	History of ARVC in a first-degree relative or premature sudden death (<35 years) due to suspected ARVC or ARVC confirmed pathologically, or by Task Force Criteria in second-degree relative

RV right ventricle, *PLAX* parasternal long axis, *RVOT* right ventricular outflow tract, *PSAX* parasternal short axis, *MRI* magnetic resonance imaging, *BSA* body surface area, *EMB* endomyocardial biopsy, *RBBB* right bundle-branch block, *LBB* left bundle branch, *SAECG* signal averaged electrocardiograph, *ARVC* arrhythmogenic right ventricular cardiomyopathy (Modified from Marcus et al. [9])

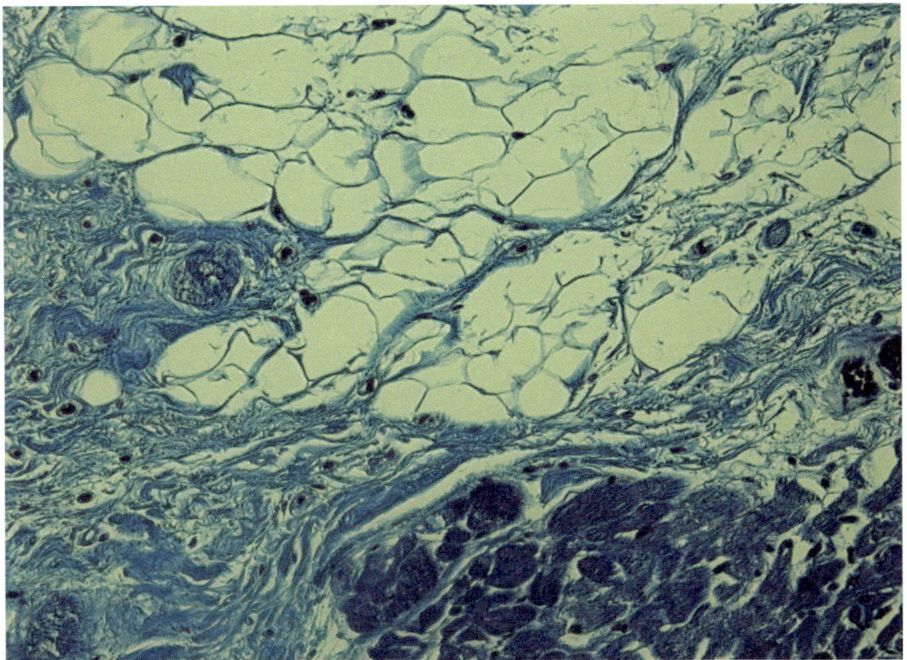

Fig. 14.2 Histologic specimen (Azan Mallory, ×20) at the right ventricular level in a case of arrhythmogenic right ventricular cardiomyopathy (ARVC). Severe fatty infiltration associated with patchy and interstitial fibrosis (*blue*) is present

and intramyocardial fatty infiltration. CMR allows the clearest visualization of the RV (for dilatation, dysfunction, regional wall motion abnormalities, and aneurysm formation) [11].

Diagnosis of ARVC remains a clinical challenge, particularly in its early stages and in patients with minimal echocardiographic RV abnormalities and especially in the absence of structural changes in the typical triangle of dysplasia [subtricuspid region, RV outflow tract (OT), and RV inferoapical region] [12]. Positive endomyocardial biopsy (EMB) of the RV is a recognized gold standard, but it often yields a false-negative result (sensitivity ~67 %) because of the frequently localized fibroadipose infiltration. Consequently, the best approach in making a diagnosis of ARVC is by combining different diagnostic tests [9, 13]. The histological hallmark of the disease is fibrofatty infiltration of the RV myocardium with areas of surviving myocytes (Fig. 14.2) and sometimes inflammatory infiltration. Pathologic abnormalities can progress with time, typically starting from the epicardium and eventually extending down to reach the subendocardium and becoming transmural. This implies a weakness and thinning of the free wall, resulting in RV dilatation and aneurysm formation, bulges, and sacculations, which constitute the typical diagnostic findings on noninvasive imaging tests [14].

LV involvement, typically affecting the posterior and lateral walls, is present in more than half of ARVC cases [15, 16]. The frequent, and sometimes predominant, LV involvement suggests that ARVC is not a unique entity but a complex disease,

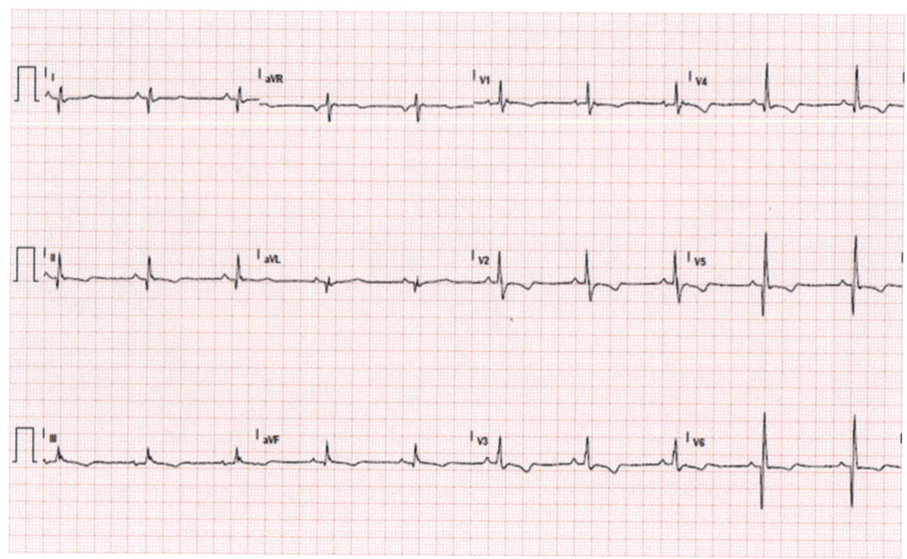

Fig. 14.3 Electrocardiogram (ECG) of a patient with arrhythmogenic right ventricular cardiomy-opathy with biventricular involvement. Sinus rhythm; epsilon waves in V1; inverted T waves in right precordial leads; negative T waves from V4 to V6 and inferior leads; deep Q waves in infero-lateral leads

with three possible patterns of expression: classic right-dominant (39 % of cases), left-dominant arrhythmogenic cardiomyopathy (LDAC) (5 %), and biventricular (56 %) forms [17, 18]. Interestingly, recent data showed that the LV may be affected not only in the late stage of the disease but may also occur in absence of alterations in RV systolic dysfunction, characterizing the LDAC form of the disease [16]. This left-dominant pattern is characterized by predominant LV involvement (dilation, systolic impairment, LGE) exceeding that of the RV or in the presence of preserved RV function [19]. Other features of this pattern are the LV origin of arrhythmias (RBBB morphology), inferolateral T-wave inversion on ECG (Fig. 14.3), and family history of LDAC.

14.3.1 Differential Diagnosis

Diagnosis of ARVC should be considered in any patient who does not have known heart disease and who presents with frequent premature ventricular contractions or symptomatic ventricular tachycardia. The main differential diagnoses include the following conditions:

1. Idiopathic RV outflow tract/ventricular tachycardia is a mostly benign condition that is not associated with structural heart disease. In its early stage, ARVC can be difficult to distinguish from this idiopathic type of ventricular arrhythmia in

Table 14.2 Clinical expressions of RVOT VT and ARVC

	RVOT VT	ARVC
Age at onset	Third or fifth decade of life	Third or fourth decade of life
Sex	Females predominantly	Males predominantly
Family history	–	+
Reports of SD	–	+
12-lead ECG	Normal	T-wave inversion in precordial leads V1–5 Prolongation of QRS complex in leads V1 or V2 Epsilon waves observed
SAECG	Normal	Late potentials observed
ECHO	Normal	Structural and wall motion abnormalities of RV
Arrhythmias	PVCs, repetitive monomorphic VT, induced/sustained VT	PVCs, SVT, NSVT, VF
Origin of arrhythmia	Septum	Parietal wall
Mechanism of arrhythmia	cAMP-mediated triggered activity	Reentrant mechanism
BNP levels	Normal	Increased

Modified from Steckman et al. [22]
RVOT right ventricular outflow tract, *VT* ventricular tachycardia, *SD* sudden death, *ECG* electrocardiogram, *SAECG* signal-averaged ECG, *ECHO* echocardiography, *BNP* brain natriuretic peptide, *PVC* polymorphic ventricular tachycardia, cAMP cyclic adenosine monophosphate, *SVT* sustained ventricular tachycardia, *NVST* nonsustained ventricular tachycardia, *VF* ventricular fibrillation

the absence of structural changes. Differential diagnosis is based on the fact that this arrhythmia is nonfamilial, and patients do not have the characteristic ECG/ signal average ECG abnormalities of ARVC (inversion T waves in V1–V3, epsilon waves, QRS duration >110 ms) (Table 14.2) [20].

2. Brugada syndrome is an inherited cardiac condition that, similarly to ARVC, is transmitted with an autosomal dominant pattern, which can lead to SD from malignant ventricular arrhythmias. Conversely, it is also characterized by a distinct typical ECG pattern, with J wave in precordial leads (Fig. 14.4) and by the absence of morphological echocardiographic features.

3. Dilated cardiomyopathy may be difficult to distinguish from ARVC, especially in its advanced stage with severe biventricular involvement. In this late phase, signs and symptoms of RV and/or LV failure can be present; finally, severe biventricular congestive HF can occur. In the absence of classic ARVC hallmarks (RV aneurysms, bulging), clinical distinction between these two CMP can be extremely difficult or impossible. Table 14.3 shows some differences between these two pathologies that are useful in differential diagnosis.

4. Myocarditis can mimic ARVC, especially when the RV is involved. Myocarditis can cause structural abnormalities, including microaneurysms, as well as the arrhythmic manifestations considered typical of ARVC. Moreover, myocardial inflammatory infiltrates, myocyte necrosis, and replacement fibrosis may lead to

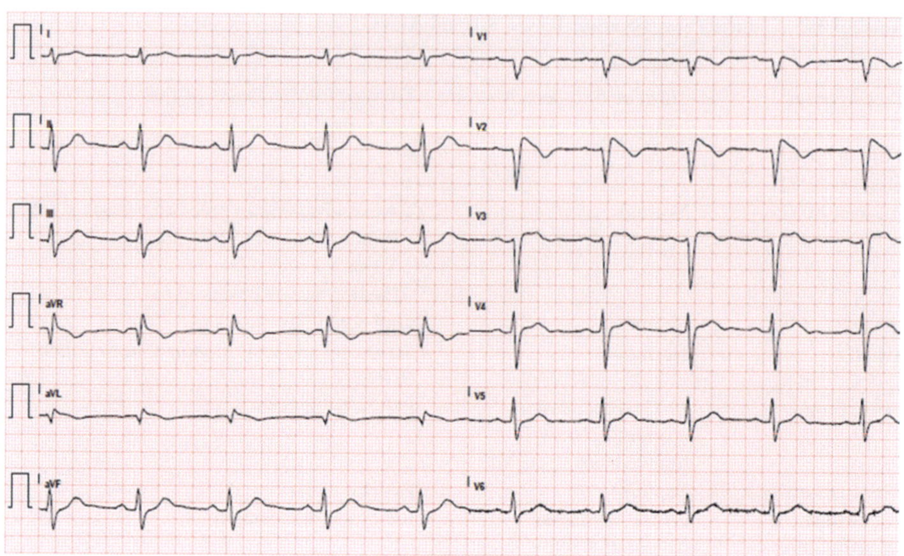

Fig. 14.4 Electrocardiogram (ECG) of a patient with Brugada syndrome: sinus rhythm. In precordial leads (V1–3), a typical type 1 pattern is present. "Coved-type" ST elevation with at least 2 mm (0.2 mV) J-point elevation, gradually descending ST segment, followed by a negative T wave

Table 14.3 Differential diagnosis between ARVC with biventricular involvement and DCM

	ARVC (biventricular)	DCM
Main dilatation	RV	LV
Main dysfunction	RV (or biventricular)	LV (or biventricular)
Aneurysm	RV (+/–LV)	Rare
Fibro-fatty tissue	RV (+/–LV)	–
Pulmonary hypertension	–	+/–
Family history	+	+/–
Epsilon waves (ECG)	+/–	–
Ventricular morphology of arrhythmias	LBBB or polymorphic morphology	RBBB or polymorphic morphology

ARVC arrhythmogenic right ventricular cardiomyopathy, *DCM* dilated cardiomyopathy, *LV* left ventricle, *RV* right ventricle, *LBBB* left bundle branch block, *RBBB* right bundle branch block

functional and structural changes in the RV myocardium, resembling those produced by ARVC fibrofatty replacement. New tools, such as 3D electroanatomic mapping, applied to the standard EMB, have been introduced to improve diagnostic accuracy in clinical practice. In a provocative study, Pieroni et al. [21] found that 50 % of patients with a diagnosis of noninvasive ARVC fulfilled Dallas histological criteria of active myocarditis. These data require confirmation in large patient populations.

5. Sarcoidosis with cardiac involvement can mimic ARVC, making accurate differential diagnosis more challenging. It must be considered if conduction defects with a high-grade atrioventricular block, respiratory, or systemic symptoms are present. Global RV hypokinesis or some regional wall motion abnormalities can be present due to the patchy nature of the granulomatous infiltration. Both sarcoidosis and ARVC can be progressive pathologies, and the accuracy of CMR could vary depending on the stage of the disease at which CMR data are acquired. The absence of myocardial fat infiltrates at CMR could be a useful distinguishing feature by which to suspect sarcoidosis [22].

6. Other pathologies:
   (a) Coronary artery disease and myocardial infarction can involve both ventricles and mimic aspects of ARVC.
   (b) Pulmonary hypertension (RV-pressure overload) and tricuspid regurgitation (RV-volume overload secondary to increasing stroke volume) can cause RV dilation and dysfunction.
   (c) Congenital heart diseases, such as Uhl anomaly (a rare congenital heart disease with a partial or total loss of the RV myocardial muscle) [22] and repaired tetralogy of Fallot must be considered, especially for their prevalent RV involvement.
   (d) Intracardiac shunts (e.g., atrial septal defects and anomalous pulmonary venous drainage) may cause RV volume overload. The diagnosis can be missed on standard echocardiogram, and in this cases, transesophageal echocardiography (TEE) and/or CMR (which have excellent correlation with RV angiography) can improve diagnostic accuracy.

Conclusions

ARVC is a frequently progressive disease with risk of life-threatening complications and which constitutes a clinical diagnostic challenge for physicians given the different genotypic and phenotypic variations and the wide ranges of clinical manifestations. Genetic studies indicate that ARVC should be considered a disease of desmosome dysfunction. Its diagnosis is based on the modified Task Force Criteria for ARVC [9] and should be approached with great caution. The main challenge is to improve risk stratification in relation to SD and HF and identify patients who will most benefit from early intervention involving lifestyle changes, restriction of physical sport activity, antiarrhythmic drugs, and/or ICD placement.

References

1. Corrado D, Basso C, Thiene G (2000) Arrhythmogenic right ventricular cardiomyopathy: diagnosis, prognosis, and treatment. Heart 83(5):588–595
2. Pinamonti B, Sinagra G, Camerini F (2000) Clinical relevance of right ventricular dysplasia/cardiomyopathy. Heart 83:9–11

3. Corrado D, Thiene G (2006) Arrhythmogenic right ventricular cardiomyopathy/dysplasia: clinical impact of molecular genetic studies. Circulation 113(13):1634–1637. doi:10.1161/CIRCULATIONAHA.105.616490

4. Campuzano O, Alcalde M, Allegue C, Iglesias A, Garcia-Pavia P, Partemi S, Oliva A, Pascali VL, Berne P, Sarquella-Brugada G, Brugada J, Brugada P, Brugada R (2013) Genetics of arrhythmogenic right ventricular cardiomyopathy. J Med Genet 50(5):280–289. doi:10.1136/jmedgenet-2013-101523

5. Taylor M, Graw S, Sinagra G, Barnes C, Slavov D, Brun F, Pinamonti B, Salcedo EE, Sauer W, Pyxaras S, Anderson B, Simon B, Bogomolovas J, Labeit S, Granzier H, Mestroni L (2011) Genetic variation in titin in arrhythmogenic right ventricular cardiomyopathy-overlap syndromes. Circulation 124(8):876–885. doi:10.1161/CIRCULATIONAHA.110.005405

6. Corrado D, Thiene G, Nava A, Rossi L, Pennelli N (1990) Sudden death in young competitive athletes: clinicopathologic correlations in 22 cases. Am J Med 89(5):588–596

7. Dalal D, Nasir K, Bomma C, Prakasa K, Tandri H, Piccini J, Roguin A, Tichnell C, James C, Russell SD, Judge DP, Abraham T, Spevak PJ, Bluemke DA, Calkins H (2005) Arrhythmogenic right ventricular dysplasia: a United States experience. Circulation 112(25):3823–3832. doi:10.1161/CIRCULATIONAHA.105.542266

8. Basso C, Corrado D, Marcus FI, Nava A, Thiene G (2009) Arrhythmogenic right ventricular cardiomyopathy. Lancet 373(9671):1289–1300. doi:10.1016/S0140-6736(09)60256-7

9. Marcus FI, McKenna WJ, Sherrill D, Basso C, Bauce B, Bluemke DA, Calkins H, Corrado D, Cox MG, Daubert JP, Fontaine G, Gear K, Hauer R, Nava A, Picard MH, Protonotarios N, Saffitz JE, Sanborn DM, Steinberg JS, Tandri H, Thiene G, Towbin JA, Tsatsopoulou A, Wichter T, Zareba W (2010) Diagnosis of arrhythmogenic right ventricular cardiomyopathy/dysplasia: proposed modification of the task force criteria. Circulation 121(13):1533–1541. doi:10.1161/CIRCULATIONAHA.108.840827

10. Scheinman MM, Crawford MH (2005) Echocardiographic findings and the search for a gold standard in patients with arrhythmogenic right ventricular dysplasia. J Am Coll Cardiol 45(6):866–867. doi:10.1016/j.jacc.2004.12.021

11. Tandri H, Saranathan M, Rodriguez ER, Martinez C, Bomma C, Nasir K, Rosen B, Lima JA, Calkins H, Bluemke DA (2005) Noninvasive detection of myocardial fibrosis in arrhythmogenic right ventricular cardiomyopathy using delayed-enhancement magnetic resonance imaging. J Am Coll Cardiol 45(1):98–103. doi:10.1016/j.jacc.2004.09.053

12. Basso C, Thiene G (2005) Adipositas cordis, fatty infiltration of the right ventricle, and arrhythmogenic right ventricular cardiomyopathy. Just a matter of fat? Cardiovasc Pathol 14(1):37–41. doi:10.1016/j.carpath.2004.12.001

13. Angelini A, Basso C, Nava A, Thiene G (1996) Endomyocardial biopsy in arrhythmogenic right ventricular cardiomyopathy. Am Heart J 132(1 Pt 1):203–206

14. Fisher NG, Gilbert TJ (2000) Arrhythmogenic right ventricular dysplasia. An illustrated review highlighting developments in the diagnosis and management of this potentially fatal condition. Postgrad Med J 76(897):395–398

15. Corrado D, Basso C, Thiene G, McKenna WJ, Davies MJ, Fontaliran F, Nava A, Silvestri F, Blomstrom-Lundqvist C, Wlodarska EK, Fontaine G, Camerini F (1997) Spectrum of clinico-pathologic manifestations of arrhythmogenic right ventricular cardiomyopathy/dysplasia: a multicenter study. J Am Coll Cardiol 30(6):1512–1520

16. Pinamonti B, Sinagra G, Salvi A, Di Lenarda A, Morgera T, Silvestri F, Bussani R, Camerini F (1992) Left ventricular involvement in right ventricular dysplasia. Am Heart J 123(3):711–724

17. Sen-Chowdhry S, Syrris P, Ward D, Asimaki A, Sevdalis E, McKenna WJ (2007) Clinical and genetic characterization of families with arrhythmogenic right ventricular dysplasia/cardiomyopathy provides novel insights into patterns of disease expression. Circulation 115(13):1710–1720. doi:10.1161/CIRCULATIONAHA.106.660241

18. Sen-Chowdhry S, Lowe MD, Sporton SC, McKenna WJ (2004) Arrhythmogenic right ventricular cardiomyopathy: clinical presentation, diagnosis, and management. Am J Med 117(9):685–695. doi:10.1016/j.amjmed.2004.04.028

19. Sen-Chowdhry S, Syrris P, Prasad SK, Hughes SE, Merrifield R, Ward D, Pennell DJ, McKenna WJ (2008) Left-dominant arrhythmogenic cardiomyopathy: an under-recognized clinical entity. J Am Coll Cardiol 52(25):2175–2187. doi:10.1016/j.jacc.2008.09.019
20. Pamuru PR, Dokuparthi MV, Remersu S, Calambur N, Nallari P (2010) Comparison of Uhl's anomaly, right ventricular outflow tract ventricular tachycardia (RVOT VT) & arrhythmogenic right ventricular dysplasia/cardiomyopathy (ARVD/C) with an insight into genetics of ARVD/C. Indian J Med Res 131:35–45
21. Pieroni M, Dello Russo A, Marzo F, Pelargonio G, Casella M, Bellocci F, Crea F (2009) High prevalence of myocarditis mimicking arrhythmogenic right ventricular cardiomyopathy differential diagnosis by electroanatomic mapping-guided endomyocardial biopsy. J Am Coll Cardiol 53(8):681–689. doi:10.1016/j.jacc.2008.11.017
22. Steckman DA, Schneider PM, Schuller JL, Aleong RG, Nguyen DT, Sinagra G, Vitrella G, Brun F, Cova MA, Pagnan L, Mestroni L, Varosy PD, Sauer WH (2012) Utility of cardiac magnetic resonance imaging to differentiate cardiac sarcoidosis from arrhythmogenic right ventricular cardiomyopathy. Am J Cardiol 110(4):575–579. doi:10.1016/j.amjcard.2012.04.029

Basic Echocardiography in Arrhythmogenic Right Ventricular Cardiomyopathy

15

Andreea M. Dragos, Bruno Pinamonti, and Elena Abate

15.1 Introduction

Two-dimensional echocardiography is the first-line imaging tool in the diagnosis and follow-up of patients with arrhythmogenic right ventricular cardiomyopathy (ARVC) due to its widespread use and availability. When a patient is referred to the echocardiography laboratory for a suspected diagnosis of ARVC, particular care must be taken to assess right ventricular (RV) morphology and function using both standard and specific RV views in order to gain as much information as possible. Furthermore, left ventricular (LV) evaluation is fundamental, as LV involvement is relatively frequent in ARVC either in the more advanced forms of the disease with biventricular involvement, or in a recently described form of the disease called left-dominant arrhythmogenic cardiomyopathy (LDAC) [1].

15.2 Assessment of Right Ventricular Dimension, Function, and Morphology

Two-dimensional echocardiographic assessment of the RV is somehow more problematic than of the LV due to the complex half-moon-shaped geometry of the RV chamber, which is wrapped around the LV and has separate infundibulum and prominent trabeculations. Until the publication of the latest Revised Task Force Criteria for

---

Electronic supplementary material The online version of this chapter (doi: 10.1007/978-3-319-06019-4_15) contains supplementary material, which is available to authorized users. Videos can also be accessed at http://www.springerimages.com/videos/978-3-319-06018-7.

A.M. Dragos, MD (✉) • B. Pinamonti, MD • E. Abate, MD
Department of Cardiology, University Hospital of Trieste,
Via P. Valdoni 7, Trieste 34139, Italy
e-mail: dragosandreea82@yahoo.com; bruno.pinamonti@gmail.com;
abate.elena@gmail.com

B. Pinamonti, G. Sinagra (eds.), *Clinical Echocardiography and Other Imaging Techniques in Cardiomyopathies*, DOI 10.1007/978-3-319-06019-4_15,
© Springer International Publishing Switzerland 2014

Table 15.1 Revised echocardiographic Task Force Criteria for the diagnosis of ARVC

Major criteria	Minor criteria
Regional RV akinesia, dyskinesia, or aneurysm *and* 1 of the following (end-diastole):	Regional RV akinesia or dyskinesia *and* 1 of the following (end-diastole):
PLAX RV OT >32 mm [corrected for body size (PLAX/BSA) >19 mm/m^2]	PLAX RV OT ≥29 to <32 mm [corrected for body size (PLAX/BSA) ≥16 to <19 mm/m^2]
PSAX RV OT ≥36 mm [corrected for body size (PSAX/BSA) ≥21 mm/m^2]	PSAX RV OT ≥32 to <36 mm [corrected for body size (PSAX/BSA) ≥18 to <21 mm/m^2]
Or RV fractional area change ≤33 %	*Or* RV fractional area change >33 to ≤40 %

Adapted from Marcus et al. [2], with permission
ARVC arrhythmogenic right ventricular cardiomyopathy, *BSA* body surface area, *OT* outflow tract, *PLAX* parasternal long-axis, *PSAX* parasternal short-axis, *RV* right ventricular

ARVC [2], the detection of impaired RV function and RV morphological assessment were mainly based on qualitative parameters that were highly dependent on operator experience and therefore, less reproducible. The New Revised Task Force Criteria [2] propose a more quantitative approach for RV morphological and functional assessment in order to improve diagnostic accuracy and specificity. Specific cutoff values were defined to characterize RV enlargement and systolic dysfunction, and regional wall motion abnormalities (WMA) were considered diagnostically important only in the presence of akinesia, dyskinesia, or aneurismal bulges. The conjunction of these parameters resulted in major and minor diagnostic criteria, as shown in Table 15.1.

15.3 Right Ventricular Dimensions

In ARVC, an enlarged RV is a common finding. RV outflow and inflow can be involved, but a short-axis dimension of >30 mm of the RV outflow tract (OT) had the highest sensitivity and specificity (89 and 86 %, respectively) for ARVC diagnosis) [3], and therefore RV OT measurement has become an integral part of the new diagnostic criteria. RV OT dimensions can be measured either in the parasternal long-axis view or in parasternal short-axis view (Figs. 15.1 and 15.2, Clip 15.1a, b). Measurements of RV basal and midcavity minor dimensions, longitudinal dimension, and end-diastolic and end-systolic areas (all obtained from a four-chamber apical view focused on the RV) are recommended by the RV echocardiographic guidelines [4], but such measurements correlate poorly with ARVC [3] and therefore are not ordinarily used for diagnostic assessment in ARVC patients.

15.4 Right Ventricular Systolic Function

Quantitative echocardiographic assessment of RV systolic function is problematic due to its complex geometry, which precludes imaging the inflow and outflow tracts in a single 2D plane and lack of standard methods for assessing RV volumes. Nonetheless, 2D echocardiography represents the first-line imaging technique available for

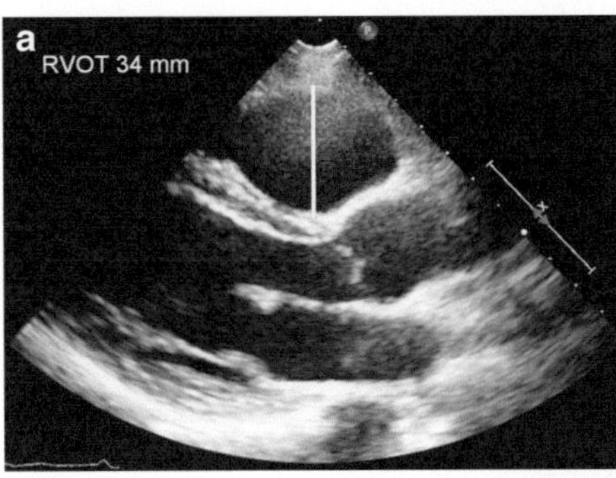

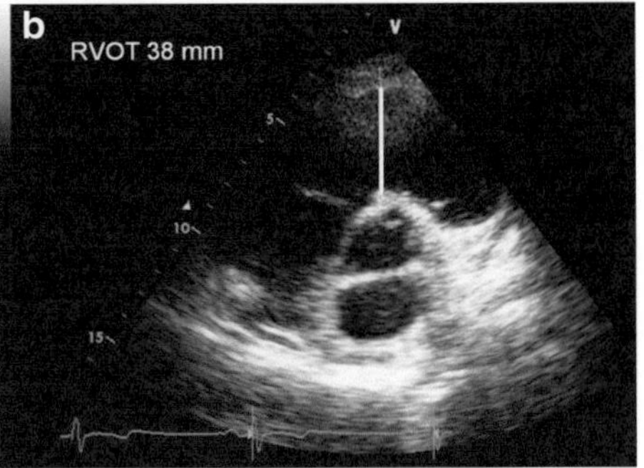

Fig. 15.1 Right ventricular outflow tract (RVOT) dimensions measured in parasternal long-axis view (34 mm) (**a**) and in parasternal short-axis view (38 mm) (**b**) in a patient with arrhythmogenic RV cardiomyopathy

Fig. 15.2 Patient with arrhythmogenic right ventricular (RV) cardiomyopathy and severely dilated RV. The RV outflow tract diameter measured in parasternal short axis view is 55.8 mm

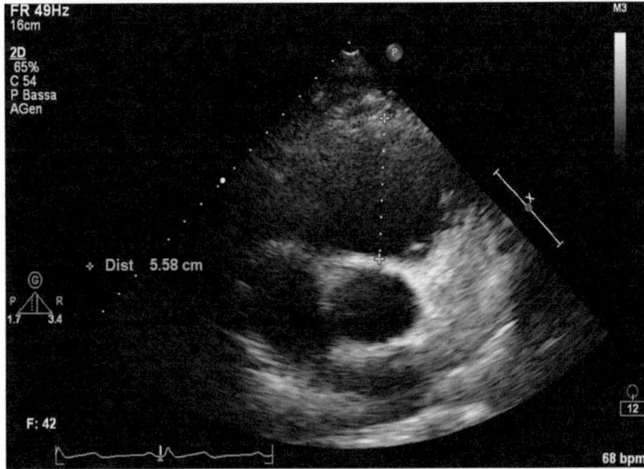

screening patients with suspected ARVC and is of utmost importance when studying these patients, as cardiac magnetic resonance (CMR) is not highly available in most centers. CMR is considered the gold-standard technique for thorough evaluation of RV dimensions and function; however, its use is mainly reserved for equivocal cases (Chap. 22).

RV fractional area change (FAC) is one of the most commonly used 2D echocardiographic method to assess RV systolic function, as it correlates well with RV ejection fraction (EF) determined by CMR volumetric analysis and is superior to other 2D parameters [5, 6]. RV FAC is obtained in the four-chamber apical view (focused on the RV) by tracing the RV endocardium both in end diastole and end-systole from the annulus, along the free wall to the apex, and then back to the annulus, along the interventricular septum. Care must be taken to trace the free wall beneath the trabeculations. Impaired RV function, defined as RV FAC < 33 %, has been described in approximately two thirds of patients with ARVC and represents an important diagnostic parameter (Fig. 15.3, Clip 15.2a) [7, 8].

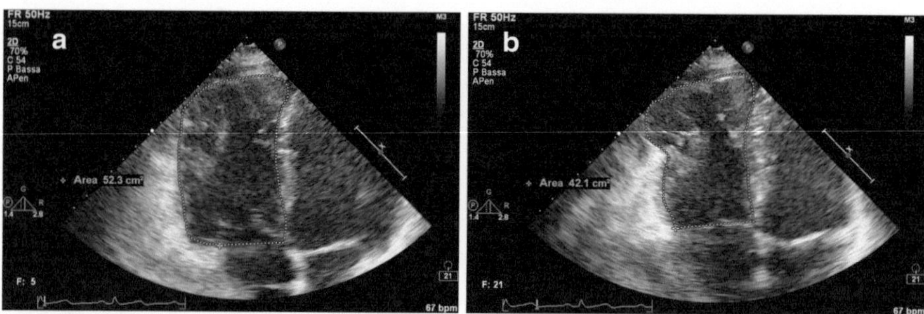

Fig. 15.3 Right ventricular (RV) fractional area change measurement from an apical four-chamber view in a patient with arrhythmogenic RV cardiomyopathy with severe RV dilation and pronounced aneurysms in the RV apex. RV end-diastolic area is 52.3 cmq (**a**), end-systolic area is 42.1 cmq (**b**), and fractional area change is 19 %

15.5 Right Ventricular Regional Assessment

RV localized WMA are a landmark of ARVC and reflect the patchy infiltration and substitution of normal myocardium with fibrofatty tissue. In the Revised Diagnostic Criteria of ARVC [2], the presence of localized akinetic, dyskinetic, or aneurysmal RV segments represents a major diagnostic criterion, emphasizing the importance of their recognition. Of note, with respect to the original 1994 International Task Force Criteria [9], hypokinesis is no longer considered a morphological diagnostic criteria due to its low specificity.

The typical echocardiographic appearance consists of localized aneurysmal bulges of the RV wall classically described in the "triangle of dysplasia," namely the RV OT, apex, and basal subtricuspid area (Fig. 15.3 and Clips 15.2a, b, 15.3a–c, and 15.4a, b) [10]. However, in clinical practice, regional WMA may be found in all RV segments; therefore a complete assessment of RV using conventional and off-axis views must be conducted [11]. Parasternal RV inflow and outflow views are particularly useful for exploring the anterior wall of the RV OT and inferior and anterior walls of the RV inflow tract (Clip 15.5). RV free wall is better assessed from the RV-focused four- and two-chamber apical views and the four-chamber subcostal view.

A panoramic view of the RV apex can be obtained by combining the apical RV-focused four- or two-chamber views and subcostal four-chamber view. If considerable LV enlargement coexists, apical kinesis is more difficult to assess because of the translational movement of the RV wall during the cardiac cycle. The presence of hypokinesia of this particular segment in the absence of wall thinning or deformity is not a specific finding and should not be considered pathological, as it may be seen also in normal and athletic individuals [12].

In patients with poor acoustic window, the use of contrast echocardiography (also simply using an agitated saline intravenous infusion) improved visualization of the RV endocardial border [13] and may be particularly useful in enhancing regional WMA assessment as well as RV measurements.

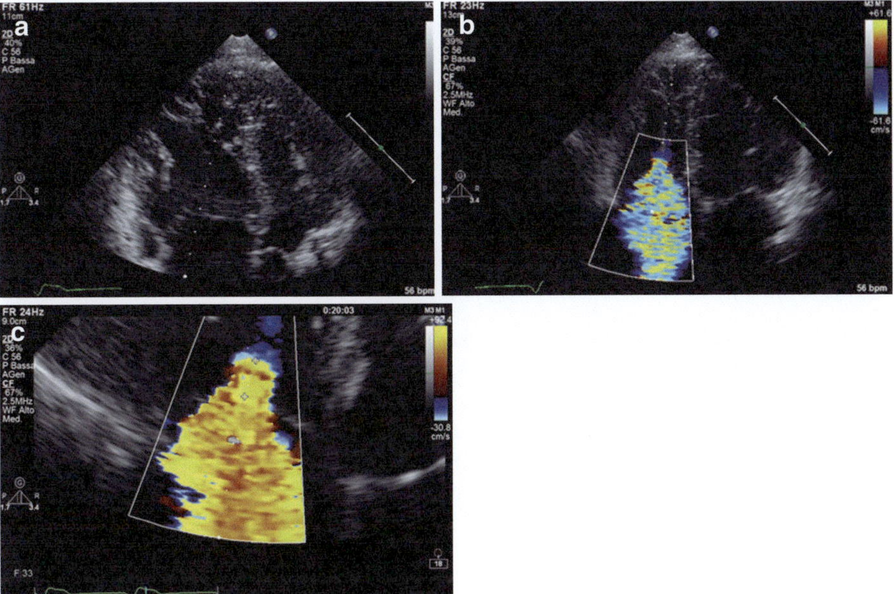

Fig. 15.4 Arrhythmogenic right ventricular (RV) cardiomyopathy with moderately dilated RV (end-diastolic area 33 cmq) with diffuse hypokinesis (**a**) and severe tricuspid regurgitation (**b, c**). The area of the tricuspid regurgitation jet assessed with color Doppler is 15 cmq (**b**), and the effective regurgitant orifice area [proximal isovelocity surface area (PISA) method] is 0.63 cmq (**c**)

15.6 Tricuspid Valve Function

Tricuspid regurgitation (TR) is often present in ARVC and is usually secondary to RV enlargement and annulus dilation and remodeling (Fig. 15.4, Clip 15.6a, b). Assessing TR severity is clinically important, as moderate to severe TR plays an adverse prognostic role in the natural history of ARVC patients [8].

15.7 Left Ventricular Morphology and Function

LV involvement is a relatively common finding in ARVC patients, ranging from 30 to 76 % of cases [14, 15]. WMA can be present in both the septum and LV free wall, with a predilection for inferoseptal and posterolateral areas [15]. LV aneurysms are rarely reported (Clip 15.7a–d) [16]. LV enlargement and systolic dysfunction may also occur, but usually, RV abnormalities predominate (Clip 15.8a, b). Accurate assessment of LV dimensions and EF should be routinely performed, as the presence of LV dysfunction identifies a subgroup of patients at high risk of death or heart transplant [8]. Conversely, in the recently described entity of LDAC, structural abnormalities are exclusively or predominantly found in the LV, with no or only mild RV involvement. The LV may show localized WMA, chamber dilation

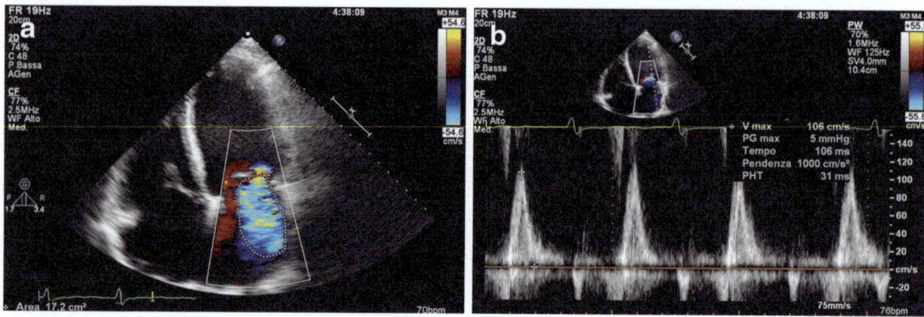

Fig. 15.5 Advanced arrhythmogenic right ventricular cardiomyopathy with biventricular involvement, functional severe mitral regurgitation (**a**), and restrictive left ventricular filling pattern (**b**)

(usually not severe), and/or systolic impairment [1]. However, no systematic reports on echocardiographic features of this pathology are available.

15.8 Follow-up Data

Few data are available on the echocardiographic assessment of ARVC evolution [17]. In our experience, progressive RV enlargement, with widespread wall bulgings and severe RV dysfunction, can be observed in some cases (Clip 15.9a), sometimes associated with progressive worsening of functional TR (typically without signs of pulmonary hypertension). Progressive LV involvement and dysfunction (usually without severe chamber enlargement) can also be observed during the long-term course of the disease (Clip 15.9b). RV as well as LV restrictive filling pattern and functional mitral regurgitation can be seen in advanced, end-stage ARVC with biventricular involvement (Fig. 15.5, Clip 15.8c, d). Intracavitary thrombi can be found within all four cardiac chambers, sometimes despite the presence of sinus rhythm, exposing patients to a potential embolic risk (Clip 15.7b, c). These echocardiographic findings are usually associated with a progressive clinical deterioration and high risk of refractory heart failure which may eventually require heart transplantation.

References

1. Sen-Chowdhry S, Syrris S, Prasad SK et al (2008) Left-dominant arrhythmogenic cardiomyopathy: an under-recognized clinical entity. J Am Coll Cardiol 52:2175–2187
2. Marcus FI, McKenna WJ, Sherrill D et al (2010) Diagnosis of arrhythmogenic right ventricular cardiomyopathy/dysplasia: proposed modification of the Task Force Criteria. Eur Heart J 31:806–814
3. Yoerger DM, Marcus F, Sherrill D et al (2005) Echocardiographic findings in patients meeting task force criteria for arrhythmogenic right ventricular dysplasia: new insights from the multidisciplinary study of right ventricular dysplasia. J Am Coll Cardiol 45:860–865

4. Rudski LG, Lai WW, Afilalo L et al (2010) Guidelines for the echocardiographic assessment of the right heart in adults: a report from the American Society of Echocardiography endorsed by the European Association of Echocardiography, a registered branch of the European Society of Cardiology, and the Canadian Society of Echocardiography. J Am Soc Echocardiogr 23:685–713; quiz 786–788
5. Anavekar NS, Gerson D, Skali H et al (2007) Two-dimensional assessment of right ventricular function: an echocardiographic-MRI correlative study. Echocardiography 24:452–456
6. Anavekar NS, Skali H, Bourgoun M et al (2008) Usefulness of right ventricular fractional area change to predict death, heart failure, and stroke following myocardial infarction (from the VALIANT ECHO Study). Am J Cardiol 101:607–612
7. Hulot JS, Jouven X, Emoana JP et al (2004) Natural history and risk stratification of arrhythmogenic right ventricular dysplasia/cardiomyopathy. Circulation 110:1879–1884
8. Pinamonti B, Dragos AM, Pyxaras SA et al (2011) Prognostic predictors in arrhythmogenic right ventricular cardiomyopathy: results from a 10-year registry. Eur Heart J 32:1105–1113
9. McKenna WJ, Thiene G, Nava A et al (1994) Diagnosis of arrhythmogenic right ventricular dysplasia/cardiomyopathy. Task Force of the Working Group Myocardial and Pericardial Disease of the European Society of Cardiology and of the Scientific Council on Cardiomyopathies of the International Society and Federation of Cardiology. Br Heart J 71:215–218
10. Marcus FI, Fontaine GH, Guiraudon G et al (1982) Right ventricular dysplasia: a report of 24 adult cases. Circulation 65:384–398
11. Scognamiglio R, Fasoli G, Nava A et al (1989) Contribution of cross-sectional echocardiography to the diagnosis of right ventricular dysplasia at the asymptomatic stage. Eur Heart J 10:538–542
12. Sievers B, Marvin A, Ulrich F et al (2004) Right ventricular wall motion abnormalities found in healthy subjects by cardiovascular magnetic resonance imaging and characterized with a new segmental model. J Cardiovasc Magn Reson 6:601–608
13. Van den Bosch AE, Meijiboom FJ, McGhie JS et al (2004) Enhanced visualization of the right ventricle by contrast echocardiography in congenital heart disease. Eur J Echocardiogr 5:104–110
14. Pinamonti B, Sinagra G, Salvi A et al (1992) Left ventricular involvement in right ventricular dysplasia. Am Heart J 123:711–724
15. Corrado D, Basso C, Thiene G et al (1997) Spectrum of clinicopathologic manifestations of arrhythmogenic right ventricular cardiomyopathy/dysplasia: a multicenter study. J Am Coll Cardiol 30:1512–1520
16. Pinamonti B, Pagnan L, Bussani R et al (1998) Images in cardiovascular medicine: right ventricular dysplasia with biventricular involvement. Circulation 98:1943–1945
17. Pinamonti B, Di Lenarda A, Sinagra G et al (1995) Long-term evolution of right ventricular dysplasia-cardiomyopathy. Am Heart J 129:412–415

Advanced Echocardiographic Techniques in Arrhythmogenic Right Ventricular Cardiomyopathy

16

Andreea M. Dragos, Elena Abate, and Bruno Pinamonti

16.1 Introduction

Basic echocardiography has significant limitations in assessing patients with arrhyrhmogenic right ventricular cardiomyopathy (ARVC). Substantial research has been made in the last years regarding the possible diagnostic role of advanced echocardiographic techniques.

16.2 Three-Dimensional Echocardiography

Three-dimensional echocardiography has emerged as a highly promising technique for studying right ventricular (RV) morphology and function. This technique is of great interest, as it seems to overcome the major limitations of 2D echocardiography for assessing RV volumes and ejection fraction (EF). It does not depend on geometric assumptions, and RV volumes and EF assessment with 3D echocardiography has been validated against cardiac magnetic resonance (CMR), which is considered the gold-standard technique and demonstrates quite good accuracy [1].

Three-dimensional RV data are usually acquired as a full-volume data set from the four-chamber apical view adapted to maximize visualization of the RV and are subsequently postprocessed using dedicated software. RV volumes are obtained by tracing both end-diastolic and end-systolic endocardial borders in distinct

Electronic supplementary material The online version of this chapter (doi: 10.1007/978-3-319-06019-4_16) contains supplementary material, which is available to authorized users. Videos can also be accessed at http://www.springerimages.com/videos/978-3-319-06018-7.

A.M. Dragos, MD (✉) • E. Abate, MD • B. Pinamonti, MD
Department of Cardiology, University Hospital of Trieste,
via P. Valdoni 7, Trieste 34139, Italy
e-mail: dragosandreea82@yahoo.com;
abate.elena@gmail.com; bruno.pinamonti@gmail.com

B. Pinamonti, G. Sinagra (eds.), *Clinical Echocardiography and Other Imaging Techniques in Cardiomyopathies*, DOI 10.1007/978-3-319-06019-4_16,
© Springer International Publishing Switzerland 2014

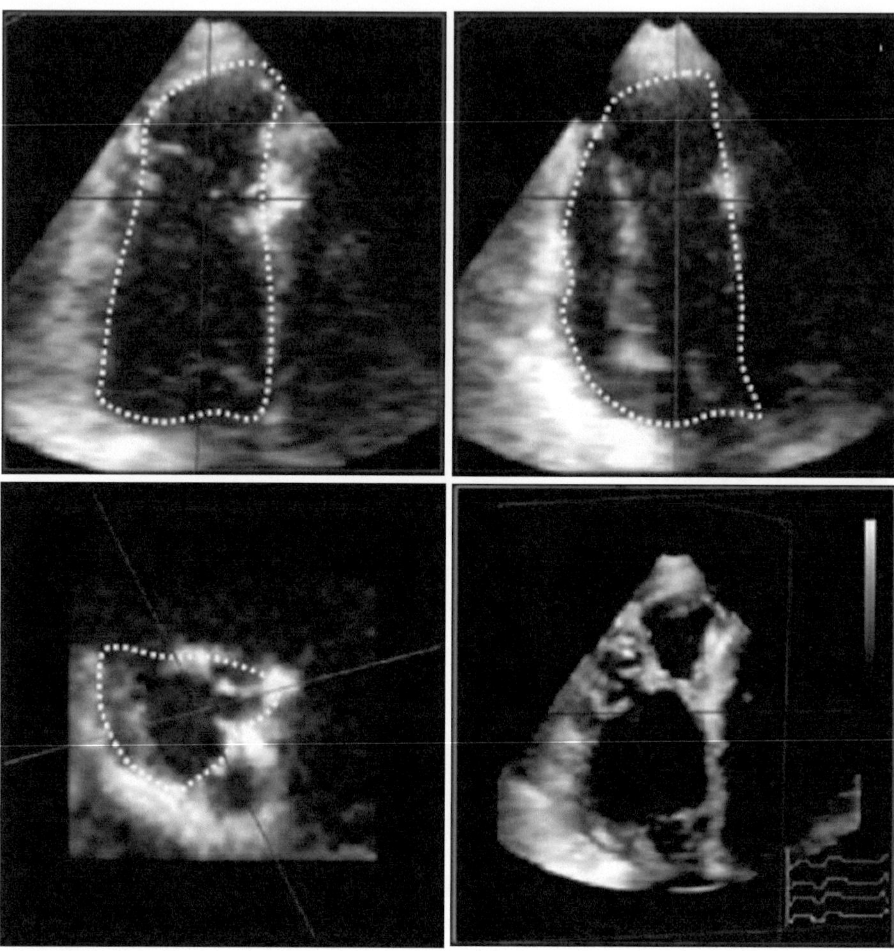

Fig. 16.1 Representative 3D images of the right ventricle of a patient with arrhythmogenic right ventricular cardiomyopathy (ARVC). Orthogonal long-axis views of the right ventricle (*top*), short-axis view (*bottom left*), 3D view (*bottom right*) (Modified from Prakasa et al. [4], with permission)

cross-sectional planes aimed at visualizing the three components of the RV: inflow (sagittal plane), apex (four-chamber), and RV outflow tract (coronal view), as suggested by the European Association of Echocardiography/American Society of Echocardiography recommendations for 3D echocardiography image acquisition and display [2]. End-systolic and -diastolic volumes are then generated by summing the three components, and EF is automatically calculated. Normal 3D echocardiography reference values for RV volumes and EF are reported by Tamborini et al. [3].

The feasibility of 3D echocardiography in ARVC was proven by Prakasa et al. [4], who showed good correlation between 3D and CMR for RV volumes and EF assessment, with a systematic underestimation of volumes calculated with 3D echocardiography (Fig. 16.1). Three-dimensional echocardiography data demonstrated high to moderate reproducibility, indicating it may be a reliable tool for follow-up studies in ARVC patients. However, in patients with severe RV enlargement, repeated image acquisitions with frequent off-axis views are needed in order to include the entire RV in the 3D data set. Furthermore, 3D echocardiography is capable of detecting structural abnormalities typical of ARVC, such as thinning of the RV free wall, excessive trabeculations, and localized apical aneurysms [5]. Although 3D echocardiography was not included in the new ARVC diagnostic criteria [6], the good accuracy of RV volumes and EF measurements with respect to CMR makes it clinically attractive and should be taken into consideration in the global evaluation of an ARVC patient.

16.3   Tissue Doppler Imaging

Tissue Doppler imaging (TDI), if applied to RV walls, allows quantitative assessment of RV longitudinal function by measuring myocardial velocities and velocity-derived deformation parameters (strain and strain rate). Owing to its theoretical ability to assess regional contractile function, TDI can provide important information in ARVC, considering the dyshomogeneous nature of myocardial involvement in this peculiar type of cardiomyopathy. Furthermore, this technique demonstrates the potential of detecting subtle impairment in a given myocardial segment, which are missed by standard echocardiographic parameters [7–9].

A simple and quick application of pulsed TDI is the measurement of tricuspid annular velocity, which reflects RV longitudinal contraction. Interestingly, in one study on ARVC patients, tricuspid annular systolic tissue velocity was the echocardiographic parameter that correlated best with RV EF assessed by CMR [10].

Regional myocardial velocities can be measured simultaneously in the three segments of the RV free wall (base, mid, and apex) using color-coded TDI images, which are usually recorded in the apical four-chamber view and subsequently processed offline. To obtain accurate myocardial velocities, sample regions of 3- to 5-mm in diameter should be placed in the basal part of the segment and on the endomyocardial side in end-systole [11].

Other potentially important information is the assessment of RV strain and strain rate by TDI. These deformation parameters have correlated closely with invasive measures of contractility [12], and reference values for both RV TDI velocities and strain are reported in normal individuals [13].

In a cohort of ARVC patients, Teske et al. [14] demonstrated that the lowest strain value in any of the three segments of the RV free wall had the best diagnostic accuracy when using a cutoff value of −18.2 % (Fig. 16.2). This parameter was superior to all conventional echocardiographic measures for functional and structural RV alterations. Furthermore, this method seems to eliminate almost entirely the false-positive findings on visual assessment of regional function, primarily due to the presence of hypokinesis in the basal or mid segment of the RV free wall or dyskinesis in the apical region.

Nevertheless, although this technique seems to offer a more accurate assessment of regional function over standard 2D echocardiography and has been applied

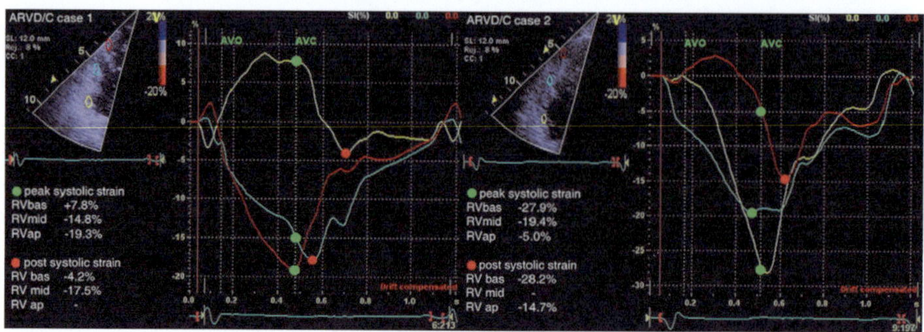

Fig. 16.2 Tissue-Doppler-imaging assessment of right ventricular (*RV*) strain in two cases of arrhythmogenic right ventricular cardiomyopathy (*ARVC*). In case 1 (*left*), RV basal segment (*RVBAS*) (*yellow curve*) is most affected (dyskinetic), with a normal function in the RV apical segment (*RVAP*) (*red curve*). In case 2 (*right*), normal peak systolic values are found in RVBAS (*yellow curve*) and RV mid segment (*RVMID*) (*blue curve*), but RV apical segment (*RVAP*) (*red curve*) shows an abnormal deformation pattern. *AVC* arterial (pulmonic) valve closure, *AVO* arterial (pulmonic) valve opening (Adapted from Teske et al. [14], with permission)

extensively for research purposes, its use in clinical practice is limited by a variety of factors. One of the most important is that TDI is an angle-dependent technique, and appropriate alignment with the vector of contraction is needed in order to obtain reliable measurements. Furthermore, acquisition is conditioned by a series of artifacts, and processing is time consuming.

16.4 Speckle-Tracking Echocardiography

Speckle-tracking echocardiography can be used for quantitative functional assessment of both LV and RV. As longitudinal RV shortening is a more important contributor to RV systolic function compared with circumferential shortening [15], most experience with RV speckle-tracking echocardiography is with regional and global longitudinal strain and strain-rate assessment (Fig. 16.3, Clips 16.1).

RV data acquisition for speckle-tracking analysis is performed with a 2D echocardiographic probe in the apical four-chamber view, and data are subsequently processed offline. Different software allow endocardial border tracing in a semiautomatic or manual mode, usually at end-systole. RV is automatically divided into six segments: base, mid, and apex of the RV free wall and septum, respectively, and segmental and global longitudinal strain and strain rate are calculated (Fig. 16.3, Clips 16.1).

Speckle-tracking echocardiography applied in ARVC shows significantly reduced RV global longitudinal strain in the affected population compared with normal controls [14]. A cutoff value of −18.1 % for the lowest strain value in any RV segment demonstrates a sensitivity and specificity of 91.2 % in identifying patients with ARVC [14].

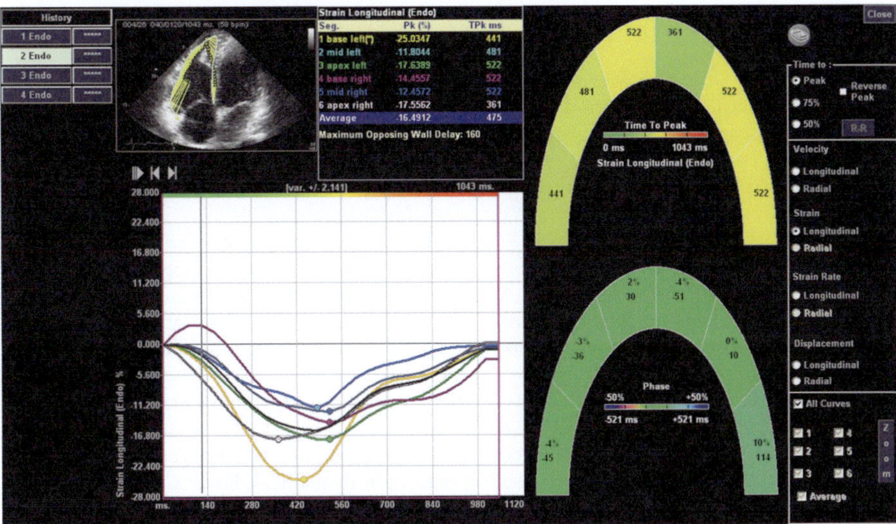

Fig. 16.3 Assessment of right ventricular (RV) longitudinal strain and strain rate by speckle-tracking echocardiography in a patient with arrhythmogenic right ventricular cardiomyopathy (ARVC) using a six-segment model from an apical four-chamber view. Regional longitudinal strain and strain-rate values are shown for each segment, and average values are automatically provided. Of note, global longitudinal strain results are significantly reduced (−16 %) in this patient

In a series of asymptomatic ARVC gene carriers, abnormal deformation, mainly localized in the basal segment of the lateral RV free wall, was found in 71 % of cases. These data suggest a possible role of deformation parameters assessed by speckle-tracking echocardiography for early detection of regional functional abnormalities in this peculiar group of patients [16]. This finding was subsequently confirmed by Sarvari et al. [17], who demonstrated significantly reduced global strain of both ventricles in asymptomatic gene carriers, indicating subclinical myocardial abnormalities [17]. Moreover, the same authors demonstrated that RV mechanical dispersion, defined as the standard deviation of contraction duration in a six-segment RV model, was an independent predictor of ventricular arrhythmia among ARVC patients. Therefore, mechanical dispersion assessed by speckle-tracking echocardiography might be a useful tool for risk stratification of affected patients as well as asymptomatic mutation carriers.

Although speckle-tracking echocardiography offers great potential with high accuracy for quantitative assessment of myocardial function [18, 19] and good reproducibility [20], it still has considerable limitations due to technical issues (image quality, proper tracing of the endocardial border, out-of-plane motion) and lack of standardization between different software algorithms. Further prospective longitudinal studies are needed to elucidate the real additional value of speckle-tracking echocardiography with respect to standard echocardiography in diagnosis and risk stratification of ARVC patients.

References

1. Shimada YJ, Shiota M, Siegel RJ et al (2010) Accuracy of right ventricular volumes and function determined by three-dimensional echocardiography in comparison with magnetic resonance imaging: a meta-analysis study. J Am Soc Echocardiogr 23:943–953
2. Lang RM, Badano LP, Tsang W et al (2012) EAE/ASE recommendations for image acquisition and display using three-dimensional echocardiography. Eur Heart J Cardiovasc Imaging 13:1–46
3. Tamborini G, Marsan NA, Gripari P et al (2010) Reference values for right ventricular volumes and ejection fraction with real-time three-dimensional echocardiography: evaluation in a large series of normal subjects. J Am Soc Echocardiogr 23:109–115
4. Prakasa KR, Dalal D, Wang J et al (2006) Feasibility and variability of three dimensional echocardiography in arrhythmogenic right ventricular dysplasia/cardiomyopathy. Am J Cardiol 97:703–709
5. Goland S, Czer LS, Luthringer D et al (2008) A case of arrhythmogenic right ventricular cardiomyopathy. Can J Cardiol 24:61–62
6. Marcus FI, McKenna WJ, Sherrill D et al (2010) Diagnosis of arrhythmogenic right ventricular cardiomyopathy/dysplasia: proposed modification of the Task Force Criteria. Eur Heart J 31:806–814
7. Weidemann F, Kowalski M, D'Hooge J et al (2001) Doppler myocardial imaging. A new tool to assess regional inhomogeneity in cardiac function. Basic Res Cardiol 96:595–605
8. Jurcut R, Wildiers H, Ganame J et al (2008) Detection and monitoring of cardiotoxicity-what does modern cardiology offer? Support Care Cancer 16:437–445
9. Voigt JU, Exner B, Schmiedehausen K et al (2003) Strain-rate imaging during dobutamine stress echocardiography provides objective evidence of inducible ischemia. Circulation 107:2120–2126
10. Wang J, Prakasa K, Bomma C et al (2007) Comparison of novel echocardiographic parameters of right ventricular function with ejection fraction by cardiac magnetic resonance. J Am Soc Echocardiogr 20:1058–1064
11. D'Hooge J, Heimdal A, Jamal F et al (2000) Regional strain and strain rate measurements by cardiac ultrasound: principles, implementation and limitations. Eur J Echocardiogr 1:154–170
12. Jamal F, Bergerot C, Argaud L et al (2003) Longitudinal strain quantitates regional right ventricular contractile function. Am J Physiol Heart Circ Physiol 285:H2842–H2847
13. Kjaergaard J, Sogaard P, Hassager C (2006) Quantitative echocardiographic analysis of the right ventricle in healthy individuals. J Am Soc Echocardiogr 19:1365–1372
14. Teske AJ, Cox MG, De Boeck BW et al (2009) Echocardiographic tissue deformation imaging quantifies abnormal regional right ventricular function in arrhythmogenic right ventricular dysplasia/cardiomyopathy. J Am Soc Echocardiogr 22:920–927
15. Kukulski T, Hubbert L, Arnold M et al (2000) Normal regional right ventricular function and its change with age: a Doppler myocardial imaging study. J Am Soc Echocardiogr 13:194–204
16. Teske AJ, Cox MG, Te Riele AS et al (2012) Early detection of regional functional abnormalities in asymptomatic ARVD/C gene carriers. J Am Soc Echocardiogr 25:997–1006
17. Sarvari SI, Haugaa KH, Anfinsen OG et al (2011) Right ventricular mechanical dispersion is related to malignant arrhythmias: a study of patients with arrhythmogenic right ventricular cardiomyopathy and subclinical right ventricular dysfunction. Eur Heart J 32:1089–1096
18. Korinek J, Kjaergaard J, Sengupta PP et al (2007) High spatial resolution speckle tracking improves accuracy of 2-dimensional strain measurements: an update on a new method in functional echocardiography. J Am Soc Echocardiogr 20:165–170
19. Amundsen BH, Helle-Valle T, Edvardsen T et al (2006) Noninvasive myocardial strain measurement by speckle tracking echocardiography: validation against sonomicrometry and tagged magnetic resonance imaging. J Am Coll Cardiol 47:789–793
20. Teske AJ, De Boeck BW, Olimulder M et al (2008) Echocardiographic assessment of regional right ventricular function: a head-to-head comparison between 2-dimensional and tissue Doppler-derived strain analysis. J Am Soc Echocardiogr 21:275–283

Other Imaging Modalities in the Assessment of Arrhythmogenic Right Ventricular Cardiomyopathy

17

Giancarlo Vitrella, Lorenzo Pagnan, and Andrea Perkan

17.1 Introduction

The clinical diagnosis of arrhythmogenic right ventricular displasia/cardiomyopathy is challenging for even the most experienced cardiologists. There is no gold standard test for the diagnosis, thus multidisciplinary criteria are used, clinical, genetic, electrocardiographic, and imaging. Cardiac magnetic resonance has gained widespread acceptance as one of the principal imaging methods in the assessment of this condition. The role of other imaging modalities such as positron emission tomography (PET), single-photon emission tomography, computed tomography and right ventriculography, is also reviewed.

17.2 Cardiac Magnetic Resonance

Cardiac magnetic resonance (CMR) abnormalities found in arrhythmogenic right ventricular cardiomyopathy (ARVC) can be divided into morphological (fibrofatty infiltration, RV wall thinning, trabecular disarray, hypertrophy) and functional [RV dilatation, aneurysms, segmental wall motion abnormalities (WMA), global systolic dysfunction] changes. Both types of abnormalities are commonly found in the triangle of dysplasia [1] and have been extensively studied.

Electronic supplementary material The online version of this chapter (doi: 10.1007/978-3-319-06019-4_17) contains supplementary material, which is available to authorized users. Videos can also be accessed at http://www.springerimages.com/videos/978-3-319-06018-7.

G. Vitrella (✉) • A. Perkan
Department of Cardiology, University Hospital of Trieste, via P. Valdoni 7, Trieste 34139, Italy
e-mail: giancarlo.vitrella@gmail.com

L. Pagnan, MD
Radiology Unit, University Hospital of Trieste, via P. Valdoni 7, Trieste 34139, Italy
e-mail: pagny@inwind.it

B. Pinamonti, G. Sinagra (eds.), *Clinical Echocardiography and Other Imaging Techniques in Cardiomyopathies*, DOI 10.1007/978-3-319-06019-4_17,
© Springer International Publishing Switzerland 2014

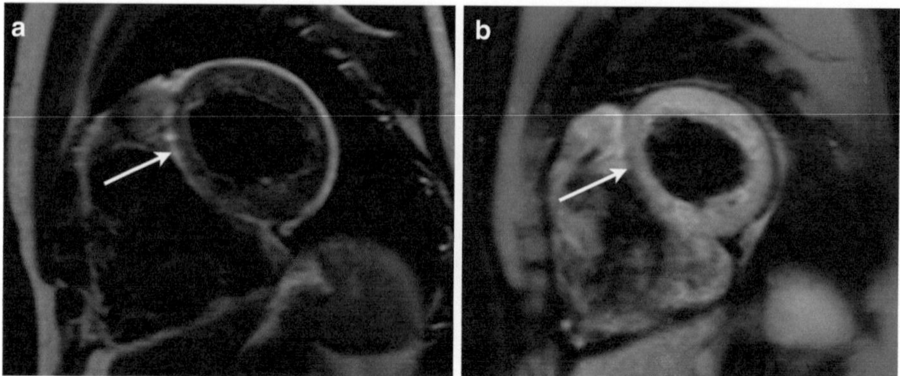

Fig. 17.1 Biventricular involvement in a patient with arrhythmogenic right ventricular cardiomyopathy (ARVC) seen as fatty infiltration of both ventricles: T1-weighted (**a**) and fat-saturated (**b**) short-axis images. Note the extensive hyperintensity of RV walls in the T1-weighted image, suppressed (*dark*) at the fat-saturation image. An area of fatty infiltration is also present at the intraventricular septum (IVS) (*arrows*), and small spotty hyperintense areas in the left ventricular (LV) free walls

17.2.1 Fatty Infiltration

The presence of fatty infiltration of the RV free wall displayed by T1-weighted images was the first-described CMR abnormality in ARVC [2]. Fatty infiltration was found to correspond to areas of WMA and to be associated with inducible ventricular tachycardia at electrophysiological studies [3, 4]. A good correlation was found between lesion location and distribution seen at CMR and ex vivo histology in an explanted heart from a patient with ARVC who was undergoing transplantation [5]. The presence of hyperintense areas at T1 CMR compatible with the presence of fat can be also found in the left ventricle (LV) and interventricular septum (IVS) in cases of ARVC with LV involvement (Fig. 17.1).

These findings were initially encouraging. However, CMR image interpretation for assessing fatty infiltration is difficult, and a significant proportion of patients have nondiagnostic scans [6]—even with state-of-the-art clinical CMR protocols—due to coil proximity and motion artifacts [7, 8], thus leading to misdiagnosis of ARVC [9]. In addition, fatty infiltration is frequently observed in CMR examinations from normal and obese individuals and in patients with clinical conditions that are not linked to ARVC [10–12]. Accordingly, fatty infiltration assessed by CMR was not included in the original [13] or revised diagnostic Task Force Criteria for ARVC [14].

17.2.2 Late Gadolinium Enhancement

Late gadolinium enhancement (LGE) of the RV wall was reported in various studies in ARVC patients and correlated with fibrofatty changes, inducible ventricular tachycardia (VT), and severe RV dysfunction confirmed on biopsy [15–19]. LGE was also described in the LV, particularly in familial forms with desmoplakin mutations, which exhibit a phenotype of left-dominant arrhythmogenic cardiomyopathy (LDAC) [20, 21].

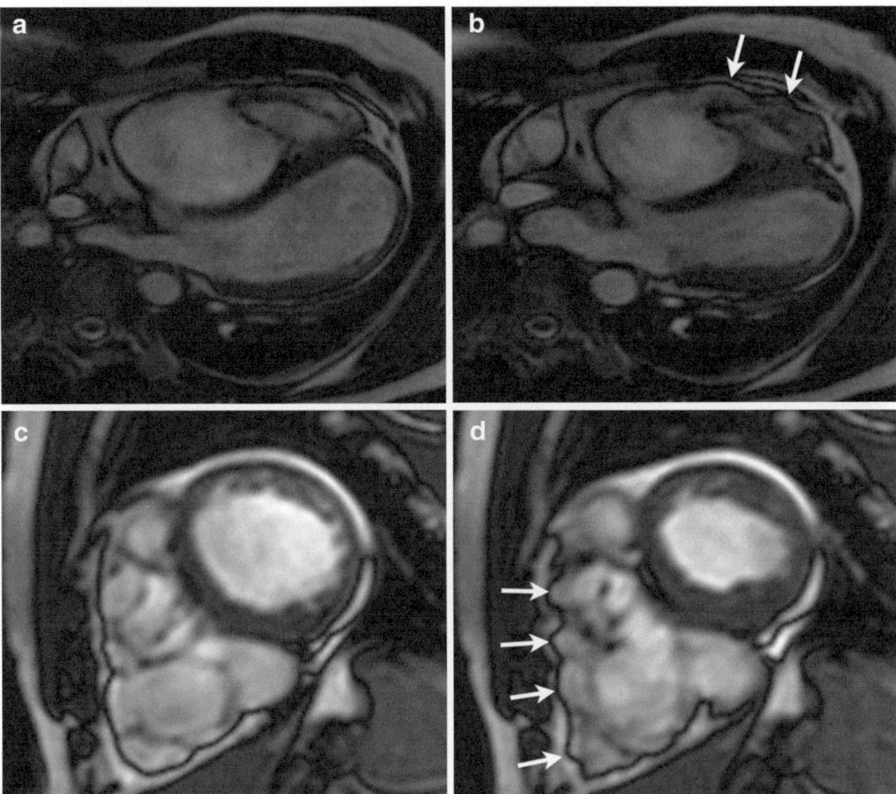

Fig. 17.2 Biventricular wall motion abnormalities (WMA) in a patient with arrhythmogenic right ventricular cardiomyopathy (ARVC) and left ventricular (LV) involvement seen at steady-state free precession (SSFP) imaging. End-diastole (**a**, **c**), end-systole (**b**, **d**). Four-chamber off-axis (**a**, **b**), and short-axis (**c**, **d**) slices. Note RV end-systolic bulging areas in b and d (*arrows*). Apical LV hypokinesis is also present

17.2.3 Cine CMR

Cine CMR with gradient recall echo (GRE) or steady-state free precession (SSFP) sequences may be used to assess RV volumes in ARVC with good interobserver correlation ($r=0.90$ for LV, and $r=0.89$ for RV volumes) [3]. Quantitative RV evaluation by CMR may have a high sensitivity and specificity for ARVC diagnosis [22]. Cine CMR is also useful in assessing wall motion. RV morphological abnormalities found at cine CMR are important findings in ARVC and are frequently found in the midcavity and basal regions of the RV [23–26] (Fig. 17.2, Clips 17.1 and 17.2). Regional functional abnormalities correlate with areas of signal abnormality, and the association of both types of abnormality is more suggestive of ARVC than either of them alone [27]. Cine-CMR-derived quantitative [end-diastolic and end-systolic volumes and ejection fraction (EF)] and qualitative (WMA) parameters are highly reproducible [28].

17.2.4 Left Ventricular Involvement

CMR assessment of LV involvement using volume analysis and LGE imaging is integral to delineation of distinct patterns of disease expression [29]. Correlation of electrocardiogram (ECG), arrhythmia, and CMR findings in ARVC patients revealed three patterns of disease expression: (1) classic, with isolated RV disease or LV involvement in association with significant RV impairment; (2) LDAC, with early and prominent LV manifestations and relatively mild right-sided disease; (3) biventricular, characterized by parallel involvement of both ventricles. In the well-recognized classic form of the disease, LV LGE is observed in the setting of global RV dysfunction, with a predilection for the inferolateral wall and the inferior wall–septal junction, consistent with reports from pathological series [29, 30]. LV dilation may also occur, but the RV is consistently more severely affected. LV LGE in ARVC is commonly found in a subepicardial or midwall distribution, in concordance with the pattern of fibrofatty substitution observed on histopathology, and is distinct from the subendocardial involvement characteristic of ischemic heart disease [29]. A study using cardiac-tagged CMR to measure regional circumferential strain showed that ARVC is associated with regional LV dysfunction, which appears to parallel the degree of RV dysfunction [31].

17.2.5 Diagnostic Accuracy of Cardiac Magnetic Resonance

CMR is a valuable component of the diagnostic workup for ARVC. Sensitivity and specificity of 100 and 29 %, respectively, are reported in patients fulfilling Task Force Criteria, and 96 and 78 %, respectively, in genotyped individuals when the exam is performed with a dedicated protocol by experienced specialists [21]. Combining multiple diagnostic criteria for ARVC yields the highest diagnostic accuracy [32].

In 2010, a revision of the Task Force Criteria for the Diagnosis of ARVC was published [14], suggesting RV dilation and severe regional WMA as imaging criteria to establish evidence for the disease. Compared with the original Task Force Criteria [33], this revision seemed to maintain a high specificity without improving sensitivity for identifying early forms of ARVC.

17.2.6 Limitations

CMR was found to be a potentially frequent cause of misdiagnosis of ARVC due to overreliance on the presence of intramyocardial fat/wall thinning assessed by this technique in the absence of other Task Force Criteria [9]. RV wall motion must also be carefully evaluated, as abnormalities have been reported in >93 % of healthy individuals undergoing CMR for RV evaluation [34]. False-positive diagnosis by CMR may primarily be related to perceived motion abnormalities not seen by RV angiography [35]. The importance of expert interpretation of the complex-shaped RV and the need for quantitation of RV structure and function were emphasized by the North American

Multidisciplinary Study of ARVC, as the authors of that study reported a high rate of high-false-positive CMR scans read by less experienced referral centers [36].

17.3 Computed Tomography

Whereas CMR is the imaging tool of choice in ARVC, computed tomography (CT) may also show the typical findings of RV dilatation, reduced EF, and fatty infiltration in the RV free wall and interventricular septum [37–41]. As with CMR, fatty infiltration of the RV free wall is not specific to ARVC and was found in 17–40 % of patients affected by other pathologies [42–44].

17.4 Single-Photon-Emission Computed Tomography

Decreased RV EF, RV dilatation, nonsynchronized contraction of the ventricles, increased RV contraction dispersion, presence of segmental RV wall motion disorders and/or phase delays, and—occasionally—regional LV abnormalities may be demonstrated in ARVC patients by gated-blood-pool single-photon-emission CT (SPECT) [45]. In addition, LV involvement in ARVC may be seen as perfusion defects at thallium-201 radiochemical thallium chloride [(^{201})Tl] SPECT [46]. Abnormal adrenergic innervation occurred frequently in ARVC patients and was associated with a higher incidence of recurrent ventricular tachyarrhythmias [47]. LV involvement may also be detected at early stages with [^{123}]I-metaiodobenzylguanidine ([^{123}]I-MIBG) SPECT [48].

17.5 Positron Emission Tomography

Positron emission tomography (PET) was scarcely used in the setting of ARVC. Reduced myocardial beta-adrenergic receptor density, and impaired hyperemic myocardial blood flow with increased coronary vascular resistance were found [49, 50].

17.6 Right Ventricular Angiography

RV angiography was initially regarded as the imaging standard for ARVC diagnosis [51–53]. However, it is now regarded as an alternative modality when CMR is contraindicated and echocardiography is nondiagnostic. A variety of structural and morphological RV angiographic features are suggestive of ARVC [54–57]. Localized morphologic and contraction abnormalities of the RV free wall, such as bulges, akinetic areas, or the so-called "stack–of-plates" sign (hypertrophic trabeculae separated by deep fissures), are commonly found [55, 58]. Computed angiography may also provide objective measurements (RV volumes and EF), which are helpful in diagnosing ARVC [59, 60].

References

1. van der Wall EE, Kayser HW, Bootsma MM et al (2000) Arrhythmogenic right ventricular dysplasia: MRI findings. Herz 25:356–364
2. Wolf JE, Rose-Pittet L, Page E et al (1989) Detection of parietal lesions using magnetic resonance imaging in arrhythmogenic dysplasia of the right ventricle. Arch Mal Coeur Vaiss 82:1711–1717
3. Auffermann W, Wichter T, Breithardt G et al (1993) Arrhythmogenic right ventricular disease: MR imaging vs angiography. AJR Am J Roentgenol 161:549–555
4. Blake LM, Scheinman MM, Higgins CB (1994) MR features of arrhythmogenic right ventricular dysplasia. AJR Am J Roentgenol 162:809–812
5. Ricci C, Longo R, Pagnan L et al (1992) Magnetic resonance imaging in right ventricular dysplasia. Am J Cardiol 70:1589–1595
6. Menghetti L, Basso C, Nava A et al (1996) Spin-echo nuclear magnetic resonance for tissue characterisation in arrhythmogenic right ventricular cardiomyopathy. Heart 76:467–470
7. Castillo E, Tandri H, Rodriguez ER et al (2004) Arrhythmogenic right ventricular dysplasia: ex vivo and in vivo fat detection with black-blood MR imaging. Radiology 232:38–48
8. Abbara S, Migrino RQ, Sosnovik DE et al (2004) Value of fat suppression in the MRI evaluation of suspected arrhythmogenic right ventricular dysplasia. AJR Am J Roentgenol 182:587–591
9. Bomma C, Rutberg J, Tandri H et al (2004) Misdiagnosis of arrhythmogenic right ventricular dysplasia/cardiomyopathy. J Cardiovasc Electrophysiol 15:300–306
10. Kimura F, Matsuo Y, Nakajima T et al (2010) Myocardial fat at cardiac imaging: how can we differentiate pathologic from physiologic fatty infiltration? Radiographics 30:1587–1602
11. Macedo R, Prakasa K, Tichnell C et al (2007) Marked lipomatous infiltration of the right ventricle: MRI findings in relation to arrhythmogenic right ventricular dysplasia. AJR Am J Roentgenol 188:W423–W427
12. Tandri H, Calkins H, Marcus FI (2003) Controversial role of magnetic resonance imaging in the diagnosis of arrhythmogenic right ventricular dysplasia. Am J Cardiol 92:649
13. McKenna WJ, Thiene G, Nava A et al (1994) Diagnosis of arrhythmogenic right ventricular dysplasia/cardiomyopathy. Task Force of the Working Group Myocardial and Pericardial Disease of the European Society of Cardiology and of the Scientific Council on Cardiomyopathies of the International Society and Federation of Cardiology. Br Heart J 71:215–218
14. Marcus FI, McKenna WJ, Sherrill D et al (2010) Diagnosis of arrhythmogenic right ventricular cardiomyopathy/dysplasia: proposed modification of the task force criteria. Circulation 121:1533–1541
15. Tandri H, Saranathan M, Rodriguez ER et al (2005) Noninvasive detection of myocardial fibrosis in arrhythmogenic right ventricular cardiomyopathy using delayed-enhancement magnetic resonance imaging. J Am Coll Cardiol 45:98–103
16. Hunold P, Wieneke H, Bruder O et al (2005) Late enhancement: a new feature in MRI of arrhythmogenic right ventricular cardiomyopathy? J Cardiovasc Magn Reson 7:649–655
17. Sen-Chowdhry S, Prasad SK, McKenna WJ (2005) Arrhythmogenic right ventricular cardiomyopathy with fibrofatty atrophy, myocardial oedema, and aneurysmal dilation. Heart 91:784
18. Nijveldt R, Beek AM, Germans T et al (2007) Arrhythmogenic right ventricular cardiomyopathy with evidence of biventricular involvement. CMAJ 176:1819–1821
19. Pfluger HB, Phrommintikul A, Mariani JA et al (2008) Utility of myocardial fibrosis and fatty infiltration detected by cardiac magnetic resonance imaging in the diagnosis of arrhythmogenic right ventricular dysplasia–a single centre experience. Heart Lung Circ 17:478–483
20. Norman M, Simpson M, Mogensen J et al (2005) Novel mutation in desmoplakin causes arrhythmogenic left ventricular cardiomyopathy. Circulation 112:636–642
21. Sen-Chowdhry S, Prasad SK, Syrris P et al (2006) Cardiovascular magnetic resonance in arrhythmogenic right ventricular cardiomyopathy revisited: comparison with task force criteria and genotype. J Am Coll Cardiol 48:2132–2140

22. Tandri H, Macedo R, Calkins H et al (2008) Role of magnetic resonance imaging in arrhythmogenic right ventricular dysplasia: insights from the North American arrhythmogenic right ventricular dysplasia (ARVD/C) study. Am Heart J 155:147–153
23. Bluemke DA, Krupinski EA, Ovitt T et al (2003) MR Imaging of arrhythmogenic right ventricular cardiomyopathy: morphologic findings and interobserver reliability. Cardiology 99:153–162
24. Tandri H, Calkins H, Nasir K et al (2003) Magnetic resonance imaging findings in patients meeting task force criteria for arrhythmogenic right ventricular dysplasia. J Cardiovasc Electrophysiol 14:476–482
25. Bomma C, Dalal D, Tandri H et al (2005) Regional differences in systolic and diastolic function in arrhythmogenic right ventricular dysplasia/cardiomyopathy using magnetic resonance imaging. Am J Cardiol 95:1507–1511
26. Molinari G, Sardanelli F, Gaita F et al (1995) Right ventricular dysplasia as a generalized cardiomyopathy? Findings on magnetic resonance imaging. Eur Heart J 16:1619–1624
27. Tandri H, Bomma C, Calkins H et al (2004) Magnetic resonance and computed tomography imaging of arrhythmogenic right ventricular dysplasia. J Magn Reson Imaging 19:848–858
28. Tandri H, Castillo E, Ferrari VA et al (2006) Magnetic resonance imaging of arrhythmogenic right ventricular dysplasia: sensitivity, specificity, and observer variability of fat detection versus functional analysis of the right ventricle. J Am Coll Cardiol 48:2277–2284
29. Sen-Chowdhry S, Syrris P, Ward D et al (2007) Clinical and genetic characterization of families with arrhythmogenic right ventricular dysplasia/cardiomyopathy provides novel insights into patterns of disease expression. Circulation 115:1710–1720
30. Corrado D, Basso C, Thiene G et al (1997) Spectrum of clinicopathologic manifestations of arrhythmogenic right ventricular cardiomyopathy/dysplasia: a multicenter study. J Am Coll Cardiol 30:1512–1520
31. Jain A, Shehata ML, Stuber M et al (2010) Prevalence of left ventricular regional dysfunction in arrhythmogenic right ventricular dysplasia: a tagged MRI study. Circ Cardiovasc Imaging 3:290–297
32. Maksimovic R, Ekinci O, Reiner C et al (2006) The value of magnetic resonance imaging for the diagnosis of arrhythmogenic right ventricular cardiomyopathy. Eur Radiol 16:560–568
33. Vermes E, Strohm O, Otmani A et al (2011) Impact of the revision of arrhythmogenic right ventricular cardiomyopathy/dysplasia task force criteria on its prevalence by CMR criteria. JACC Cardiovasc Imaging 4:282–287
34. Sievers B, Addo M, Franken U et al (2004) Right ventricular wall motion abnormalities found in healthy subjects by cardiovascular magnetic resonance imaging and characterized with a new segmental model. J Cardiovasc Magn Reson 6:601–608
35. White JB, Razmi R, Nath H et al (2004) Relative utility of magnetic resonance imaging and right ventricular angiography to diagnose arrhythmogenic right ventricular cardiomyopathy. J Interv Card Electrophysiol 10:19–26
36. Marcus FI, Zareba W, Calkins H et al (2009) Arrhythmogenic right ventricular cardiomyopathy/dysplasia clinical presentation and diagnostic evaluation: results from the North American Multidisciplinary Study. Heart Rhythm 6:984–992
37. Villa A, Di Guglielmo L, Salerno J et al (1988) Arrhythmogenic dysplasia of the right ventricle. Evaluation of 7 cases using computerized tomography. Radiol Med 75:28–35
38. Sotozono K, Imahara S, Masuda H et al (1990) Detection of fatty tissue in the myocardium by using computerized tomography in a patient with arrhythmogenic right ventricular dysplasia. Heart Vessels Suppl 5:59–61
39. Hamada S, Takamiya M, Ohe T et al (1993) Arrhythmogenic right ventricular dysplasia: evaluation with electron-beam CT. Radiology 187:723–727
40. Tada H, Shimizu W, Ohe T et al (1996) Usefulness of electron-beam computed tomography in arrhythmogenic right ventricular dysplasia. Relationship to electrophysiological abnormalities and left ventricular involvement. Circulation 94:437–444
41. Bomma C, Dalal D, Tandri H et al (2007) Evolving role of multidetector computed tomography in evaluation of arrhythmogenic right ventricular dysplasia/cardiomyopathy. Am J Cardiol 100:99–105

42. Kirsch J, Williamson EE, Glockner JF (2008) Focal macroscopic fat deposition within the right ventricular wall in asymptomatic patients undergoing screening EBCT coronary calcium scoring examinations. Int J Cardiovasc Imaging 24:223–227

43. Hori Y, Funabashi N, Uehara M et al (2010) Positive influence of aging on the occurrence of fat replacement in the right ventricular myocardium determined by multislice-CT in subjects with atherosclerosis. Int J Cardiol 142:152–158

44. Imada M, Funabashi N, Asano M et al (2007) Epidemiology of fat replacement of the right ventricular myocardium determined by multislice computed tomography using a logistic regression model. Int J Cardiol 119:410–413

45. Casset-Senon D, Philippe L, Babuty D et al (1998) Diagnosis of arrhythmogenic right ventricular cardiomyopathy by Fourier analysis of gated blood pool single-photon emission tomography. Am J Cardiol 82:1399–1404

46. Lindstrom L, Nylander E, Larsson H et al (2005) Left ventricular involvement in arrhythmogenic right ventricular cardiomyopathy – a scintigraphic and echocardiographic study. Clin Physiol Funct Imaging 25:171–177

47. Paul M, Wichter T, Kies P et al (2011) Cardiac sympathetic dysfunction in genotyped patients with arrhythmogenic right ventricular cardiomyopathy and risk of recurrent ventricular tachyarrhythmias. J Nucl Med 52:1559–1565

48. Takahashi N, Ishida Y, Maeno M et al (1997) Noninvasive identification of left ventricular involvements in arrhythmogenic right ventricular dysplasia: comparison of 123I-MIBG, 201TlCl, magnetic resonance imaging and ultrafast computed tomography. Ann Nucl Med 11:233–241

49. Wichter T, Schafers M, Rhodes CG et al (2000) Abnormalities of cardiac sympathetic innervation in arrhythmogenic right ventricular cardiomyopathy: quantitative assessment of presynaptic norepinephrine reuptake and postsynaptic beta-adrenergic receptor density with positron emission tomography. Circulation 101:1552–1558

50. Paul M, Rahbar K, Gerss J et al (2012) Microvascular dysfunction in nonfailing arrhythmogenic right ventricular cardiomyopathy. Eur J Nucl Med Mol Imaging 39:416–420

51. Marcus FI, Fontaine GH, Guiraudon G et al (1982) Right ventricular dysplasia: a report of 24 adult cases. Circulation 65:384–398

52. Reiter MJ, Smith WM, Gallagher JJ (1983) Clinical spectrum of ventricular tachycardia with left bundle branch morphology. Am J Cardiol 51:113–121

53. Robertson JH, Bardy GH, German LD et al (1985) Comparison of two-dimensional echocardiographic and angiographic findings in arrhythmogenic right ventricular dysplasia. Am J Cardiol 55:1506–1508

54. Drobinski G, Verdiere C, Fontaine GH et al (1985) Angiocardiographic diagnosis in right ventricular dysplasias. Arch Mal Coeur Vaiss 78:544–551

55. Daubert C, Descaves C, Foulgoc JL et al (1988) Critical analysis of cineangiographic criteria for diagnosis of arrhythmogenic right ventricular dysplasia. Am Heart J 115:448–459

56. Rossi P, Massumi A, Gillette P et al (1982) Arrhythmogenic right ventricular dysplasia: clinical features, diagnostic techniques, and current management. Am Heart J 103:415–420

57. Rowland E, McKenna WJ, Sugrue D et al (1984) Ventricular tachycardia of left bundle branch block configuration in patients with isolated right ventricular dilatation. Clinical and electrophysiological features. Br Heart J 51:15–24

58. Daliento L, Rizzoli G, Thiene G et al (1990) Diagnostic accuracy of right ventriculography in arrhythmogenic right ventricular cardiomyopathy. Am J Cardiol 66:741–745

59. Indik JH, Wichter T, Gear K et al (2008) Quantitative assessment of angiographic right ventricular wall motion in arrhythmogenic right ventricular dysplasia/cardiomyopathy (ARVD/C). J Cardiovasc Electrophysiol 19:39–45

60. Indik JH, Dallas WJ, Gear K et al (2012) Right ventricular volume analysis by angiography in right ventricular cardiomyopathy. Int J Cardiovasc Imaging 28:995–1001

Arrhythmogenic Right Ventricular Cardiomyopathy: Usefulness of Imaging in Prognostic Stratification and Choice of Treatment

18

Francesca Brun, Concetta Di Nora, Massimo Zecchin, Bruno Pinamonti, and Gianfranco Sinagra

18.1 Introduction

Since the first description of arrhythmogenic right ventricular cardiomyopathy (ARVC) more than 30 years ago [1], considerable progress has been made in understating its pathogenesis, genetics, and diagnosis. Nevertheless, large prospective randomized trials on risk predictors and prognostic stratification are not available yet. Consequently, therapeutic recommendations for this disease have been developed from observational studies and case series or adopted from other cardiomyopathies (CMP) [2] in which solid evidence is supported by clinical trials and clear guidelines are defined [3, 4].

The choice of treatment in ARVC, therefore, is often an individualized decision based on patient presentation, risk assessment, and physician judgment [5]. The mortality rate of ARVC patients on medical therapy is estimated to be ~1.8 % (0.08–3.6 %) per year. Of note, in a meta-analysis reporting on about 600 ARVC patients who received an implantable cardioverter defibrillator (ICD)—for both primary and secondary prevention of sudden death (SD)—the annualized cardiac mortality rate was 0.9 %, whereas the annualized appropriate ICD intervention rate was 9.5 % [6].

ICD implantation, however, incurs potential risk for complications—mostly due to lead placement and inappropriate ICD interventions—occurring at a considerably high rate (4.4 and 3.7 % per year, respectively). These data suggest that accurate patient selection is necessary in order to identify high- versus low-risk

Electronic supplementary material The online version of this chapter (doi: 10.1007/978-3-319-06019-4_18) contains supplementary material, which is available to authorized users. Videos can also be accessed at http://www.springerimages.com/videos/978-3-319-06018-7.

F. Brun (✉) • C. Di Nora • M. Zecchin • B. Pinamonti, MD • G. Sinagra, MD, FESC
Department of Cardiology, University Hospital of Trieste, Via P Valdoni, n° 7,
Trieste 34149, Italy
e-mail: frabrun77@gmail.com; concetta.dinora@gmail.com; bruno.pinamonti@gmail.com; gianfranco.sinagra@aots.sanita.fvg.it

B. Pinamonti, G. Sinagra (eds.), *Clinical Echocardiography and Other Imaging Techniques in Cardiomyopathies*, DOI 10.1007/978-3-319-06019-4_18,
© Springer International Publishing Switzerland 2014

subgroups. Thus, a multiparametric evaluation of the patient is needed, and different scoring systems have been proposed [6]. Moreover, indications for ICD therapy for primary prevention of SD in heart diseases pertain to specific inclusion criteria based on left ventricular ejection fraction (LVEF) and mainly in patients with ischemic heart disease [7–9].

As opposed to the other CMP in which the cutoff of LVEF $\leq$35 % is a marker for disease severity and is used to guide treatment decisions, ARVC lacks similar objective criteria. As known, it is not a unique entity but a complex disease with three possible patterns of presentation: the classic right dominant (39 % of cases), the left-dominant arrhythmogenic CMP (5 %), and the biventricular (56 %) form [10, 11].

The most challenging clinical dilemma is not whether to treat patients who already experienced malignant ventricular arrhythmias (secondary prevention) but to consider prophylactic treatment in patients with no or only minor symptoms (primary prevention). In this regard, current guidelines are scant, and the indications for prophylactic ICD therapy in primary prevention are still unresolved. Therefore, the actual challenge is to provide sensitive and specific clinical and imaging parameters helpful in identifying patients with a high probability of SD. Several risk factors are considered in the literature, including male gender, young age at presentation, one or more affected family member with SD, unexplained syncope, electrocardiogram (ECG) abnormalities, detection of nonsustained ventricular tachycardia (VT) on noninvasive monitoring, echocardiographic findings (severe RV dilation and LV involvement), and induction of VT during electrophysiological testing [5, 12–18].

Although it is important to consider the presence of a malignant family history, genotype information is not generally included in the decision regarding ICD implantation, as it is not known conclusively whether the disease course is influenced by genotype. Nevertheless, genetic information is prognostically useful in selected patients. For example, in ARVC5, mutation of the *TMEM43* gene causes a fully penetrant disease variant with lethal arrhythmic outcome [19]; patients with Naxos disease, also characterized by palmoplantar keratosis and woolly hair; and other recessive forms of ARVC (Chap. 19) may be at an increased risk of SD and be candidates for ICD implantation in primary prevention [5, 13, 20, 21]. In addition, in a large ARVC cohort, Rigato et al. found that to be a carrier of more than one gene mutation (compound-digenic heterozygosity) constitutes a powerful risk factor for lifetime major arrhythmic events and SD [22]; similar data were reported in HCM [23] (Chap. 9).

- Male gender and young age at onset, as confirmed in several studies, is a subgroup of patients at increased risk of SD [24–26]. Similarly, unexplained syncopal episodes suggest the presence of major ventricular arrhythmias. The value of syncope as a prognostic factor for SD was first reported by Marcus et al. [27], later considered by Turrini et al. [28], and recently further confirmed by Silvano et al. [29].
- The role of ECG in risk stratification is demonstrated in different studies. Turrini et al. [28] reported that right precordial QRS prolongation correlates with an increased arrhythmic risk in ARVC patients. Moreover, a QRS dispersion >40 ms had a good sensitivity and specificity (90 and 77 %, respectively) in predicting SD.
- Concerning ventricular arrhythmias, Bhonsale et al. [30] demonstrated that nonsustained VT or frequent premature ventricular contractions (>1,000/24 h) on

Holter monitoring were predictors of appropriate ICD discharge at univariate analysis. Furthermore nonsustained VT was the only independent predictor found on multivariable analysis. The role of electrophysiologic studies with programmed ventricular stimulation remains controversial. Indeed, in the Darvin II study [31], this test had poor accuracy in predicting appropriate ICD interventions. Contrasting data came from the study of Bhonsale et al. [30], who reported that VT inducibility was a strong predictor of appropriate ICD discharge.

In conclusion, ICD implantation is considered a reasonable choice in ARVC in the presence of one or more of the following risk factors for SD (Class IIa, level of evidence C): (1) severe RV dysfunction and/or LV involvement (*see* below); (2) one or more affected family members with SD; (3) unexplained syncope of suspected arrhythmic origin [5] (Table 18.1).

18.2   Role of Imaging in Prognostic Stratification

Imaging tests show that RV dilation and regionalized or global RV hypokinesis are traits of the disease [32], but it is well established that LV involvement may occur as well [33]. The presence of RV dysfunction at diagnosis is an independent predictor of SD or heart transplantation in ARVC patients [18]. Furthermore, data from our group and a previous study [34, 35], emphasize that long-term outcome is influenced by either the presence of RV or LV dysfunction, demonstrating the incremental prognostic value of LV involvement in the risk stratification.

Another echocardiographic finding related to an adverse prognosis seems to be the presence of moderate to severe tricuspid regurgitation (TR). Interestingly, in patients with a dilated and dysfunctioning RV, TR is usually functional and secondary to RV and right atrial (RA) remodeling, and its presence potentially contributes to worsening of HF [34]. No data are available regarding the possible prognostic value of advanced echocardiographic techniques and CMR, specifically in ARVC. Nevertheless, magnetic resonance imaging (MRI) sensitivity and specificity is debated in relation to determining ARVC prognosis due to a lack of systematic comparative studies [36].

Three-dimensional electroanatomic voltage mapping provides a reliable tool by which to identify and locate low-voltage areas in the RV, corresponding to areas of fibrofatty replacement, even in patients with very early disease who display completely normal ECG and CMR findings [37]. No data are available about the prognostic role of this test in this disease.

18.3   Role of Imaging in Pharmacologic Treatment of ARVC

Antiarrhythmic medications are used for symptomatic control in patients who are not candidates for ICD or as an adjunct therapy to reduce frequent ICD discharges due to recurrent VT. The combination of beta-blockers and amiodarone has a proven beneficial effect in suppressing nonsustained VT, in reducing the frequency and rate of sustained VT, in preventing syncope, and in promoting antitachycardia pacing termination over shock therapy. Furthermore, these drugs can suppress other

Table 18.1 Risk stratification in arrhythmogenic right ventricular cardiomyopathy (ARVC)

Subgroups	Risk markers	Recommendations	Follow-up	ICD indication
Definite ARVC: high risk	Aborted SD Sustained VT Unexplained syncope	Reduce physical exercise Avoid competitive sport β-blockers	Annually, including: Electrocardiography Cardiac imaging (echocardiography vs. CMR) Holter Exercise stress testing	Recommended
Definite ARVC: moderate risk	Extensive disease (severe RV dysfunction, large LV involvement) Nonsustained VT	Reduce physical exercise Avoid competitive sport β-blockers	Annually including: Electrocardiography Cardiac imaging (echocardiography vs. CMR) Holter Exercise stress testing	Consider
Definite ARVC: low risk	Remaining patients with definite diagnosis of ARVC	Reduce physical exercise Avoid competitive sport β-blockers	Annually including: Electrocardiography Cardiac imaging (echocardiography vs. CMR) Holter Exercise stress testing	Not recommended
Asymptomatic mutation carriers	Asymptomatic mutation-carrying relatives of ARVC	Reduce physical exercise Avoid competitive sport	Annually including: Electrocardiography Cardiac imaging (echocardiography vs. CMR) Holter Exercise stress testing	Not recommended

Modified from Epstein et al. [3]

CMR cardiac magnetic resonance, *LV* left ventricle, *RV* right ventricle, *SD* sudden death, *VT* ventricular tachycardia

arrhythmias, such as supraventricular tachycardia and atrial fibrillation, which may cause symptoms or interfere with ICD function, resulting in inappropriate discharges.

In particular, sotalol and amiodarone have been proposed as effective adjunctive therapy for sustained VT or ventricular fibrillation or in patients who are not candidates for ICD implantation (class of recommendation IIa, level of evidence C) [4, 38].

Similarly, the North American ARVC Registry demonstrated that amiodarone prevents VT [39]. Conversely, our group reported that this drug is an independent predictor of mortality [40].

As with antiarrhythmic drugs, radiofrequency ablation is not a definitive therapy for ventricular arrhythmias and should not be considered as an equivalent alternative to ICD therapy in patients at high risk of SD. It can be appropriate in selecting patients who are not candidates for an ICD or who have frequent episodes of VT and ICD shocks despite antiarrhythmic therapy. Multiple studies suggest that simultaneous epicardial and endocardial approaches for VT mapping and ablation are feasible and might even result in eliminating recurrent VT. This could be explained by the preferential subepicardial involvement of the disease [41].

Imaging data can be helpful for treatment choices in selected ARVC patients. The presence of severe RV dilation and systolic dysfunction may increase the risk of thrombosis and subsequent embolism; consequently, anticoagulant treatment should be considered in ARVC patients with dilated and hypokinetic RV and slow blood flow within the RV [42], as well as in the presence of severe biventricular involvement. Furthermore, ARVC in the advanced stage, characterized by the presence of severe biventricular dysfunction and signs and symptoms of HF, can require the introduction of standard drugs recommended in HF management, such as beta-blockers, angiotensin-converting enzyme inhibitors, and diuretics [43]. Finally, heart transplantation must be considered in patients with refractory HF and recurrent arrhythmic storms despite optimal treatment, including ICD [44].

Conclusion

In conclusion, ARVC—at least, in some affected patients—is a progressive disease with life-threatening complications that constitutes a clinical challenge for physicians given the different genotypic and phenotypic variations and the wide range of clinical manifestations of the disease. ARVC management is primarily aimed at reducing the burden of symptomatic arrhythmias and decreasing the incidence of SD. Automatic ICD significantly reduces mortality in patients with ARVC, as in patients with other heart diseases involving high arrhythmic risk.

The main unresolved challenge for physicians is to improve risk stratification to better identify those patients at high risk of SD and HF who will most benefit from early intervention with lifestyle changes, restriction of physical activity, antiarrhythmic drugs, ICD placement, new ablation approaches with simultaneous endocardial and epicardial ablation, and, if necessary, heart transplantation. Further investigations and prospective studies on genetic tests, environmental factors, molecular pathways, and refinements of imaging techniques with prognostic value are necessary for better management of the disease.

References

1. Marcus FI, Fontaine GH, Guiraudon G, Frank R, Laurenceau JL, Malergue C, Grosgogeat Y (1982) Right ventricular dysplasia: a report of 24 adult cases. Circulation 65(2):384–398
2. Hauer RN, Aliot E, Block M, Capucci A, Luderitz B, Santini M, Vardas PE (2001) Indications for implantable cardioverter defibrillator (ICD) therapy. Study Group on Guidelines on ICDs of the Working Group on Arrhythmias and the Working Group on Cardiac Pacing of the European Society of Cardiology. Eur Heart J 22(13):1074–1081. doi:10.1053/euhj.2001.2584
3. Epstein AE, DiMarco JP, Ellenbogen KA, Estes NA 3rd, Freedman RA, Gettes LS, Gillinov AM, Gregoratos G, Hammill SC, Hayes DL, Hlatky MA, Newby LK, Page RL, Schoenfeld MH, Silka MJ, Stevenson LW, Sweeney MO, Smith SC Jr, Jacobs AK, Adams CD, Anderson JL, Buller CE, Creager MA, Ettinger SM, Faxon DP, Halperin JL, Hiratzka LF, Hunt SA, Krumholz HM, Kushner FG, Lytle BW, Nishimura RA, Ornato JP, Riegel B, Tarkington LG, Yancy CW (2008) ACC/AHA/HRS 2008 guidelines for device-based therapy of cardiac rhythm abnormalities: a report of the American College of Cardiology/American Heart Association Task Force on Practice Guidelines (Writing Committee to Revise the ACC/AHA/NASPE 2002 Guideline Update for Implantation of Cardiac Pacemakers and Antiarrhythmia Devices): developed in collaboration with the American Association for Thoracic Surgery and Society of Thoracic Surgeons. Circulation 117(21):e350–e408. doi:10.1161/CIRCUALTIONAHA.108.189742
4. Zipes DP, Camm AJ, Borggrefe M, Buxton AE, Chaitman B, Fromer M, Gregoratos G, Klein G, Moss AJ, Myerburg RJ, Priori SG, Quinones MA, Roden DM, Silka MJ, Tracy C, Smith SC Jr, Jacobs AK, Adams CD, Antman EM, Anderson JL, Hunt SA, Halperin JL, Nishimura R, Ornato JP, Page RL, Riegel B, Blanc JJ, Budaj A, Dean V, Deckers JW, Despres C, Dickstein K, Lekakis J, McGregor K, Metra M, Morais J, Osterspey A, Tamargo JL, Zamorano JL (2006) ACC/AHA/ESC 2006 guidelines for management of patients with ventricular arrhythmias and the prevention of sudden cardiac death: a report of the American College of Cardiology/American Heart Association Task Force and the European Society of Cardiology Committee for Practice Guidelines (Writing Committee to Develop Guidelines for Management of Patients With Ventricular Arrhythmias and the Prevention of Sudden Cardiac Death). J Am Coll Cardiol 48(5):e247–e346. doi:10.1016/j.jacc.2006.07.010
5. Epstein AE, DiMarco JP, Ellenbogen KA, Estes NA 3rd, Freedman RA, Gettes LS, Gillinov AM, Gregoratos G, Hammill SC, Hayes DL, Hlatky MA, Newby LK, Page RL, Schoenfeld MH, Silka MJ, Stevenson LW, Sweeney MO, Smith SC Jr, Jacobs AK, Adams CD, Anderson JL, Buller CE, Creager MA, Ettinger SM, Faxon DP, Halperin JL, Hiratzka LF, Hunt SA, Krumholz HM, Kushner FG, Lytle BW, Nishimura RA, Ornato JP, Riegel B, Tarkington LG, Yancy CW (2008) ACC/AHA/HRS 2008 guidelines for device-based therapy of cardiac rhythm abnormalities: a report of the American College of Cardiology/American Heart Association Task Force on Practice Guidelines (Writing Committee to Revise the ACC/AHA/NASPE 2002 Guideline Update for Implantation of Cardiac Pacemakers and Antiarrhythmia Devices) developed in collaboration with the American Association for Thoracic Surgery and Society of Thoracic Surgeons. J Am Coll Cardiol 51(21):e1–e62. doi:10.1016/j.jacc.2008.02.032
6. Schinkel AF (2013) Implantable cardioverter defibrillators in arrhythmogenic right ventricular dysplasia/cardiomyopathy: patient outcomes, incidence of appropriate and inappropriate interventions, and complications. Circ Arrhythm Electrophysiol 6(3):562–568. doi:10.1161/CIRCEP.113.000392
7. Saxon LA, Bristow MR, Boehmer J, Krueger S, Kass DA, De Marco T, Carson P, DiCarlo L, Feldman AM, Galle E, Ecklund F (2006) Predictors of sudden cardiac death and appropriate shock in the Comparison of Medical Therapy, Pacing, and Defibrillation in Heart Failure (COMPANION) Trial. Circulation 114(25):2766–2772. doi:10.1161/CIRCULATIONAHA.106.642892
8. Buxton AE, Lee KL, Fisher JD, Josephson ME, Prystowsky EN, Hafley G (1999) A randomized study of the prevention of sudden death in patients with coronary artery disease. Multicenter Unsustained Tachycardia Trial Investigators. N Engl J Med 341(25):1882–1890. doi:10.1056/NEJM199912163412503

9. Pires LA, Hafley GE, Lee KL, Fisher JD, Josephson ME, Prystowsky EN, Buxton AE (2002) Prognostic significance of nonsustained ventricular tachycardia identified postoperatively after coronary artery bypass surgery in patients with left ventricular dysfunction. J Cardiovasc Electrophysiol 13(8):757–763

10. Sen-Chowdhry S, Syrris P, Ward D, Asimaki A, Sevdalis E, McKenna WJ (2007) Clinical and genetic characterization of families with arrhythmogenic right ventricular dysplasia/cardiomyopathy provides novel insights into patterns of disease expression. Circulation 115(13):1710–1720. doi:10.1161/CIRCULATIONAHA.106.660241

11. Sen-Chowdhry S, Lowe MD, Sporton SC, McKenna WJ (2004) Arrhythmogenic right ventricular cardiomyopathy: clinical presentation, diagnosis, and management. Am J Med 117(9):685–695. doi:10.1016/j.amjmed.2004.04.028

12. Corrado D, Leoni L, Link MS, Della Bella P, Gaita F, Curnis A, Salerno JU, Igidbashian D, Raviele A, Disertori M, Zanotto G, Verlato R, Vergara G, Delise P, Turrini P, Basso C, Naccarella F, Maddalena F, Estes NA 3rd, Buja G, Thiene G (2003) Implantable cardioverter-defibrillator therapy for prevention of sudden death in patients with arrhythmogenic right ventricular cardiomyopathy/dysplasia. Circulation 108(25):3084–3091. doi:10.1161/01.CIR.0000103130.33451.D2

13. Hodgkinson KA, Parfrey PS, Bassett AS, Kupprion C, Drenckhahn J, Norman MW, Thierfelder L, Stuckless SN, Dicks EL, McKenna WJ, Connors SP (2005) The impact of implantable cardioverter-defibrillator therapy on survival in autosomal-dominant arrhythmogenic right ventricular cardiomyopathy (ARVD5). J Am Coll Cardiol 45(3):400–408. doi:10.1016/j.jacc.2004.08.068

14. Roguin A, Bomma CS, Nasir K, Tandri H, Tichnell C, James C, Rutberg J, Crosson J, Spevak PJ, Berger RD, Halperin HR, Calkins H (2004) Implantable cardioverter-defibrillators in patients with arrhythmogenic right ventricular dysplasia/cardiomyopathy. J Am Coll Cardiol 43(10):1843–1852. doi:10.1016/j.jacc.2004.01.030

15. Tavernier R, Gevaert S, De Sutter J, De Clercq A, Rottiers H, Jordaens L, Fonteyne W (2001) Long term results of cardioverter-defibrillator implantation in patients with right ventricular dysplasia and malignant ventricular tachyarrhythmias. Heart 85(1):53–56

16. Wichter T, Paul M, Wollmann C, Acil T, Gerdes P, Ashraf O, Tjan TD, Soeparwata R, Block M, Borggrefe M, Scheld HH, Breithardt G, Bocker D (2004) Implantable cardioverter/defibrillator therapy in arrhythmogenic right ventricular cardiomyopathy: single-center experience of long-term follow-up and complications in 60 patients. Circulation 109(12):1503–1508. doi:10.1161/01.CIR.0000121738.88273.43

17. Priori SG, Aliot E, Blomstrom-Lundqvist C, Bossaert L, Breithardt G, Brugada P, Camm AJ, Cappato R, Cobbe SM, Di Mario C, Maron BJ, McKenna WJ, Pedersen AK, Ravens U, Schwartz PJ, Trusz-Gluza M, Vardas P, Wellens HJ, Zipes DP (2001) Task Force on Sudden cardiac Death of the European Society of Cardiology. Eur Heart J 22(16):1374–1450. doi:10.1053/euhj.2001.2824

18. Hulot JS, Jouven X, Empana JP, Frank R, Fontaine G (2004) Natural history and risk stratification of arrhythmogenic right ventricular dysplasia/cardiomyopathy. Circulation 110(14):1879–1884. doi:10.1161/01.CIR.0000143375.93288.82

19. Merner ND, Hodgkinson KA, Haywood AF, Connors S, French VM, Drenckhahn JD, Kupprion C, Ramadanova K, Thierfelder L, McKenna W, Gallagher B, Morris-Larkin L, Bassett AS, Parfrey PS, Young TL (2008) Arrhythmogenic right ventricular cardiomyopathy type 5 is a fully penetrant, lethal arrhythmic disorder caused by a missense mutation in the TMEM43 gene. Am J Hum Genet 82(4):809–821. doi:10.1016/j.ajhg.2008.01.010

20. Gatzoulis K, Protonotarios N, Anastasakis A, Tsatsopoulou A, Vlasseros J, Gialafos J, Toutouzas P (2000) Implantable defibrillator therapy in Naxos disease. Pacing Clin Electrophysiol 23(7):1176–1178

21. Wichter T, Breithardt G (2005) Implantable cardioverter-defibrillator therapy in arrhythmogenic right ventricular cardiomyopathy: a role for genotyping in decision-making? J Am Coll Cardiol 45(3):409–411. doi:10.1016/j.jacc.2004.11.009

22. Rigato I, Bauce B, Rampazzo A, Zorzi A, Pilichou K, Mazzotti E, Migliore F, Marra MP, Lorenzon A, De Bortoli M, Calore M, Nava A, Daliento L, Gregori D, Iliceto S, Thiene G, Basso C, Corrado D (2013) Compound and digenic heterozygosity predicts lifetime arrhythmic outcome and sudden cardiac death in desmosomal gene-related arrhythmogenic right ventricular cardiomyopathy. Circ Cardiovasc Genet 6(6):533–542. doi:10.1161/CIRCGENETICS.113.000288

23. Girolami F, Ho CY, Semsarian C, Baldi M, Will ML, Baldini K, Torricelli F, Yeates L, Cecchi F, Ackerman MJ, Olivotto I (2010) Clinical features and outcome of hypertrophic cardiomyopathy associated with triple sarcomere protein gene mutations. J Am Coll Cardiol 55(14):1444–1453. doi:10.1016/j.jacc.2009.11.062

24. Bauce B, Frigo G, Marcus FI, Basso C, Rampazzo A, Maddalena F, Corrado D, Winnicki M, Daliento L, Rigato I, Steriotis A, Mazzotti E, Thiene G, Nava A (2008) Comparison of clinical features of arrhythmogenic right ventricular cardiomyopathy in men versus women. Am J Cardiol 102(9):1252–1257. doi:10.1016/j.amjcard.2008.06.054

25. Daliento L, Turrini P, Nava A, Rizzoli G, Angelini A, Buja G, Scognamiglio R, Thiene G (1995) Arrhythmogenic right ventricular cardiomyopathy in young versus adult patients: similarities and differences. J Am Coll Cardiol 25(3):655–664. doi:10.1016/0735-1097(94)00433-Q

26. McRae AT 3rd, Chung MK, Asher CR (2001) Arrhythmogenic right ventricular cardiomyopathy: a cause of sudden death in young people. Cleve Clin J Med 68(5):459–467

27. Marcus FI, Fontaine GH, Frank R, Gallagher JJ, Reiter MJ (1989) Long-term follow-up in patients with arrhythmogenic right ventricular disease. Eur Heart J 10(Suppl D):68–73

28. Turrini P, Corrado D, Basso C, Nava A, Bauce B, Thiene G (2001) Dispersion of ventricular depolarization-repolarization: a noninvasive marker for risk stratification in arrhythmogenic right ventricular cardiomyopathy. Circulation 103(25):3075–3080

29. Silvano M, Corrado D, Kobe J, Monnig G, Basso C, Thiene G, Eckardt L (2013) Risk stratification in arrhythmogenic right ventricular cardiomyopathy. Herzschrittmacherther Elektrophysiol 24(4):202–208. doi:10.1007/s00399-013-0291-5

30. Bhonsale A, James CA, Tichnell C, Murray B, Gagarin D, Philips B, Dalal D, Tedford R, Russell SD, Abraham T, Tandri H, Judge DP, Calkins H (2011) Incidence and predictors of implantable cardioverter-defibrillator therapy in patients with arrhythmogenic right ventricular dysplasia/cardiomyopathy undergoing implantable cardioverter-defibrillator implantation for primary prevention. J Am Coll Cardiol 58(14):1485–1496. doi:10.1016/j.jacc.2011.06.043

31. Corrado D, Calkins H, Link MS, Leoni L, Favale S, Bevilacqua M, Basso C, Ward D, Boriani G, Ricci R, Piccini JP, Dalal D, Santini M, Buja G, Iliceto S, Estes NA 3rd, Wichter T, McKenna WJ, Thiene G, Marcus FI (2010) Prophylactic implantable defibrillator in patients with arrhythmogenic right ventricular cardiomyopathy/dysplasia and no prior ventricular fibrillation or sustained ventricular tachycardia. Circulation 122(12):1144–1152. doi:10.1161/CIRCULATIONAHA.109.913871

32. Marcus FI, McKenna WJ, Sherrill D, Basso C, Bauce B, Bluemke DA, Calkins H, Corrado D, Cox MG, Daubert JP, Fontaine G, Gear K, Hauer R, Nava A, Picard MH, Protonotarios N, Saffitz JE, Sanborn DM, Steinberg JS, Tandri H, Thiene G, Towbin JA, Tsatsopoulou A, Wichter T, Zareba W (2010) Diagnosis of arrhythmogenic right ventricular cardiomyopathy/dysplasia: proposed modification of the task force criteria. Circulation 121(13):1533–1541. doi:10.1161/CIRCULATIONAHA.108.840827

33. Pinamonti B, Sinagra G, Salvi A, Di Lenarda A, Morgera T, Silvestri F, Bussani R, Camerini F (1992) Left ventricular involvement in right ventricular dysplasia. Am Heart J 123(3):711–724

34. Pinamonti B, Dragos AM, Pyxaras SA, Merlo M, Pivetta A, Barbati G, Di Lenarda A, Morgera T, Mestroni L, Sinagra G (2011) Prognostic predictors in arrhythmogenic right ventricular cardiomyopathy: results from a 10-year registry. Eur Heart J 32(9):1105–1113. doi:10.1093/eurheartj/ehr040

35. Lemola K, Brunckhorst C, Helfenstein U, Oechslin E, Jenni R, Duru F (2005) Predictors of adverse outcome in patients with arrhythmogenic right ventricular dysplasia/cardiomyopathy: long term experience of a tertiary care centre. Heart 91(9):1167–1172. doi:10.1136/hrt.2004.038620

36. Deac M, Alpendurada F, Fanaie F, Vimal R, Carpenter JP, Dawson A, Miller C, Roussin I, di Pietro E, Ismail TF, Roughton M, Wong J, Dawson D, Till JA, Sheppard MN, Mohiaddin RH, Kilner PJ, Pennell DJ, Prasad SK (2013) Prognostic value of cardiovascular magnetic resonance in patients with suspected arrhythmogenic right ventricular cardiomyopathy. Int J Cardiol 168(4):3514–3521. doi:10.1016/j.ijcard.2013.04.208

37. Santangeli P, Pieroni M, Dello Russo A, Casella M, Pelargonio G, Macchione A, Camporeale A, Smaldone C, Bartoletti S, Di Biase L, Bellocci F, Natale A (2010) Noninvasive diagnosis of electroanatomic abnormalities in arrhythmogenic right ventricular cardiomyopathy. Circ Arrhythm Electrophysiol 3(6):632–638. doi:10.1161/CIRCEP.110.958116

38. Wichter T, Borggrefe M, Haverkamp W, Chen X, Breithardt G (1992) Efficacy of antiarrhythmic drugs in patients with arrhythmogenic right ventricular disease. Results in patients with inducible and noninducible ventricular tachycardia. Circulation 86(1):29–37

39. Marcus GM, Glidden DV, Polonsky B, Zareba W, Smith LM, Cannom DS, Estes NA 3rd, Marcus F, Scheinman MM (2009) Efficacy of antiarrhythmic drugs in arrhythmogenic right ventricular cardiomyopathy: a report from the North American ARVC Registry. J Am Coll Cardiol 54(7):609–615. doi:10.1016/j.jacc.2009.04.052

40. Pinamonti B, Di Lenarda A, Sinagra G, Silvestri F, Bussani R, Camerini F (1995) Long-term evolution of right ventricular dysplasia-cardiomyopathy. The Heart Muscle Disease Study Group. Am Heart J 129(2):412–415

41. Garcia FC, Bazan V, Zado ES, Ren JF, Marchlinski FE (2009) Epicardial substrate and outcome with epicardial ablation of ventricular tachycardia in arrhythmogenic right ventricular cardiomyopathy/dysplasia. Circulation 120(5):366–375. doi:10.1161/CIRCULATIONAHA.108.834903

42. Corrado D, Basso C, Nava A, Thiene G (2001) Arrhythmogenic right ventricular cardiomyopathy: current diagnostic and management strategies. Cardiol Rev 9(5):259–265

43. Yancy CW, Jessup M, Bozkurt B, Butler J, Casey DE Jr, Drazner MH, Fonarow GC, Geraci SA, Horwich T, Januzzi JL, Johnson MR, Kasper EK, Levy WC, Masoudi FA, McBride PE, McMurray JJ, Mitchell JE, Peterson PN, Riegel B, Sam F, Stevenson LW, Tang WH, Tsai EJ, Wilkoff BL (2013) 2013 ACCF/AHA guideline for the management of heart failure: a report of the American College of Cardiology Foundation/American Heart Association Task Force on practice guidelines. Circulation 128(16):e240–e319. doi:10.1161/CIR.0b013e31829e8776

44. Lacroix D, Lions C, Klug D, Prat A (2005) Arrhythmogenic right ventricular dysplasia: catheter ablation, MRI, and heart transplantation. J Cardiovasc Electrophysiol 16(2):235–236. doi:10.1046/j.1540-8167.2005.40495.x

Part V

Restrictive, Infiltrative/Storage and Other Cardiomyopathies

Restrictive Cardiomyopathy: Clinical Assessment and Imaging in Diagnosis and Patient Management

19

Marco Merlo, Elena Abate, Bruno Pinamonti,
Giancarlo Vitrella, Enrico Fabris, Francesco Negri,
Francesca Brun, Manuel Belgrano, Rossana Bussani,
and Gianfranco Sinagra

19.1 Introduction

In this chapter, clinical and imaging features of restrictive cardiomyopathy (RCM) are described. The differential diagnosis with constrictive pericarditis (CP) and the distinguishing features from infiltrative and storage cardiomyopathies (CMP) are also considered.

Electronic supplementary material The online version of this chapter (doi: 10.1007/978-3-319-06019-4_19) contains supplementary material, which is available to authorized users. Videos can also be accessed at http://www.springerimages.com/videos/978-3-319-06018-7.

M. Merlo (✉) • E. Abate • B. Pinamonti, MD • G. Vitrella
E. Fabris • F. Negri • F. Brun •
G. Sinagra, MD, FESC
Department of Cardiology, University Hospital of Trieste,
Via P. Valdoni 7, Trieste 34139, Italy
e-mail: supermerloo@libero.it; abate.elena@gmail.com; bruno.pinamonti@gmail.com;
giancarlo.vitrella@gmail.com; enrico.fabris@hotmail.it; francesco_negri@yahoo.it;
frabrun77@gmail.com; gianfranco.sinagra@aots.sanita.fvg.it

M. Belgrano, MD
Radiology Unit, University Hospital of Trieste, Via P. Valdoni 7, Trieste 34139, Italy
e-mail: belgranom@gmail.com

R. Bussani
Department of Pathology and Morbid Anatomy,
University Hospital of Trieste, Via P. Valdoni 7, Trieste 34139, Italy
e-mail: bussani@univ.trieste.it

B. Pinamonti, G. Sinagra (eds.), *Clinical Echocardiography and Other Imaging Techniques in Cardiomyopathies*, DOI 10.1007/978-3-319-06019-4_19,
© Springer International Publishing Switzerland 2014

19.2 Restrictive Cardiomyopathy

19.2.1 Clinical Assessment

The main difference between RCM and the other CMP is how they are classified: morphological criteria are used for the diagnosis of dilated (DCM), hypertrophic (HCM), and arrhythmogenic (ARVC) CMP, whereas a functional definition is used in RCM [1]. The recognition of this entity by the clinician can be a challenge because the restrictive filling pattern (RFP)—considered in the past as the typical and pathognomonic sign of RCM [2]—can be also present in patients affected by other CMP [3, 4].

Idiopathic RCM is a rare CMP characterized by myocardial fibrosis and diastolic dysfunction of one or both ventricles in the absence of significant ventricular dilatation and/or hypertrophy [1–8]. At the time of diagnosis, RCM patients are usually in an advanced functional New York Heart Association (NYHA) class. The disease can be observed at any age. Ventricular sizes are small compared with the atria, which are markedly enlarged. The left ventricle (LV) generally has preserved systolic function. No specific histologic patterns are reported in this CMP; usually, severe and widespread myocardial interstitial fibrosis is present. Genetic forms of RCM are reported with mutations in sarcomeric protein genes, similarly to other forms of CMP [5, 9]. The most important differential diagnoses that must be made are with CP and with infiltrative and storage CMP [3–5].

The distinction between these pathologies is made possible by considering clinical clues and using imaging tools and cardiac catheterization data. Clinical suspicion is fundamental and must orient the diagnostic workup and interpretation of imaging and hemodynamic data (*see* below). RCM is usually characterized by the typical dip-plateau pattern of LV diastolic pressure tracing at cardiac catheterization. In RCM—a pathologic condition that typically increases pulmonary as well as systemic capillary pressures—common clinical signs are jugular venous distention, peripheral edema, and—in the more advanced stage—ascites. No specific electrocardiographic (ECG) findings are reported. Enlargement of the P waves and atrioventricular block can be observed. Generally, the QRS voltage is normal in RCM, whereas in amyloidosis, it is usually low, especially compared with ventricular wall thickness. Chest radiography can be normal in the early stage, whereas cardiomegaly and pulmonary vascular congestion are present in the more advanced cases.

RCM is a very rare disease and, as a consequence, data on long-term survival are lacking in the literature. The disease might have a protracted course in the early phase, when patients are younger and symptoms are mild; however, older patients, with increasing symptoms and signs of systemic and pulmonary venous congestion, have the worst prognosis [6]. No specific treatment for RCM is available. Supportive therapy includes diuretics, heart-rate control to increase diastolic filling time, and maintenance of sinus rhythm. In the presence of atrial fibrillation (AF), long-term anticoagulation therapy is mandatory. The only effective intervention in patients with advanced RCM and refractory heart failure (HF) is heart transplantation [6].

Desmin CMP is a rare genetic disease that results from mutations in the intermediate filament desmin gene. Clinical presentation is heterogeneous. Cardiac phenotypes related to Desmin CMP include DCM, RCM, and, occasionally, ARVC-like

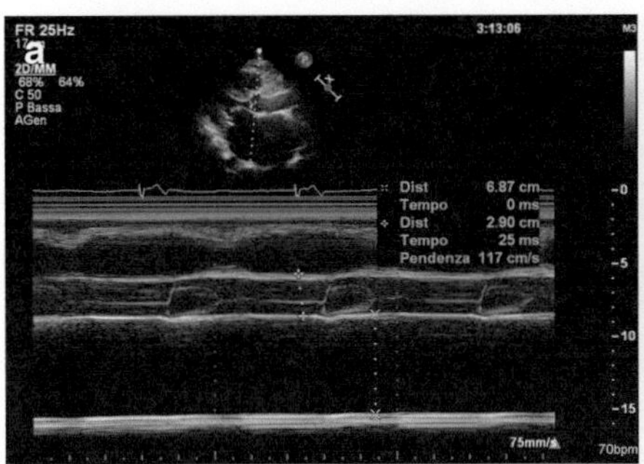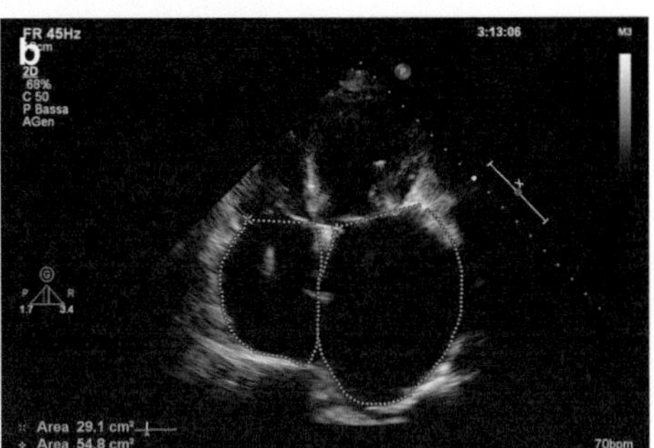

Fig. 19.1 (**a**, **b**) Echocardiographic findings in a patient with idiopathic restrictive cardiomyopathy. Severe left atrial and moderate right atrial dilation with normal ventricular dimensions and function. M-mode tracing on the left atrium (end-systolic diameter=6.87 cm) (**a**); apical four-chamber view (**b**)

forms. In cases with Desmin CMP and RCM phenotype, restriction to diastolic ventricular filling is only part of the disease, and patients usually present clinical or subclinical skeletal myopathy and varying degrees of atrioventricular blocks [10].

Some CMP, characterized by myocardial interstitial infiltration or intracellular deposition by various substances, frequently present as predominant diastolic HF and RFP, and, accordingly, are considered among RCM in some classifications [1, 5]. However, as clinical, pathologic, and imaging features of these diseases are peculiar, they are addressed in this book in a separate chapter (Chap. 20).

19.2.2 Echocardiographic Features

Echo-Doppler findings of idiopathic RCM are characterized by abnormal ventricular filling due to severe diastolic dysfunction (RFP) in the presence of normal or reduced ventricular volumes and in the absence of significant wall hypertrophy [1–3, 9]; ventricular systolic function is usually preserved, even though contractility is not totally normal, as demonstrated using advanced echocardiographic techniques (*see* below).

Echocardiographic characteristics of RCM might not be specific, particularly in the initial phases of the disease, showing only a mild left atrial (LA) dilatation [7]. In more advanced forms, both atria are severely dilated, in contrast with the normal or reduced ventricular size (Fig. 19.1, Clip 19.1a, b). In the presence of a severely dilated LA, it is rather common to identify a thrombosis in the LA appendage during transesophageal echocardiography (TEE), particularly in patients with atrial fibrillation (AF) [7].

The disease can involve both the LV and RV [11]. Wall thickness is usually normal, but in some cases, it is possible to detect mild LV or RV wall hypertrophy [12]. Various degrees of systolic dysfunction with diffuse hypokinesis can be found in more advanced disease [11] (Clip 19.2). Functional mild-to-moderate mitral (MR) and tricuspid (TR) regurgitation are frequent (Clip 19.3) [8]. The inferior vena cava is dilated with reduced inspiratory collapse, the consequence of elevated right atrial (RA) pressure (Clip 19.4).

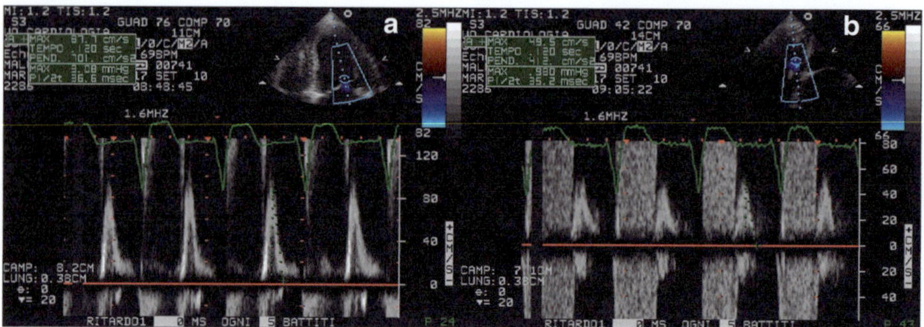

Fig. 19.2 (**a, b**) Doppler interrogation of transmitral (**a**) and tricuspid (**b**) flow showing restrictive filling pattern in a patient with restrictive cardiomyopathy and atrial fibrillation. In both cases, E-wave deceleration time was reduced to 120 ms

Typical echo-Doppler characteristics of the disease are severe diastolic dysfunction, with RFP interrogation of transmitral and/or tricuspid flow: there is a high, early diastolic E wave; a low, late diastolic A wave; and a short E-wave deceleration time, indicative of increased ventricular chamber stiffness (Fig. 19.2) [2–4, 11–13]. This transmitral and tricuspid flow pattern corresponds to the dip-plateau appearance (square root sign) of diastolic ventricular pressure curves at cardiac catheterization, i.e., abrupt, early diastolic increase of ventricular pressure followed by persistent high pressure during mid- and end-diastole (plateau) [7].

Pulmonary venous-flow Doppler shows reduced systolic wave peak velocity, increased diastolic wave peak velocity with reduced deceleration time, and accentuated and prolonged end-diastolic retrograde wave due to LA contraction against high end-diastolic ventricular pressure [14]. A similar pattern can be observed at the level of hepatic vein flow, with reverse systolic waves in the presence of severe TR, and prolonged end-diastolic retrograde flow due to increased RV end-diastolic pressure [13].

Transmitral and pulmonary vein flow Doppler patterns demonstrate good correlation with LV end-diastolic and pulmonary-wedge pressure at cardiac catheterization [3, 13], providing a semiquantitative assessment of the hemodynamic severity of the disease.

In clinical practice, it is important to recall that in some patients with RCM, treatment with diuretics may normalize the filling pattern. In this situation, RFP can be unmasked after a fluid challenge.

Tissue Doppler imaging (TDI) can be useful in the diagnostic workup of patients with suspected RCM. TDI curves on the septal or lateral mitral annulus and basal LV segments typically show low velocities of both the systolic (S′) and the early diastolic (E′) wave (Fig. 19.3). The ratio of transmitral E velocity to mitral annular E′ velocity (E/E′) is therefore high, and this is an additional marker of elevated ventricular filling pressures. Furthermore, global reduction of TDI-derived annular velocities in RCM is a sign of intrinsic myocardial disease. However, it must be remembered that these abnormalities are nonspecific.

The value of TDI in identifying initial alterations in myocardial contractility through reduced systolic velocities has been studied in RCM patients. In fact, TDI

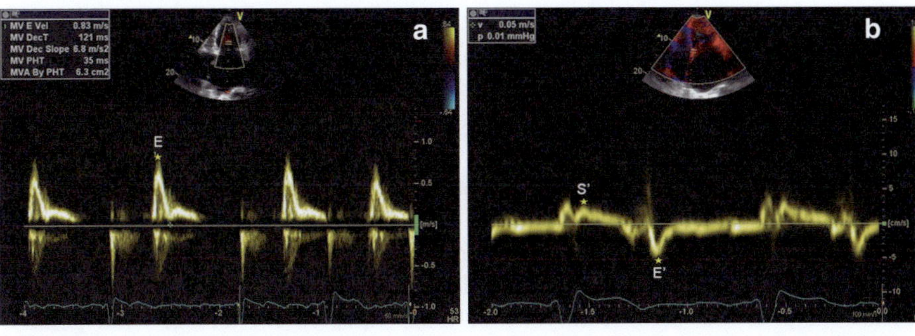

Fig. 19.3 (**a**, **b**) Patient with idiopathic restrictive cardiomyopathy. Doppler interrogation of transmitral valve (**a**) shows a restrictive filling pattern (E-wave velocity = 83 cm/s, E-wave deceleration time = 121 ms). Tissue Doppler imaging curve on the septal mitral valve annulus (**b**) shows low velocities of the systolic (S′ wave = 4 cm/s) and early diastolic (E′ wave = 5 cm/s) waves. E/E′ ratio is 16

imaging was employed to evaluate longitudinal velocities at the LV lateral wall, interventricular septum (IVS), and RV in children with RCM and normal LV ejection fraction (EF): TDI peak velocities were significantly lower at the septum in RCM patients and could therefore identify global subclinical systolic dysfunction in this setting [15].

19.2.3 Other Imaging Techniques

To our knowledge, extensive and systematic studies on cardiac magnetic resonance (CMR) or other imaging techniques in this specific CMP are lacking in published literature considering the extreme rarity of this pathology. However, some information can be obtained from of studies on distinctive features between RCM and CP. RCM is characterized at CMR and computed tomography (CT) studies by small, nonhypertrophied ventricles with preserved systolic function, enlarged atria, and severe myocardial fibrosis in the absence of pericardial abnormalities. CMR late gadolinium enhancement (LGE) and/or T1 analyses can be employed to identify myocardial fibrosis, which is the histologic hallmark of this CMP.

19.2.4 Imaging in Prognosis and Patient Management

In RCM, prognosis mainly depends on the clinical stage of the disease, which can range from an early subclinical phase to the severe advanced stage. Early recognition and a correct and specific diagnosis are essential for prognostic stratification and choice of treatment, as there is no specific therapy for idiopathic RCM; pharmacologic therapy of certain underlying diseases (such as sarcoidosis and hemochromatosis) may be beneficial. Furthermore, the differential diagnosis with CP is crucial because pericardiectomy can be the definitive treatment in this pathologic condition when it is refractory to medical treatment [16].

Treatment of idiopathic RCM is aimed at reducing pulmonary and systemic congestion. This is best achieved by lowering venous pressure, controlling heart rate, increasing filling time, maintaining atrial contractions, correcting atrioventricular conduction disturbances, and avoiding anemia, nutritional deficiency, calcium overload, and electrolyte imbalance.

In idiopathic RCM, echocardiographic evaluation can contribute to prognostic stratification of patients. In fact, patients with severe LA enlargement (dimension >60 mm) have a poor prognosis, particularly if >70 years and with advanced NYHA class [8]. In a series of 94 patients [8] followed for a mean of 68 months, estimated overall survival was significantly lower than expected for an age- and gender-matched group (64 % vs 85 % at 5 years, and 37 % vs 70 % at 10 years). Approximately two-thirds of deaths were cardiovascular, primarily due to HF, SD, or cerebrovascular accident. Survival was not related to the presence of AF, LV systolic dysfunction, or findings on endomyocardial biopsy (EMB).

Another echocardiographic feature that is important in patient management is identifying, particularly in the advanced phase of the disease and in AF, thrombi within the atrial appendages [7] due to the risk of embolic stroke and indication of prophylactic anticoagulant therapy.

19.3 Differential Diagnosis Between Restrictive Cardiomyopathy and Constrictive Pericarditis

The clinical problem of distinction between RCM and CP is one of the most challenging in cardiology and in internal medicine, despite the advances in diagnostics and imaging techniques [17–19]. The first step in the diagnostic workup is clinical suspicion. RCM or, alternatively, CP must be hypothesized if a patient shows signs of congestive HF in the absence of significant LV systolic dysfunction or valvular heart disease. Clinical history may provide important clues for the correct diagnosis. In fact, the possibility of CP must be considered in patients with a history of tuberculosis, past cardiac surgery, mediastinal irradiation, or previous pericarditis. Physical examination and ECG are usually nonspecific, and the described clinical signs of CP are extremely subtle. Chest X-ray can be useful only when it shows pericardial calcifications, which are particularly frequent in tubercular CP but rare in the other forms.

Hemodynamically, CP is characterized by impaired diastolic filling caused by the outer restriction of the pericardium, which is rigid from fibrosis and/or inflammation. Consequently, an increase in ventricular interdependence is present, as is a dissociation between intrathoracic and intracardiac pressures, thus isolating the heart from normal respiratory changes in intrathoracic pressure [19].

Doppler echocardiography can help in CP diagnosis in its differentiation from RCM. Both RCM and CP show RFP, but in CP, peak early diastolic filling velocities (E waves) of the two ventricles change and are reciprocal with respiration: tricuspid E wave velocity increases in inspiration; mitral velocity E wave decreases (Fig. 19.4) [13, 20]. This is a sign of increased ventricular interaction due to the presence of an abnormally stiff pericardium, typical of this disease and absent in RCM [13, 20].

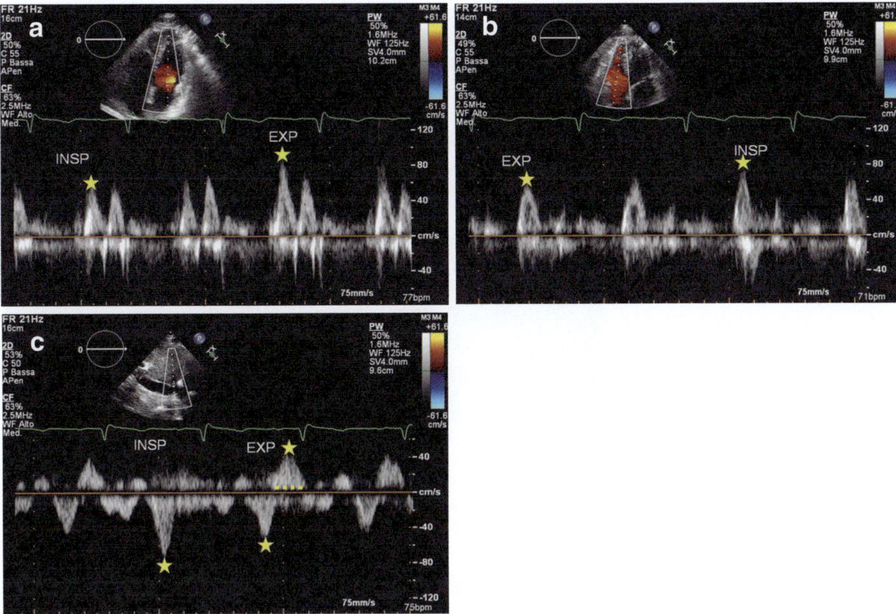

Fig. 19.4 (**a–c**) Patient with constrictive pericarditis. Mitral (**a**) and tricuspid (**b**) flow Doppler patterns show reciprocal respiratory variations: E-wave transmitral peak velocity increases with expiration; tricuspid E-wave peak velocity increases with inspiration. The hepatic vein flow Doppler (**c**) shows an increase in early diastolic wave velocity in inspiration and a prominent and prolonged end-diastolic reversal wave in expiration. *INSP* inspiration, *EXP* expiration

Furthermore, pulmonary vein flow evaluation by Doppler shows reduced forward flow during inspiration with a prominent systolic component in CP, whereas in RCM, the diastolic component is prevalent [21]. Finally, in CP hepatic vein flow on Doppler displays increase during inspiration and reduction in expiration, when there is a more prominent and prolonged end-diastolic flow reversal (Fig. 19.4) [20]. Conversely, in RCM, this flow reversal increases during inspiration.

It is important to keep in mind that some patients with CP do not demonstrate marked respiratory variations in Doppler velocities, particularly in the presence of very high filling pressure [22]. This abnormality can be unmasked by studying the patient in the upright position in order to decrease preload.

Additional echocardiographic indices have been proposed for the differential diagnosis between RCM and CP. For example, quantification of flow propagation in the LV cavity on color M-mode can be informative, and slope velocity >100 cm/s shows good accuracy in distinguishing between these two pathologies [23]. Moreover, pulmonary hypertension and diastolic MR are more likely found in RCM than in CP. On the other hand, typical characteristics of CP are abnormal diastolic septal motion with a leftward shift in inspiration, and flattening of the posterior wall in mid-diastole (Fig. 19.5, Clip 19.5) [24].

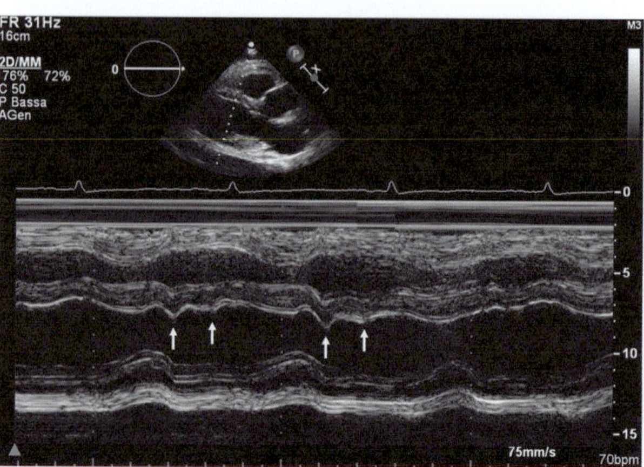

Fig. 19.5 M-mode trace in a patient with constrictive pericarditis. The posterior wall is flat during diastole, and the ventricular septum shows abnormal motion in inspiration (*double arrows*)

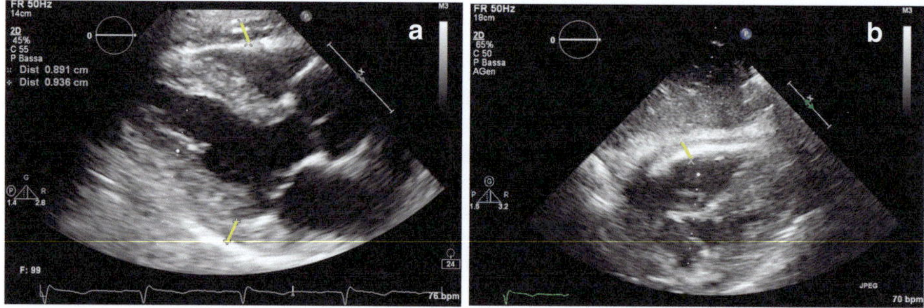

Fig. 19.6 (**a**, **b**) Echocardiographic assessment of pericardial thickening (9 mm) throughout ventricles. Parasternal long-axis (**a**) and subcostal (**b**) views in the same patient with constrictive pericarditis as in Figs. 19.4 and 19.5

Pericardial thickness assessment is another useful feature in the differential diagnosis between RCM and CP (Fig. 19.6, Clip 19.6). In particular, measuring pericardial thickness using TEE shows good correlation with that performed by CMR [25].

Novel echocardiographic techniques are particularly useful in the differential diagnosis between RCM and CP. In contrast to the global reduction in TDI-derived annular velocities seen in RCM, CP is distinguished by preserved TDI annular velocities of the LV and RV free walls, as well as of the IVS (Fig. 19.7) [26]. Peak E′ wave velocity ≥8 cm/s (in either case the septal or lateral wall) has an excellent accuracy in differentiating CP from RCM [27]. Ha et al. [28] identified a condition called annulus paradoxus in patients with CP, i.e., a paradoxical inverse correlation between low E/E′ and elevated LV filling pressures. Furthermore, other authors demonstrated that in patients with CP, E′ at the lateral mitral annulus was lower than E′ at the medial or septal mitral annulus; this condition is called *annulus reversus*, ascribed to LV free wall tethering to the pericardium [29].

However, the diagnostic value of TDI-derived annular velocities may be limited to annular-based constriction [30]. Furthermore, TDI annular velocities are reduced

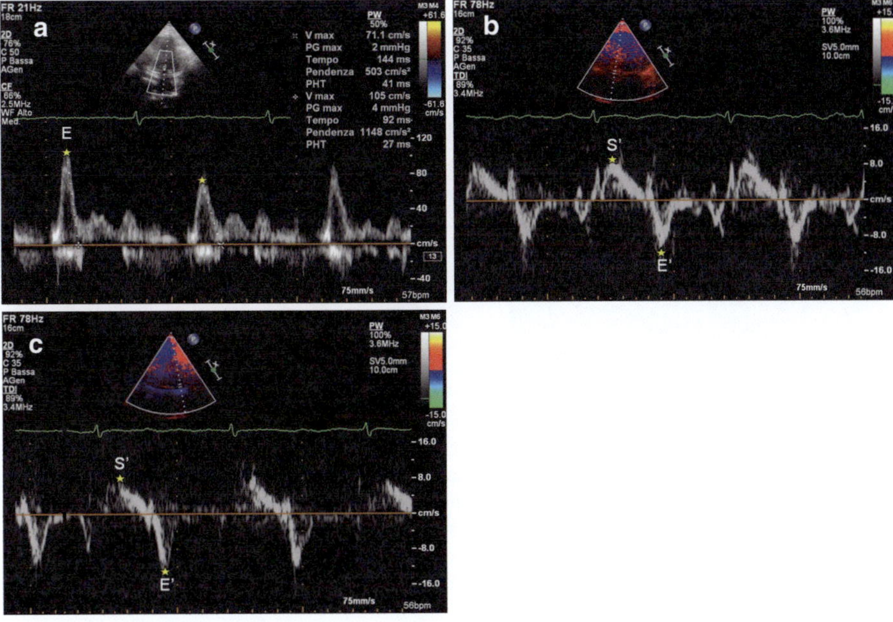

Fig. 19.7 (**a–c**) Patient with constrictive pericarditis. Doppler interrogation of transmitral valve (**a**) shows a restrictive filling pattern (E-wave velocity = 85 cm/s, E-wave deceleration time = 120 ms), with marked respiratory variations. Tissue Doppler imaging curve on the septal mitral valve annulus (**b**) shows normal systolic (S′ wave = 9 cm/s) and early diastolic (E′ wave = 10.1 cm/s) wave velocities. E/E′ ratio is 8. Tissue Doppler imaging curve on the lateral mitral valve annulus (**c**) shows normal systolic (S′ wave = 8 cm/s) and early diastolic (E′ wave = 11.3 cm/s) wave velocities. E/E′ ratio is 7

in the presence of surgical annular rings, prosthetic mitral valves, and mitral annular calcification.

In this subset of patients, evaluation of segmental myocardial deformation using 2D speckle-tracking echocardiography might add useful information to discriminate between constrictive from restrictive physiology [18]. In a study evaluating myocardial mechanics using 2D speckle-tracking echocardiography in patients with CP and RCM, CP patients had reduced depressed longitudinal strain in the LV anterolateral wall and RV free wall but preserved strain in the LV septal wall. There was a significant inverse correlation between pericardial thickness detected by CMR and ventricular strain in adjacent segments [31]. Sengupta et al. [32] demonstrated that in RCM the prominent endocardial dysfunction with sparing of epicardial function causes abnormal longitudinal mechanics with relative sparing of circumferential and twist mechanics, whereas patients with CP have relatively preserved longitudinal LV mechanics and markedly abnormal circumferential deformation, torsion, and untwisting velocity (Fig. 19.8).

CMR and/or CT play a major role in the diagnostic workup of suspected CP or RCM (Fig. 19.9) [17–19]. Volume analysis in RCM reveals normal-sized ventricles with enlarged atria and normal pericardial thickness with normal myocardial contours. CP, on the other hand, is characterized by tubular or indented, smaller-sized

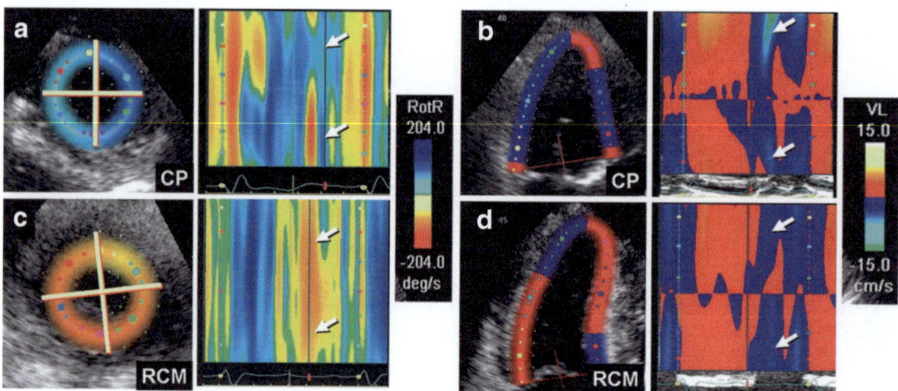

Fig. 19.8 (**a–d**) Color M-mode display of apical untwisting velocity [rotational rate of the left ventricular apex (*RotR*)], obtained from speckle-tracking imaging in short-axis view, demonstrates reduced early diastolic rate of untwisting in constrictive pericarditis (**a**, *arrows*), whereas longitudinal early diastolic velocities (*VL*) from the left ventricular base in apical four-chamber view (**b**, *arrows*) are normal. In contrast, patients with restrictive cardiomyopathy show a normal early diastolic rate of untwisting (**c**, *arrows*) and reduced longitudinal early diastolic velocities from the left ventricular base (**d**, *arrows*). *CP* constrictive pericarditis, *RCM* restrictive cardiomyopathy (From Sengupta et al. [32], with permission)

ventricles, normal myocardial thickness, and increased pericardial thickness, which can be generalized or localized [17].

Black-blood T1-weighed sequences are used to assess pericardial thickness [33]. Hyperintensity at T2-weighed black-blood sequences [34] and T1-weighted sequences after gadolinium administration [35] are indicative of active myocardial and pericardial inflammation, whereas hyperintensity at LGE sequences alone is indicative of pericardial fibrosis [36]. Calcification in CP is usually seen as a profound hypointensity on all pulse sequences.

In CP, CMR tagging sequences are used to show pericardial adhesions [37], whereas real-time cine CMR sequences during deep inspiration are used to assess ventricular interdependence. Typically, leftward movement of the IVS is seen in deep inspiration, and a rightward movement is seen in expiration, which is a pathognomonic sign of pericardial constriction [38]. Septal flattening, another sign of increase interventricular interdependence, may be observed with CMR in CP, with a reported sensitivity of 80 % and specificity of 100 % [39].

Cardiac CT provides excellent imaging of the pericardium, allowing accurate measurement of pericardial thickness. However, the demonstration of pericardial thickening (>4 mm) is not completely sensitive or specific for CP. Findings that suggest CP on CT include diffusely thickened or calcified pericardium, tubular LV and RV, and a sigmoid IVS [40]. The choice between CMR and CT depends upon the clinical setting and the available technologies. If the diagnosis is unclear, CMR study may be preferable, whereas CT is probably the best imaging modality in cases with a high suspicion of CP at clinical and echo-Doppler assessment [19].

A problem-oriented invasive hemodynamic study could be performed, particularly in the most severe cases with a surgical option or in the presence of conflicting results of noninvasive tests. CP is classically characterized by elevation and

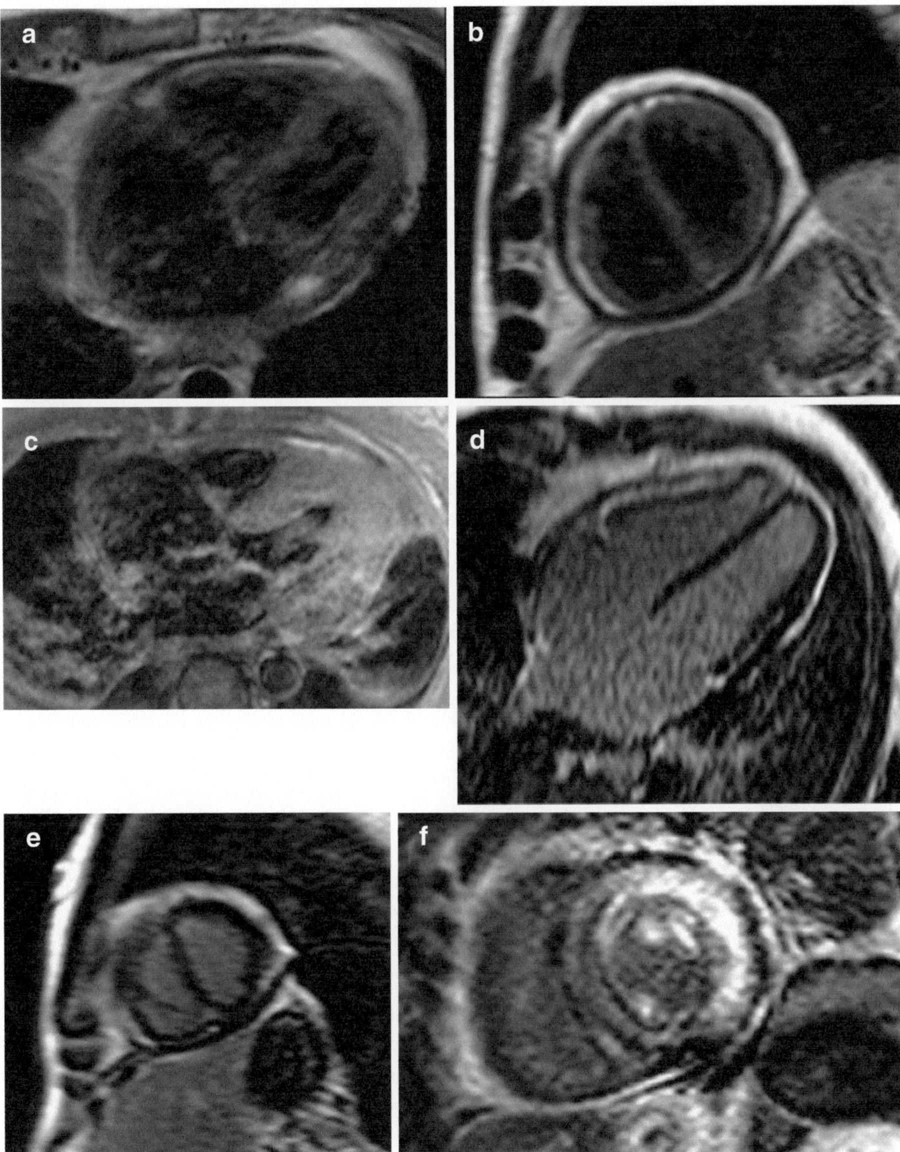

Fig. 19.9 (a–e) Examples of cardiac magnetic resonance (CMR) in differential diagnosis between restrictive cardiomyopathy (RCM) and constrictive pericarditis (CP). T1-weighted imaging showing pericardial thickening in CP axial (**a**) and short axis (**b**) and absence of pericardial thickening (**c**) in a case of RCM secondary to amyloid; axial image. Late gadolinium enhancement (LGE) imaging of CP showing absence of fibrosis in four-chamber (**c**) and short-axis (**d**) views. LGE imaging short-axis view, of RCM secondary to amyloid showing diffuse gadolinium infiltration; note septal flattening (in end-diastole) in short-axis views (**b**, **e**) in CP

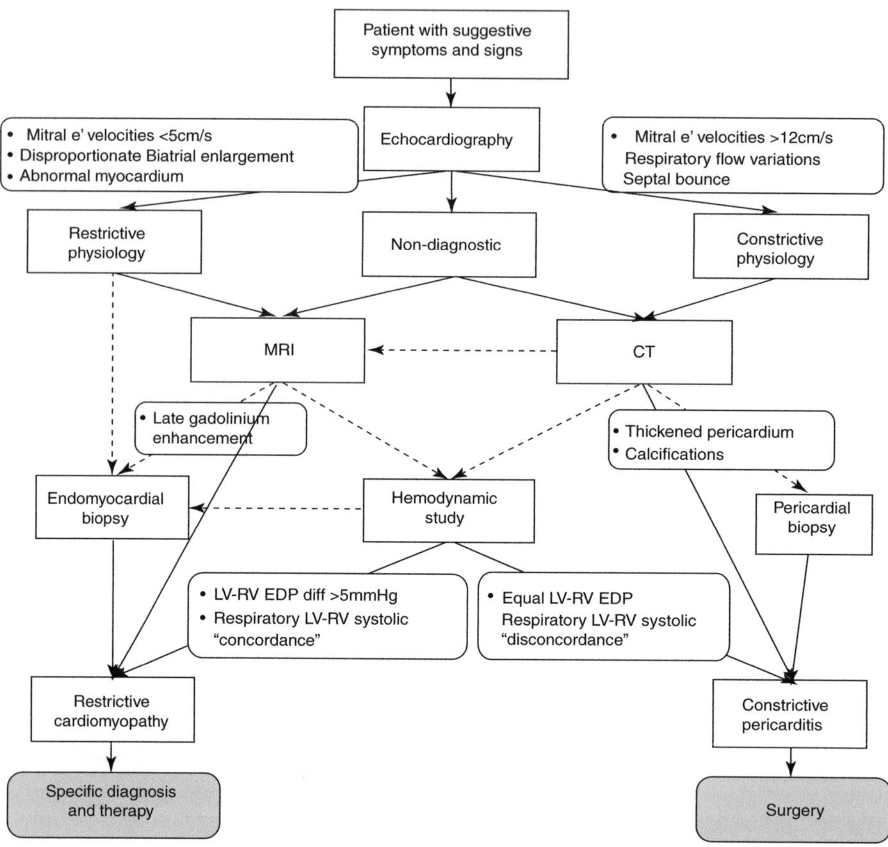

Fig. 19.10 Algorithm for evaluating patients with restrictive cardiomyopathy vs constrictive pericarditis. *Dotted arrows* denote optional choices (From Zwas et al. [19], with permission)

equalization of filling pressures [17, 19]. However, this finding is not very sensitive or specific, because it can be observed in RCM also. Furthermore, in CP, an inspiratory fall in pulmonary capillary wedge pressure (PCWP), contrasting with a fixed systemic venous pressure, is present. Reciprocal pressure variations in the two ventricles during respiratory phases is a useful sign of CP and is characterized by discordance between RV and LV systolic pressures, which increase and decrease, respectively, during inspiration. Conversely, a concordant respiratory behavior in systolic pressures in both ventricles is present in RCM [19].

In selected cases with refractory HF and nondiagnostic or discrepant imaging and hemodynamic data, an EMB and/or pericardial biopsy may be indicated [19, 41].

Finally, the intriguing possibility of mixed constrictive/restrictive physiology must be considered, particularly in patients without typical respiratory changes in flow velocities and ventricular size. These patients, however, may be less likely to benefit from pericardiectomy [42]. A useful diagnostic algorithm for a patient with suspected RCM vs CP is shown in Fig. 19.10 [19].

19.4 Eosinophilic Endomyocardial Disease and Endomyocardial Fibrosis

The definition of hypereosinophilic syndrome requires a sustained peripheral blood eosinophilia, $>1.5 \times 10^9$/L [43]. There are two types of hypereosinophilic syndromes [5, 43]. The most common is secondary hypereosinophilia, which occurs as a result of certain tumors, lymphoma, vasculitis, or parasitic or infectious diseases, as well as the hypereosinophilia that follows hypersensitivity reaction. The other form is primary hypereosinophilic syndrome that was first described by Loeffler in 1936 as "endocarditis parietalis fibroplastica." In this form, there is evidence of eosinophil-mediated end-organ damage. The disease can affect all organs, including the heart, lungs, and nervous system, leading to neurological deficits [5, 43]. The cardiac pathology of hypereosinophilic syndrome has traditionally been divided into three stages: acute necrosis, thrombosis, and fibrosis [44]. The acute necrotic stage is characterized by myocardial necrosis due to progressive degranulation of eosinophils; acute myonecrosis is followed by formation of mural thrombi, often involving both ventricles; ventricular outflow tracts (OT); and subvalvular regions. This process may lead to atrioventricular valvular incompetence. The third phase is characterized by fibrotic replacement, leading to an RCM or a DCM phenotype.

Endomyocardial fibrosis (EMF) is an idiopathic disorder common mostly in tropical and subtropical regions (predominantly in Africa), but possibly present worldwide, characterized by the development of RCM [45]. EMF is sometimes considered part of a single disease process that includes Loeffler disease. Clinical presentation of the disease includes HF with preserved LV EF, reduced LV EF in advanced stages, tricuspid and/or mitral regurgitation, hyper- or hypokinetic arrhythmias, and, rarely, angina. Therapy comprises medical drugs (mostly diuretics, angiotensin-converting enzyme (ACE) inhibitors, beta-blockers, and anticoagulant agents in the presence of thrombi and/or AF), and surgery (endocardiectomy combined with mitral/tricuspid repair/replacement) in order to resolve RFP and HF [45].

Both Loeffler eosinophilic endocarditis and EMF are characterized at echocardiography in the early stage by endocardial hyperechogenicity due to eosinophilic infiltration with necrosis and mural thrombus formation, particularly in the apex of both ventricles (Fig. 19.11) [46–49]. Notably, wall motion adjacent to this deposition is normal. The use of contrast agents permits better evaluation not only of the extend of the thrombotic mass but also of the continuity of the mass with the infiltrated endocardium [50]. A highly echogenic line in the endocardial border [attributable to areas of fibrosis (Fig. 19.11)] can be found—particularly at the level of the RV free wall or the LV posterolateral wall—that can be hypokinetic [46]. In the late stage, mural thrombosis is replaced by fibrosis, which progresses to the endomyocardium, leading to RCM with typical apical obliteration [5, 46–49]. The fibrotic mass can also involve the atrioventricular (mitral and/or tricuspid) subvalvular apparatus and leaflets, causing leaflet restriction and valvular regurgitation, which can often be severe [49].

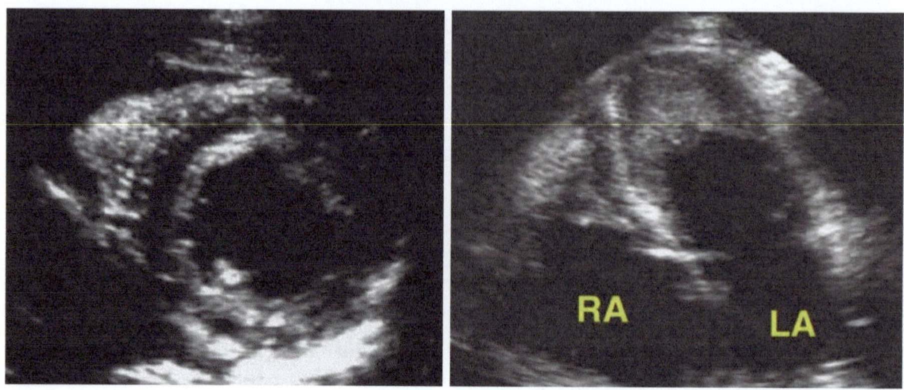

Fig. 19.11 Parasternal short-axis (*left*) and four-chamber (*right*) views from a patient with hypereosinophilic syndrome. A bright echogenic line surrounds the left ventricular endocardial border. The apical four-chamber view shows mural thrombi in the apex of both ventricles. *LA* left atrium, *RA* right atrium (From Nihoyannopoulos and Dawson [5], with permission)

Loeffler endocarditis usually involves the LV, whereas EMF shows a biventricular involvement in 50 % of cases and LV involvement in 40 %; the remaining 10 % has RV involvement [51]. Ventricles typically are normal in size and systolic function is preserved, whereas there is RFP due to interstitial fibrosis. There is usually prominent biatrial dilation [46, 47]. Finally, pericardial effusion is frequently present in EMF.

The feasibility of 3D contrast echocardiography has been proven in the diagnosis and follow-up evaluation of Loeffler disease complicated by thrombus formation and neoangiogenesis of the LV apex [52]. A preliminary report shows how 3D transthoracic echocardiography can provide substantial information in right-sided EMF concerning the region of RV involvement, as well as the various characteristics of RA thrombi [53].

Endocardial fibrous tissue deposition, the hallmark of EMF, can be assessed with LGE at contrast-enhanced CMR. A typical LGE pattern was described, with a V sign at the ventricular apex, characterized by a three-layer appearance of the myocardium, thickened fibrotic endomyocardium, and superimposed thrombus [54, 55] (Fig. 19.12). Electron-beam CT allows direct visualization of EMF, which is depicted as linear calcifications and/or a thin tissue band of low attenuation within the endomyocardium; CT enables differential diagnosis with CP [56]. In patients with hypereosinophilic syndrome undergoing CMR, a 29 % prevalence of LGE was reported, typically confined to the endocardium, located circumferentially within the RV and LV apexes [57]. A marked regression of LGE was seen after adequate therapy. Other authors report extensive myocardial hyperintensity at T2-weighted imaging during the acute phase of eosinophilic myocarditis [58].

Considering the role of imaging in prognostic assessment and management of patients with Loeffler/EMF, available data are limited because the natural history of this rare disease is not fully defined; also there are few data to guide therapeutic decisions. AF is associated with worse prognosis, particularly if associated with severe tricuspid regurgitation [59]. Although EMB is still considered part of the

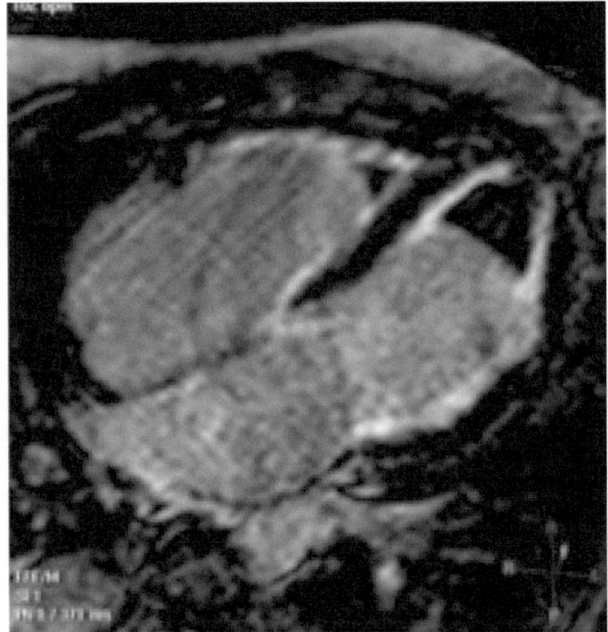

Fig. 19.12 Characteristic aspect of endomyocardial fibrosis at late gadolinium enhancement cardiac magnetic resonance imaging. Note the three layers (outermost to innermost) of hypointense myocardium, hyperintense endomyocardial fibrosis, and hypointense superimposed thrombus with biventricular involvement (Reproduced from Kharwar et al. [53], with permission)

diagnostic workup [60], a serum eosinophilic count associated with a diagnostic CMR study might replace this procedure in patients with RCM coming from endemic regions. In early disease stages, in which there is suspicion for active inflammation, CMR may be useful in identifying patients who may benefit from steroid therapy, whereas in the advanced phases, it might be helpful to provide information to the managing physician regarding the feasibility of cardiac surgery. In fact, regional EMF resection with tricuspid- and/or mitral valve replacement in patients with severe HF has resulted in functional improvement [56].

19.5 Systemic Sclerosis

Systemic sclerosis (or scleroderma) can involve any organ, including the heart [61, 62]. Extensive fibrosis, vascular alterations, and autoantibodies against various cellular antigens can be present in the organ affected. Endocardium, myocardium, and pericardium, separately or concomitantly, can be involved. As a consequence, pericardial effusion, atrial and/or ventricular arrhythmias, conduction disease, valvular regurgitation, myocardial ischemia, myocardial hypertrophy, and HF have been reported. Microvascular coronary abnormalities and dysfunction are described that can result in ether angina pectoris or acute myocardial infarction [61].

ECG can show premature atrial and ventricular beats, right bundle-branch block (RBBB), and other conduction abnormalities [5]. In this disease, the prevalence of LV systolic dysfunction is relatively low, and the most common causes of LV systolic function impairment are coronary artery disease, systemic hypertension, and acute myocarditis. Conversely, LV diastolic dysfunction is very common and is usually induced by primary myocardial involvement (RCM) or involvement secondary to hypertension, pulmonary hypertension, and pericardial disease. RV dysfunction can be also present as a consequence of pressure overload related to pulmonary hypertension. It can also occur due to myocardial fibrosis alone or be associated with microvascular disease. Pericardial involvement is described in several studies and include fibrinous pericarditis, chronic fibrous pericarditis, pericardial adhesions, and pericardial effusions [62].

The echocardiographic abnormalities observed in systemic sclerosis with cardiac involvement are secondary to diffuse myocardial fibrosis and fiber degeneration, with consequent segmental and global systolic dysfunction and restriction of ventricular filling [63]. In this setting, LV strain analysis by speckle-tracking echocardiography has been employed to detect subclinical LV dysfunction, which portends a higher risk of cardiovascular complications [64]. Furthermore, TDI and speckle-tracking-derived strain can discern early RV systolic dysfunction, even in the absence of pulmonary hypertension [65]. CMR study can also be employed in this setting. Subclinical primary cardiac involvement, characterized by decreased RV EF, was demonstrated at CMR in all patients affected by systemic sclerosis without clinical signs or symptoms of cardiac involvement [66]. Another interesting finding at CMR study was the demonstration of reduced myocardial perfusion reserve [67]. Reduced myocardial perfusion reserve may also contribute to RV dysfunction in patients with pulmonary artery hypertension [68].

LV LGE, usually seen with a basal and midcavity midwall linear pattern, was reported in a varying proportion of patients with systemic sclerosis [67, 69, 70]; in another study, 75 % of patients with systemic sclerosis had at least one of the above quoted abnormalities [71].

Stress-induced defects are often found at exercise thallium single-positron-emission CT (SPECT) scan despite minor or absent clinical evidence of cardiac involvement. Lower RV and LV EF are found in patients with defects [72]. Depressed RV EF in asymptomatic patients is also demonstrated by radionuclide ventriculography [73]. An increased calcium score on chest CT was evident in systemic sclerosis patients compared with controls, progressively increasing with disease duration [74].

Considering prognostic implications of imaging, echocardiographic evaluation can be useful, first because in patients affected by systemic sclerosis, signs of cardiac involvement are related with worse prognosis [75]. A simple two-variable-weighted cardiac score, derived from routine ECG and echocardiography, is a useful predictor of survival: left-axis deviation or large pericardial effusion independently predicted mortality [76].

Assessing microcirculation impairment with abnormal vasoreactivity with or without associated structural abnormalities of the small coronary arteries or arterioles may have prognostic and therapeutic implications in systemic sclerosis with cardiac involvement [77, 78]. Studies [79, 80] using contrast enhanced transthoracic Doppler before and after adenosine infusion show impaired coronary flow reserve in patients without clinical evidence of cardiac involvement. High-resolution perfusion CMR techniques can identify small subendocardial defects highly suggestive of microvascular alteration. Imaging can also be useful for guiding therapy, showing the beneficial effects on myocardial perfusion of vasodilators such as calcium-channel blockers. After 14 days of treatment with nifedipine, CMR showed improvement, with a mean 38 % increase in the global perfusion index [81]. Similar results were demonstrated using positron emission tomography (PET) [82] and thallium-201 SPECT [83].

19.6   Radiation Cardiomyopathy

Irradiation of the heart, incidental to mediastinal radiation therapy of malignancies such as Hodgkin's disease, breast cancer, or chest wall tumors, can induce a wide spectrum of cardiovascular complications, increasing in frequency and severity with higher radiation doses, larger volume exposed, younger age at time of exposure, and greater time elapsed since treatment [84, 85]. These complications include effusive or constrictive pericarditis, myocardial fibrosis with systolic and/or diastolic ventricular dysfunction (RCM), coronary artery disease (with frequent involvement of coronary ostia), valvular abnormalities, and conduction electrical disturbances. Cardiac damage associated with radiotherapy rarely manifest acutely, whereas it is frequently progressive. In particular, RCM, as well as CP, induced by radiotherapy is evident several years after treatment [5]. Differentiating between constriction and restriction may be particularly difficult in these patients, because the two conditions may coexist and clinical history and physical examination are often not sufficient [42]. In this field, thoracic CT and/or CMR scan could be useful in patient management.

Echocardiographic study in a patient treated with radiotherapy can rarely show pericardial effusion in the acute stage and, on very rare occasions, cardiac tamponade. In a later stage, chronic pericarditis with pericardial thickening and possible constriction can be observed. Myocardial dysfunction with a restrictive ventricular physiology secondary to interstitial fibrosis can also be present [5]. Valvular abnormalities are usually left sided and include anterior mitral valve leaflet and aortic valve thickening (due to tissue fibrosis and/or calcification), with associated regurgitation and, less commonly, stenosis. Finally, myocardial ischemia with consequent dysfunction and scar compatible with myocardial infarction can be present secondary to microvascular and/or macrovascular injury [84].

Speckle-tracking analysis can be used to identify reduced LV regional function related to radiation dose distribution not demonstrable by conventional echocardiographic parameters [86]. A number of SPECT studies evaluating myocardial perfusion after breast or mediastinum irradiation document the onset of both fixed (possibly indicating direct damage) and reversible (possibly indicating progression of atherosclerotic disease) regional perfusion defects [87–89].

Microvascular insufficiency and ischemia can result in diffuse and patchy interstitial myocardial fibrosis [90] that may contribute to impaired diastolic distensibility of the ventricles seen in this group of patients. Demonstration of the negative effects of radiation therapy on LV diastolic function by Doppler assessment is useful from a prognostic point of view. In a series of 294 patients receiving at least 35 Gy to the mediastinum, patients with LV diastolic dysfunction had worse event-free survival than patients with normal function (hazard ratio 1.66, 95 % confidence interval 1.06–2.4) over a 3.2-year follow-up. In addition, these patients more frequently had stress-induced ischemia, and E-wave velocity and pulmonary systolic to diastolic velocity ratio were independent predictors of survival [91].

After mediastinal radiation therapy, CMR can show fibrosis that does not correspond to a coronary territory or to a pattern consistent with other CMP, such as amyloidosis or sarcoidosis. This information can be used before considering revascularization in patients with potential nonischemic causes of HF, such as those with previous mediastinal radiation therapy [92].

References

1. Elliott P, Andersson B, Arbustini E et al (2008) Classification of the cardiomyopathies: a position statement from the European Society Of Cardiology Working Group on Myocardial and Pericardial Diseases. Eur Heart J 29:270–276
2. Appleton CP, Hatle LK, Popp RL (1988) Demonstration of restrictive ventricular physiology by Doppler echocardiography. J Am Coll Cardiol 22:757–768
3. Appleton CP, Hatle LK, Popp RL (1988) Relation of transmitral flow velocity patterns to left ventricular diastolic function: new insights from a combined hemodynamic and Doppler echocardiographic study. J Am Coll Cardiol 12:426–440
4. Pinamonti B, Finocchiaro G, Moretti M, Merlo M, Sinagra G (2011) Diastolic dysfunction in cardiomyopathies. J Cardiovasc Echogr 21:157–165
5. Nihoyannopoulos P, Dawson D (2009) Restrictive cardiomyopathies. Eur J Echocardiogr 10:23–33
6. Schutte DP, Essop MR (2001) Clinical profile and outcome of idiopathic restrictive cardiomyopathy. Circulation 103:E83
7. Siegel RJ, Shah PK, Fishbein MC (1984) Idiopathic restrictive cardiomyopathy. Circulation 70:165–169
8. Ammash NM, Seward JB, Bailey KR et al (2000) Clinical profile and outcome of idiopathic restrictive cardiomyopathy. Circulation 101:2490–2496
9. Daneshvar DA, Kedia G, Fishbein MC et al (2012) Familial restrictive cardiomyopathy with 12 affected family members. Am J Cardiol 109:445–447
10. Arbustini E, Morbini P, Grasso M et al (1998) Restrictive cardiomyopathy, atrioventricular block and mild to subclinical myopathy in patients with desmin-immunoreactive material deposits. J Am Coll Cardiol 31:645–653
11. Fernando Guadalajara J, Vera-Delgado A, Gaspar-Hernandez J et al (1998) Echocardiographic aspects of restrictive cardiomyopathy: their relationship with pathophysiology. Echocardiography 15:297–314
12. Keren A, Popp RL (1992) Assignment of patients into the classification of cardiomyopathies. Circulation 86:1622–1633
13. Nishimura RA, Abel MD, Hatle LK et al (1989) Assessment of diastolic function of the heart: background and current applications of Doppler echocardiography. Part II. Clinical studies. Mayo Clin Proc 64:181–204
14. Rossvoll O, Hatle LK (1993) Pulmonary venous flow velocities recorded by transthoracic Doppler ultrasound: relation to left ventricular diastolic pressures. J Am Coll Cardiol 21:1687–1696

15. Sasaki N, Garcia M, Lytrivi I et al (2011) Utility of Doppler tissue imaging-derived indices in identifying subclinical systolic ventricular dysfunction in children with restrictive cardiomyopathy. Pediatr Cardiol 32:646–651
16. Tiruvoipati R, Naik RD, Loubani M, Billa GN (2003) Surgical approach for pericardiectomy: a comparative study between median sternotomy and left anterolateral thoracotomy. Interact Cardiovasc Thorac Surg 2(3):322–326. doi:10.1016/S1569-9293(03)00074-4
17. Hancock EW (2001) Differential diagnosis of restrictive cardiomyopathy and constrictive pericarditis. Heart 86:343–349
18. Sengupta PP, Eleid MF, Khandheria BK (2008) Constrictive pericarditis. Circ J 72: 1555–1562
19. Zwas DR, Gotsman I, Admon D, Keren A (2012) Advances in the differentiation of constrictive pericarditis and restrictive cardiomyopathy. Herz 37:664–674
20. Oh JK, Hatle LK, Seward JB et al (1994) Diagnostic role of Doppler echocardiography in constrictive pericarditis. J Am Coll Cardiol 23:154–162
21. Klein AL, Cohen GI, Pietrolungo JF et al (1993) Differentiation of constrictive pericarditis from restrictive cardiomyopathy by Doppler transesophageal echocardiographic measurements of respiratory variations in pulmonary venous flow. J Am Coll Cardiol 22:1935–1943
22. Oh JK, Tajik AJ, Appleton CP et al (1997) Preload reduction to unmask the characteristic Doppler features of constrictive pericarditis. A new observation. Circulation 95:796–799
23. Rajagopalan N, Garcia MJ, Rodriguez L et al (2001) Comparison of new Doppler echocardiographic methods to differentiate constrictive pericardial heart disease and restrictive cardiomyopathy. Am J Cardiol 87:86–94
24. Candell-Riera J, Garcia del Castillo H, Permanyer-Miralda G et al (1978) Echocardiographic features of the interventricular septum in chronic constrictive pericarditis. Circulation 57:1154–1158
25. Ling LH, Oh JK, Tei C et al (1997) Pericardial thickness measured with transesophageal echocardiography: feasibility and potential clinical usefulness. J Am Coll Cardiol 29:1317–1323
26. Choi JH, Choi JO, Ryu DR et al (2011) Mitral and tricuspid annular velocities in constrictive pericarditis and restrictive cardiomyopathy: correlation with pericardial thickness on computed tomography. JACC Cardiovasc Imaging 4:567–575
27. Sengupta PP, Mohan JC, Mehta V et al (2004) Accuracy and pitfalls of early diastolic motion of the mitral annulus for diagnosing constrictive pericarditis by tissue Doppler imaging. Am J Cardiol 93:886–890
28. Ha JW, Oh JK, Ling LH et al (2001) Annulus paradoxus: transmitral flow velocity to mitral annular velocity ratio is inversely proportional to pulmonary capillary wedge pressure in patients with constrictive pericarditis. Circulation 104:976–978
29. Reuss CS, Wilansky SM, Lester SJ et al (2009) Using mitral 'annulus reversus' to diagnose constrictive pericarditis. Eur J Echocardiogr 10:372–375
30. Klein AL, Dahiya A (2011) Annular velocities in constrictive pericarditis: annulus and beyond JACC Cardiovasc Imaging 4:576–579
31. Kusunose K, Dahiya A, Popovic ZB et al (2013) Biventricular mechanics in constrictive pericarditis comparison with restrictive cardiomyopathy and impact of pericardiectomy. Circ Cardiovasc Imaging 6:399–406
32. Sengupta PP, Krishnamoorthy VK, Abhayaratna WP et al (2008) Disparate patterns of left ventricular mechanics differentiate constrictive pericarditis from restrictive cardiomyopathy. JACC Cardiovasc Imaging 1:29–38
33. Misselt AJ, Harris SR, Glockner J et al (2008) MR imaging of the pericardium. Magn Reson Imaging Clin N Am 16:185–199, vii
34. Smith WH, Beacock DJ, Goddard AJ et al (2001) Magnetic resonance evaluation of the pericardium. Br J Radiol 74:384–392
35. Taylor AM, Dymarkowski S, Verbeken EK et al (2006) Detection of pericardial inflammation with late-enhancement cardiac magnetic resonance imaging: initial results. Eur Radiol 16:569–574
36. Zurick AO, Bolen MA, Kwon DH et al (2011) Pericardial delayed hyperenhancement with CMR imaging in patients with constrictive pericarditis undergoing surgical pericardiectomy: a case series with histopathological correlation. JACC Cardiovasc Imaging 4:1180–1191

37. Kojima S, Yamada N, Goto Y (1999) Diagnosis of constrictive pericarditis by tagged cine magnetic resonance imaging. N Engl J Med 341:373–374
38. Francone M, Dymarkowski S, Kalantzi M et al (2006) Assessment of ventricular coupling with real-time cine MRI and its value to differentiate constrictive pericarditis from restrictive cardiomyopathy. Eur Radiol 16:944–951
39. Giorgi B, Mollet NR, Dymarkowski S et al (2003) Clinically suspected constrictive pericarditis: MR imaging assessment of ventricular septal motion and configuration in patients and healthy subjects. Radiology 228:417–424
40. Rajiah P, Kanne JP (2010) Computed tomography of the pericardium and pericardial disease. J Cardiovasc Comput Tomogr 4:3–18
41. Leone O, Veinot JP, Angelini A et al (2012) 2011 consensus statement on endomyocardial biopsy from the Association for European Cardiovascular Pathology and the Society for Cardiovascular Pathology. Cardiovasc Pathol 21:245–274
42. Yamada H, Tabata T, Jaffer SJ, Drinko JK, Jasper SE, Lauer MS, Thomas JD, Klein AL (2007) Clinical features of mixed physiology of constriction and restriction: echocardiographic characteristics and clinical outcome. Eur J Echocardiogr 8(3):185–194
43. Roufosse FE, Goldman M, Cogan E (2007) Hypereosinophilic syndromes. Orphanet J Rare Dis 2:37
44. Ogbogu PU, Rosing DR, Horne MK 3rd (2007) Cardiovascular manifestations of hypereosinophilic syndromes. Immunol Allergy Clin North Am 27:457–475
45. Mocumbi AO, Falase AO (2013) Recent advances in the epidemiology, diagnosis and treatment of endomyocardial fibrosis in Africa. Heart 99:1481–1487
46. Davies J, Gibson DG, Foale R et al (1982) Echocardiographic features of eosinophilic endomyocardial disease. Br Heart J 48:434–440
47. Acquatella H, Schiller NB, Puigbo JJ, Gomez-Mancebo JR, Suarez C, Acquatella G (1983) Value of two-dimensional echocardiography in endomyocardial disease with and without eosinophilia. A clinical and pathologic study. Circulation 67:1219–1226
48. Ommen SR, Seward JB, Tajik AJ (2000) Clinical and echocardiographic features of hypereosinophilic syndromes. Am J Cardiol 86:110–113
49. Hassan WM, Fawzy ME, Al Helaly S, Hegazy H, Malik S (2005) Pitfalls in diagnosis and clinical, echocardiographic, and hemodynamic findings in endomyocardial fibrosis: a 25-year experience. Chest 128:3985–3992
50. D'Errico A, Galderisi M, Pollio G et al (2003) A case of hypereosinophilic cardiomyopathy: additional value of the myocardial contrast agent SonoVue for the differential diagnosis of a cardiac mass. Ital Heart J 4:571–574
51. Chew CY, Ziady GM, Raphael MJ et al (1977) Primary restrictive cardiomyopathy. Non-tropical endomyocardial fibrosis and hypereosinophilic heart disease. Br Heart J 39:399–413
52. Del Bene MR, Cappelli F, Rega L et al (2012) Characterization of Loeffler eosinophilic myocarditis by means of real time three-dimensional contrast-enhanced echocardiography. Echocardiography 29:E62–E66
53. Kharwar RB, Sethi R, Narain VS (2013) Right-sided endomyocardial fibrosis with a right atrial thrombus: three-dimensional transthoracic echocardiographic evaluation. Echocardiography 30(10):E322–5
54. Salemi VM, Rochitte CE, Shiozaki AA et al (2011) Late gadolinium enhancement magnetic resonance imaging in the diagnosis and prognosis of endomyocardial fibrosis patients. Circ Cardiovasc Imaging 4:304–311
55. Gonçalves LF, Souto FM, Faro FN et al (2012) Biventricular thrombus and endomyocardial fibrosis in antiphospholipid syndrome. Arq Bras Cardiol 99:162–165
56. Mousseaux E, Hernigou A, Azencot M et al (1996) Endomyocardial fibrosis: electron-beam CT features. Radiology 198:755–760
57. Ibrahim T, Blanke F, Huss-Marp J et al (2011) Gadolinium-enhanced cardiovascular magnetic resonance for the detection and characterization of Loeffler endocarditis in patients with hypereosinophilic syndrome. Int J Cardiol 153:105–108

58. Tani H, Amano Y, Tachi M et al (2012) T2-weighted and delayed enhancement MRI of eosino-philic myocarditis: relationship with clinical phases and global cardiac function. Jpn J Radiol 30:824–831
59. Barretto AC, Mady C, Nussbacher A, Ianni BM, Oliveira SA, Jatene A, Ramires JA (1998) Atrial fibrillation in endomyocardial fibrosis is a marker of worse prognosis. Int J Cardiol 67(1):19–25
60. Gonzalez-Lavin L, Friedman JP, Hecker SP, McFadden PM (1983) Endomyocardial fibrosis: diagnosis and treatment. Am Heart J 105(4):699–705
61. Ngian GS, Sahhar J, Wicks IP et al (2011) Cardiovascular disease in systemic sclerosis–an emerging association? Arthritis Res Ther 13:237
62. Ferri C, Giuggioli D, Sebastiani M et al (2005) Heart involvement and systemic sclerosis. Lupus 14:702–707
63. Eggebrecht RF, Kleiger RE (1977) Echocardiographic patterns in scleroderma. Chest 71:47–51
64. Cusma Piccione M, Zito C, Bagnato G et al (2013) Role of 2D strain in the early identification of left ventricular dysfunction and in the risk stratification of systemic sclerosis patients. Cardiovasc Ultrasound 11:6
65. Schattke S, Knebel F, Grohmann A et al (2010) Early right ventricular systolic dysfunction in patients with systemic sclerosis without pulmonary hypertension: a Doppler Tissue and Speckle Tracking echocardiography study. Cardiovasc Ultrasound 8:3
66. Bezante GP, Rollando D, Sessarego M et al (2007) Cardiac magnetic resonance imaging detects subclinical right ventricular impairment in systemic sclerosis. J Rheumatol 34: 2431–2437
67. Kobayashi H, Yokoe I, Hirano M et al (2009) Cardiac magnetic resonance imaging with phar-macological stress perfusion and delayed enhancement in asymptomatic patients with sys-temic sclerosis. J Rheumatol 36:106–112
68. Vogel-Claussen J, Skrok J, Shehata ML et al (2011) Right and left ventricular myocardial perfusion reserves correlate with right ventricular function and pulmonary hemodynamics in patients with pulmonary arterial hypertension. Radiology 258:119–127
69. Tzelepis GE, Kelekis NL, Plastiras SC et al (2007) Pattern and distribution of myocardial fibrosis in systemic sclerosis: a delayed enhanced magnetic resonance imaging study. Arthritis Rheum 56:3827–3836
70. Nassenstein K, Breuckmann F, Huger M et al (2008) Detection of myocardial fibrosis in sys-temic sclerosis by contrast-enhanced magnetic resonance imaging. Rofo 180:1054–1060
71. Hachulla AL, Launay D, Gaxotte V et al (2009) Cardiac magnetic resonance imaging in sys-temic sclerosis: a cross-sectional observational study of 52 patients. Ann Rheum Dis 68: 1878–1884
72. Follansbee WP, Curtiss EI, Medsger TA Jr et al (1984) Physiologic abnormalities of cardiac func-tion in progressive systemic sclerosis with diffuse scleroderma. N Engl J Med 310:142–148
73. Meune C, Allanore Y, Devaux JY et al (2004) High prevalence of right ventricular systolic dysfunction in early systemic sclerosis. J Rheumatol 31:1941–1945
74. Mok MY, Lau CS, Chiu SS et al (2011) Systemic sclerosis is an independent risk factor for increased coronary artery calcium deposition. Arthritis Rheum 63:1387–1395
75. Ioannidis JP, Vlachoyiannopoulos PG, Haidich AB, Medsger TA Jr, Lucas M, Michet CJ, Kuwana M, Yasuoka H, van den Hoogen F, Te Boome L, van Laar JM, Verbeet NL, Matucci-Cerinic M, Georgountzos A, Moutsopoulos HM (2005) Mortality in systemic sclerosis: an international meta-analysis of individual patient data. Am J Med 118(1):2–10. doi:10.1016/j.amjmed.2004.04.031
76. Clements PJ, Lachenbruch PA, Furst DE, Paulus HE, Sterz MG (1991) Cardiac score. A semi-quantitative measure of cardiac involvement that improves prediction of prognosis in systemic sclerosis. Arthritis Rheum 34(11):1371–1380
77. Kahan A, Allanore Y (2006) Primary myocardial involvement in systemic sclerosis. Rheumatology (Oxford) 45 Suppl 4:iv14–17. doi:10.1093/rheumatology/kel312
78. Allanore Y, Meune C (2010) Primary myocardial involvement in systemic sclerosis: evidence for a microvascular origin. Clin Exp Rheumatol 28(5 Suppl 62):S48–S53

79. Montisci R, Vacca A, Garau P, Colonna P, Ruscazio M, Passiu G, Iliceto S, Mathieu A (2003) Detection of early impairment of coronary flow reserve in patients with systemic sclerosis. Ann Rheum Dis 62(9):890–893

80. Sulli A, Ghio M, Bezante GP, Deferrari L, Craviotto C, Sebastiani V, Setti M, Barsotti A, Cutolo M, Indiveri F (2004) Blunted coronary flow reserve in systemic sclerosis. Rheumatology (Oxford) 43(4):505–509. doi:10.1093/rheumatology/keh087

81. Vignaux O, Allanore Y, Meune C, Pascal O, Duboc D, Weber S, Legmann P, Kahan A (2005) Evaluation of the effect of nifedipine upon myocardial perfusion and contractility using cardiac magnetic resonance imaging and tissue Doppler echocardiography in systemic sclerosis. Ann Rheum Dis 64(9):1268–1273. doi:10.1136/ard.2004.031484

82. Duboc D, Kahan A, Maziere B, Loc'h C, Crouzel C, Menkes CJ, Amor B, Strauch G, Guerin F, Syrota A (1991) The effect of nifedipine on myocardial perfusion and metabolism in systemic sclerosis. A positron emission tomographic study. Arthritis Rheum 34(2):198–203

83. Kahan A, Devaux JY, Amor B, Menkes CJ, Weber S, Nitenberg A, Venot A, Guerin F, Degeorges M, Roucayrol JC (1986) Nifedipine and thallium-201 myocardial perfusion in progressive systemic sclerosis. N Engl J Med 314(22):1397–1402. doi:10.1056/NEJM198605293142201

84. Lancellotti P, Nkomo VT, Badano LP et al (2013) Expert consensus for multi-modality imaging evaluation of cardiovascular complications of radiotherapy in adults: a report from the European Association of Cardiovascular Imaging and the American Society of Echocardiography. Eur Heart J Cardiovasc Imaging 14:721–740

85. Darby SC, Cutter DJ, Boerma M et al (2010) Radiation-related heart disease: current knowledge and future prospects. Int J Radiat Oncol Biol Phys 76:656–665

86. Jurcut R, Ector J, Erven K et al (2007) Radiotherapy effects on systolic myocardial function detected by strain rate imaging in a left-breast cancer patient. Eur Heart J 28:2966

87. Gyenes G, Fornander T, Carlens P et al (1996) Myocardial damage in breast cancer patients treated with adjuvant radiotherapy: a prospective study. Int J Radiat Oncol Biol Phys 36: 899–905

88. Seddon B, Cook A, Gothard L et al (2002) Detection of defects in myocardial perfusion imaging in patients with early breast cancer treated with radiotherapy. Radiother Oncol 64:53–63

89. Prosnitz RG, Hubbs JL, Evans ES et al (2007) Prospective assessment of radiotherapy-associated cardiac toxicity in breast cancer patients: analysis of data 3 to 6 years after treatment. Cancer 110:1840–1850

90. Veinot JP, Edwards WD (1996) Pathology of radiation-induced heart disease: a surgical and autopsy study of 27 cases. Hum Pathol 27(8):766–773

91. Heidenreich PA, Hancock SL, Vagelos RH, Lee BK, Schnittger I (2005) Diastolic dysfunction after mediastinal irradiation. Am Heart J 150(5):977–982. doi:10.1016/j.ahj.2004.12.026

92. OHI D, Garot J (2011) Radiation-induced heart disease. Circ Heart Fail 4(1):e1–2. doi:10.1161/CIRCHEARTFAILURE.110.958454

Infiltrative/Storage Cardiomyopathies: Clinical Assessment and Imaging in Diagnosis and Patient Management

Michele Moretti, Enrico Fabris, Gherardo Finocchiaro, Bruno Pinamonti, Elena Abate, Giancarlo Vitrella, Marco Merlo, Francesca Brun, Lorenzo Pagnan, and Gianfranco Sinagra

20.1 Introduction

Infiltrative/storage cardiomyopathies (CMP) are characterized by the pathological deposition of abnormal substances in the heart muscle that cause myocardial hypertrophy, progressive stiffening, and diastolic and systolic dysfunction. They can result from a broad spectrum of inherited or acquired conditions and are usually associated with several systemic manifestations. It must be noted that the term infiltrative specifically refers to intercellular deposition, whereas storage refers to intracellular myocardial accumulation. The combination of clinical presentation and morphofunctional features often provides the clinician with enough insights (red flags) [1] to establish a working diagnostic hypothesis and thus correctly target further examinations. Noninvasive imaging, especially echocardiography [2] (Table 20.1) and cardiac magnetic resonance (CMR) (Table 20.2), plays a crucial role in the diagnosis and follow-up of these rare diseases. In some cases, serological, histological, and/or genetic examinations are required to confirm the diagnosis. Infiltrative and storage CMP are often characterized by a poor prognosis, although

Electronic supplementary material The online version of this chapter (doi: 10.1007/978-3-319-06019-4_20) contains supplementary material, which is available to authorized users. Videos can also be accessed at http://www.springerimages.com/videos/978-3-319-06018-7.

M. Moretti (✉) • E. Fabris • G. Finocchiaro • B. Pinamonti, MD • E. Abate • G. Vitrella
M. Merlo • F. Brun • G. Sinagra
Department of Cardiology, University Hospital of Trieste,
via P. Valdoni 7, Trieste 34139, Italy
e-mail: michele.moretti@gmail.com; enrico.fabris@hotmail.it; gherardobis@yahoo.it; bruno.pinamonti@gmail.com; abate.elena@gmail.com; giancarlo.vitrella@gmail.com; supermerloo@libero.it; frabrun77@gmail.com; gianfranco.sinagra@aots.sanita.fvg.it

L. Pagnan, MD
Radiology Unit, University Hospital of Trieste, via P. Valdoni 7, Trieste 34139, Italy
e-mail: pagny@inwind.it

B. Pinamonti, G. Sinagra (eds.), *Clinical Echocardiography and Other Imaging Techniques in Cardiomyopathies*, DOI 10.1007/978-3-319-06019-4_20,
© Springer International Publishing Switzerland 2014

Table 20.1 Echocardiographic features of infiltrative, storage, and mitochondrial cardiomyopathies (CMP)

Disease	Echocardiographic features
Infiltrative cardiomyopathies	
Amyloidosis	Left and right ventricle hypertrophy with preserved ventricular size
	Granular left ventricle appearance
	Biatrial dilatation
	Thickened interatrial septum and valve leaflets
	Pericardial effusion
	Restrictive physiology
	Decreased ejection fraction in advanced cases
Sarcoidosis	Variable wall thickness
	Normal to dilated ventricular chambers
	Scar retraction, aneurysms in the left ventricle
	Focal or global hypokinesis
	Pulmonary hypertension
Wegener granulomatosis	Wall motion abnormalities
	Pericardial effusion
Storage cardiomyopathies	
Fabry disease	Predominant concentric hypertrophy of left ventricle
	Right ventricular and papillary muscle hypertrophy also common
	Mild valve abnormalities
	Mild dilatation of the aortic root
	Possible binary appearance of the endocardial border
Danon disease	Marked symmetrical increase in left ventricular wall thickness (range 20–60 mm)
PRKAG2 cardiac syndrome	Left ventricle hypertrophy ranging between asymmetric septal hypertrophy, concentric hypertrophy, and distal hypertrophy
Glycogenoses	Pompe disease: severe thickening of the intraventricular septum, free wall, and posterior left ventricular wall, with a tumor-like appearance of the papillary muscles
	Cori-Forbes disease: concentric left ventricle thickening, increased refractile pattern, and granular appearance of the myocardium
Friedreich ataxia	Increase in left ventricular septal and posterior wall thickness
	Cavity size and ejection fraction usually normal
Oxalosis	Biventricular symmetrically thickened walls
	Myocardium characterized by patchy, echo-dense speckled reflection
Mucopolysaccharidoses	Asymmetrical septal hypertrophy
	Thickening of the valves
	Mitral and the aortic valves with insufficiency and/or stenosis
Hemochromatosis	Increase in left and right wall thickness
	Dilated left ventricle with global systolic dysfunction
	Restrictive physiology
Mitochondrial cardiomyopathy	
	Left ventricular hypertrophy
	In the late stage of disease, left ventricular dilatation and systolic dysfunction (hypokinetic end-stage evolution)

Table 20.2 Role of different imaging techniques in the assessment of infiltrative/storage cardiomyopathies

	Echocardiography	CMR	PET	SPECT	CT
Cardiac amyloidosis	++	+++	+	++	
Anderson-Fabry disease	++	+++	+		+
Cardiac hemochromatosis	+	+++			+
Cardiac sarcoidosis	+	+++	+++	++	

CMR cardiac magnetic resonance, *PET* positron emission tomography, *SPECT* single-photon-emission computed tomography, *CT* computed tomography

in some cases (e.g., Fabry disease), an early diagnosis can lead to specific treatment with potentially good results.

Heart failure (HF) is a common finding in infiltrative/storage CMP. However, as HF represents the final clinical pathway of many cardiac diseases, the recognition of many other multi-system manifestations (e.g., renal failure, peripheral neuropathy, skeletal myopathy, mental retardation, hepatosplenomegaly, etc.) is crucial to correctly direct the diagnosis [1] (Table 20.3). Moreover, it is important to emphasize that, especially in infiltrative CMP, evidence of a left ventricular (LV) hypertrophy on electrocardiography (ECG) is not a reliable indicator of increased LV mass. Indeed, infiltrative disorders mainly cause increased wall thickness by accumulation of abnormal substances in the interstitium and not within the myocytes (pseudohypertrophy). Consequently, increased wall thickness does not consistently correlate with high QRS complex voltages at ECG, and paradoxical low voltages or normal QRS voltages at ECG, contrasting with the significant LV hypertrophy, can be the first diagnostic clue of infiltrative CMP (typically amyloidosis) [1]. On the other hand, storage CMP, characterized by intracellular myocardial accumulation, frequently show very high QRS voltages at ECG, sometimes associated with ventricular pre-excitation, which can be the ECG hallmark of these disorders (e.g., Fabry disease, Danon disease).

Echocardiographic features are quite similar in most of infiltrative and storage CMP [2] (Table 20.1), frequently mimicking hypertrophic cardiomyopathy (HCM) in morphologic abnormalities and restrictive cardiomyopathy (RCM) from the hemodynamic point of view.

A final important point is that the use of advanced echocardiographic techniques, as well as CMR (Table 20.2), can be helpful in differential diagnosis, identifying early cardiac involvement, and quantifying the severity of cardiac damage in systemic infiltrative or storage diseases, with a favorable effect on treatment and outcome.

20.2 Infiltrative Cardiomyopathies

20.2.1 Cardiac Amyloidosis

Cardiac amyloidosis (CA) can be considered the prototype of infiltrative CMP. It results from pathological accumulation of insoluble extracellular fibrils derived by an abnormal folding of heterogeneous proteins [3] (Table 20.4). Regardless of

Table 20.3 Infiltrative and storage cardiomyopathies (CMP): clinical features and electrocardiograph (ECG) profile

	Age at presentation	Incidence/prevalence	ECG profile	Clinical features
Cardiac amyloidosis	>30 years	Depending on amyloidosis subtype	Low QRS voltages, pseudoinfarction pattern in anterior leads, AV and IV blocks	Multiple myeloma, dysphonia, macroglossia, skin alterations, peripheral neuropathy, carpal tunnel syndrome, renal failure with proteinuria
Cardiac sarcoidosis	>30–40 years	10.9/100,000 population	AV blocks, IV conduction defects, VT, SVT	Multiple granulomas (lungs, lymphatic system, liver, skin, eyes, nervous system)
Wegener granulomatosis	45 years (infantile and senile forms have been described)	2–12/1,000,000 live births	Aspecific	Necrotizing vascular granulomas involving multiple organs. Upper and lower airways chronic inflammation. Skin lesions, peripheral neuropathy, ocular abnormalities
Primary cardiac lymphoma	>40 years	Rare (<1/1,000,000 population/year)	Low voltages, AV blocks	Usually affects immunocompromised patients. Paraneoplastic syndrome, cardioembolic strokes
Fabry disease	Male: childhood/ adolescence Female: late adolescence/ adulthood	1/100,000 live births/ year (probably underestimated)	LVH (++), ventricular pre-excitation Can develop AV or IV conduction defects	Angiokeratomas, acroparesthesias, pain crises, fever, fatigue, hearing loss, juvenile TIA/ictus, renal failure
Danon disease	Male: ~16 years Female: ~30 years	Rare (<1/1,000,000)	LVH (++), ventricular pre-excitation/WPW syndrome May present VT or SVT	Skeletal myopathy (proximal), mental retardation, optical atrophy and retinal dysfunction, visual impairment
PRKAG2-gene-related CMP	>30 years	Unknown	LVH (++), ventricular pre-excitation/WPW syndrome. May present conduction abnormalities	May be associated with skeletal muscle glycogenosis
Glycogenoses	0–1 years	1/100,000 live births	LVH (++), ventricular pre-excitation, conduction defects	Skeletal myopathy with hypotonia and elevated CK levels, hepatomegaly, metabolic disorders

Friedreich ataxia	10–15 years	1/100,000 live births	Normal QRS voltages or mild LVH/VT.	Progressive gait ataxia followed by slurred speech and upper-limb ataxia; optic atrophy, hearing loss
Cardiac oxalosis	From infancy (severe forms) to adulthood (mild forms)	1/100,000 live births	AV blocks	Nephrocalcinosis, progressive renal failure, vascular calcifications, visual impairment
Mucopolysaccharidoses	<10 years	1/100,000 live births	May present low QRS voltages. Sudden death	Globally: mental retardation, coarse facies, skeletal abnormalities, macrocephaly, hypertrichosis, hepatosplenomegaly, upper airways obstructions, visual impairment, hearing loss Heart: valvular thickening, mitral prolapse, coronary artery disease, myocardial hypertrophy
Mucolipidoses	<10 years	Rare (<1/1,000,000)	*See* MPS	*See* MPS
Gangliosidoses	<10 years	1/200,000 live births	*See* MPS	*See* MPS
Hemochromatosis	>30 years	Depending on hemochromatosis subtype	Normal QRS; can develop low voltages and repolarization abnormalities in advanced stages	Liver cirrhosis, diabetes mellitus, hypogonadotropic hypogonadism, arthritis
Wilson disease	3–50 years	1/100,000 live births	LVH or biventricular hypertrophy, early repolarization, ST depression and T inversion	Liver cirrhosis, neurologic disorders (movement disorders or rigid dystonia), psychiatric manifestations (depression, phobias, compulsive behaviors, aggression or antisocial behavior, intellectual deterioration), Kayser-Fleischer rings (result from copper deposition in Descemet's membrane of the cornea)

(continued)

Table 20.3 (continued)

	Age at presentation	Incidence/prevalence	ECG profile	Clinical features
Mitochondrial diseases (CPEO, Kearns-Sayre syndrome, Leigh syndrome, LHON, MELAS, MERRF, NARP, Pearson's marrow-pancreas syndrome)	Variable	9.2/100,000 adults aged <65 years	Ventricular pre-excitation/ WPW syndrome, conduction disorders (AV blocks)	Encephalopathy, stroke-like episodes, seizures, cognitive impairment, depression, ataxia, sensorineural hearing loss, skeletal myopathy, palpebral ptosis, external ophthalmoplegia, optic atrophy, diabetes mellitus, hypothyroidism, hypogonadism, hypoparathyroidism, hepatic failure, renal tubulopathy

AV atrioventricular, *IV* intraventricular, *LVH* left ventricular hypertrophy, *VT* ventricular tachycardia, *SVT* supraventricular tachycardia, *WPW* Wolff-Parkinson-White, *MPS* mucopolysaccharidoses, *CK* creatine-kinase, *CPEO* chronic progressive external ophthalmoplegia, *LHON* Leber's hereditary optic neuropathy, *MELAS* myopathy, encephalopathy, and lactic acidosis with stroke-like episodes, *MERRF* mitochondrial encephalopathy with ragged red fibres, *NARP* neurogenic ataxia and retinitis pigmentosa, *TIA* transient ischemic attack

Table 20.4 Amyloidosis subtypes

Type	Precursor protein	Systems/organs involved	Notes
Primary amyloidosis (AL)	Immunoglobulin light chains λ (75 %) κ (25 %)	Heart, kidney, liver, gastrointestinal system, peripheral nervous system, autonomic nervous system	Most common form in Western countries. Associated with multiple myeloma or lymphoma.
Secondary amyloidosis (AA)	Serum amyloid A protein	Kidney, autonomic nervous system, heart (uncommon)	Chronic inflammatory disorders
Senile systemic amyloidosis (SSA)	Transthyretin (wild-type)	Heart	Advanced age (>80 years). Slowly progressive course, relatively benign prognosis.
Hereditary systemic amyloidosis (ATTR, AApoA1)	Mutated transthyretin, mutated apolipoprotein A1 (or other rare variants)	Heart, kidney, nervous system	Autosomal dominant inheritance
Atrial isolated amyloidosis	Atrial natriuretic peptide	Heart (atrium 100 %)	Increased risk of atrial fibrillation
Dialysis-related amyloidosis (Aβ2M)	β2-microglobulin	Osteoarticular system	Long-lasting hemodialysis

ATTR transthyretin, *AApo A1* apolipoprotein A1, *Aβ2M* β2-microglobulin-derived

which precursor protein causes the disease, the deposits are indistinguishable with light microscopy and invariably stain with Congo red staining (Fig. 20.2). The spectrum of organ involvement can include kidneys, blood vessels, nervous system, liver, lungs, gastrointestinal system, skin, eyes, joints, bones, and the heart.

Cardiac involvement is common and represents the most frequent cause of morbidity and mortality [4]. Symptoms include HF (dyspnea, peripheral edema, ascites), angina, hypotension, syncope, and palpitations. Supraventricular arrhythmias, especially atrial fibrillation (AF), can occur in 10–15 % of cases [3]; typical ECG pattern includes (Fig. 20.1):

- Low QRS voltages (46 % of cases)
- Pseudonecrosis Q waves in anterior leads (64 %)
- Abnormal QRS axis deviation (66 %)
- Atrioventricular blocks (35 %)
- Intraventricular blocks (16 %)
- AF or flutter (20 %)

The presence of coexisting systemic manifestations, such as a multiple myeloma, dysphonia, macroglossia, skin alterations, peripheral neuropathy, carpal tunnel syndrome, renal failure, and proteinuria, can strengthen the suspicion of systemic amyloidosis.

CA is usually indirectly diagnosed using noninvasive cardiac imaging and a bioptic confirmation of amyloid presence in an extracardiac tissue (typically abdominal fat, rectal submucosa, or salivary glands). Endomyocardial biopsy (EMB)

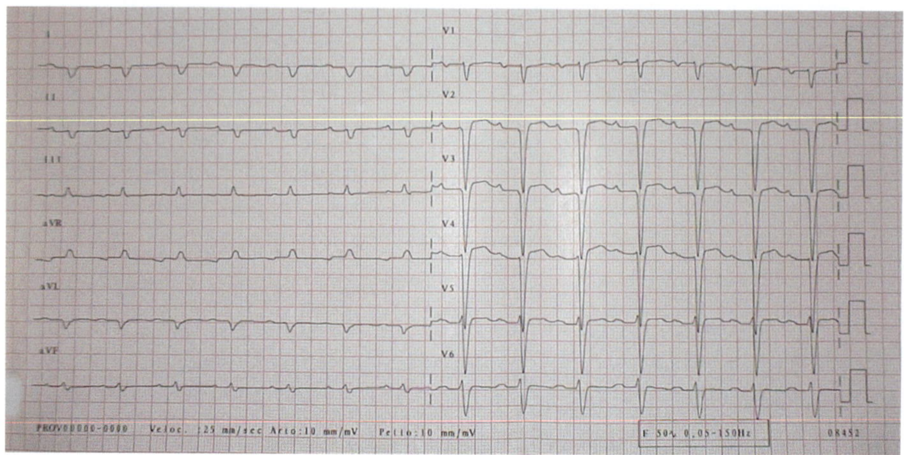

Fig. 20.1 Typical electrocardiogram (ECG) in a patient with cardiac amyloidosis. Low QRS voltages in peripheral leads and marked axis deviation are evident. Pathologic Q waves are also present

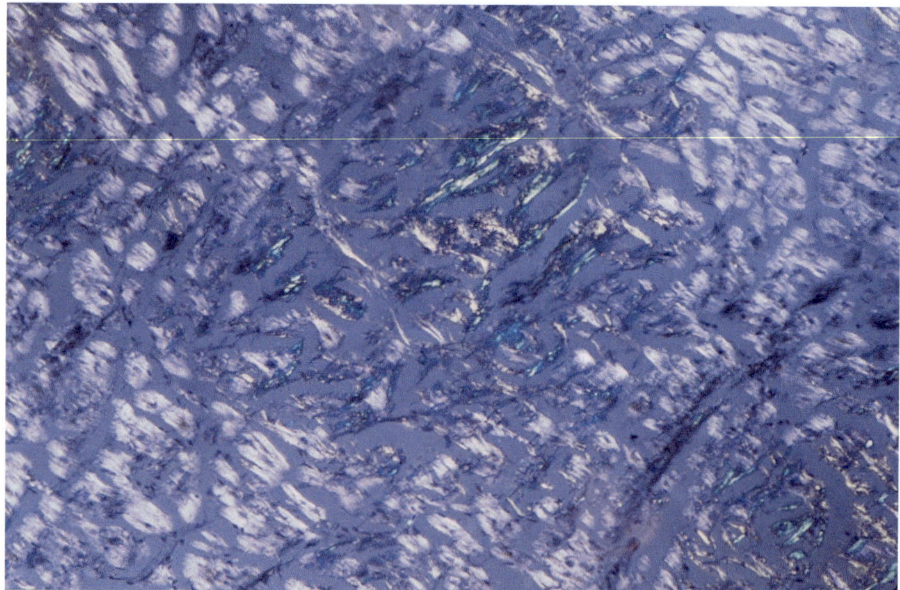

Fig. 20.2 Typical histologic pattern of cardiac amyloidosis. Interstitial depositions of amyloid are evident at Congo red staining, appearing as green birefringence under polarized light (×40)

(Fig. 20.2) may be necessary in cases with a high clinical suspicion but nondiagnostic extracardiac histology [4]. Clinical phenotype, prognosis, and treatment are highly variable, depending on the type of amyloidosis (Table 20.4). The most common form is amyloid light-chain (AL) amyloidosis, which has an estimated incidence of six to ten cases per million population per year [5]. The precursor protein is an immunoglobulin light-chain (λ or κ) and is sometimes related to multiple myeloma or lymphoma. Median survival of patients with AL amyloidosis is around 48 months [6], and the presence of symptomatic cardiac involvement at diagnosis represents a significantly negative prognostic marker [7]. Other forms include hereditary amyloidosis [transthyretin (ATTR), apolipoprotein A1 (AApo A1)], senile systemic amyloidosis (SSA), secondary amyloidosis (AA), dialysis-related amyloidosis [β2-microglobulin-derived (Aβ2M)] and isolated atrial amyloidosis (for details, *see* Table 20.4) [8].

Echocardiography represents a main diagnostic tool in CA. HF is frequently the result of the stiff-heart syndrome characterized by severe impairment of diastolic function secondary to amyloid infiltration of the myocardium, with relatively preserved systolic function and without cardiac remodelling [3, 4, 8–15]. However, it is important to realize that echocardiography cannot make the diagnosis in isolation, and images should be interpreted in the context of the clinical picture and other investigations. Moreover, the different types of amyloidosis that affect the heart (i.e., AL and variant/wild-type TTR types) cannot be distinguished by echocardiographic features, and this differential diagnosis is dependent on the recognition of some clinical and humoral clues and must be confirmed by immunohistochemical analysis from biopsy specimen [8]. Identifying the specific type of amyloidosis is compulsory in this setting, because therapeutic options are very different.

The most common echocardiographic feature is a concentric thickening of the left ventricular (LV) walls (Fig. 20.3, Clips 20.1 and 20.2), particularly in the absence of secondary causes. The combined presence of increased LV mass and low voltages at ECG (Fig. 20.1) may be more specific for infiltrative disease [4, 9, 16, 17]. Rahman et al. [9] studied 196 patients referred for EMB because of clinical suspicion of CA. The diagnosis was confirmed in 58 patients and, in multivariate logistic regression models, a combination of a low voltages and measures of myocardial thickness produced the most statistically useful model.

LV systolic function is usually preserved until the late stages of the disease process. However, despite a normal LV ejection fraction (EF), longitudinal systolic function may be altered early during disease progression. In the presence of segmental wall-motion abnormalities (WMA) or global LV systolic dysfunction, a concomitant involvement of coronary arteries (due to atherosclerotic heart disease and/or coronary infiltration by amyloid) should be suspected [18].

The echocardiographic appearance of CA can closely mimic several other diseases. Asymmetric hypertrophy of the septum due to amyloid deposition, even if rare, may occur, simulating HCM. Increased echogenicity of the myocardium (granular sparkling appearance) is not specific for CA and can also be found in myocarditis with severe fibrosis; it is quite common in HCM, as well as in other infiltrative and storage CMP [19]. Cardiac valves, papillary muscles, and intra-atrial septum are also frequently thickened, and pericardial effusion is frequently observed (Fig. 20.3, Clips 20.1 and 20.2). Mild valvular dysfunction is quite common, but severe dysfunction is rare [20]. Both atria are often enlarged, in keeping with

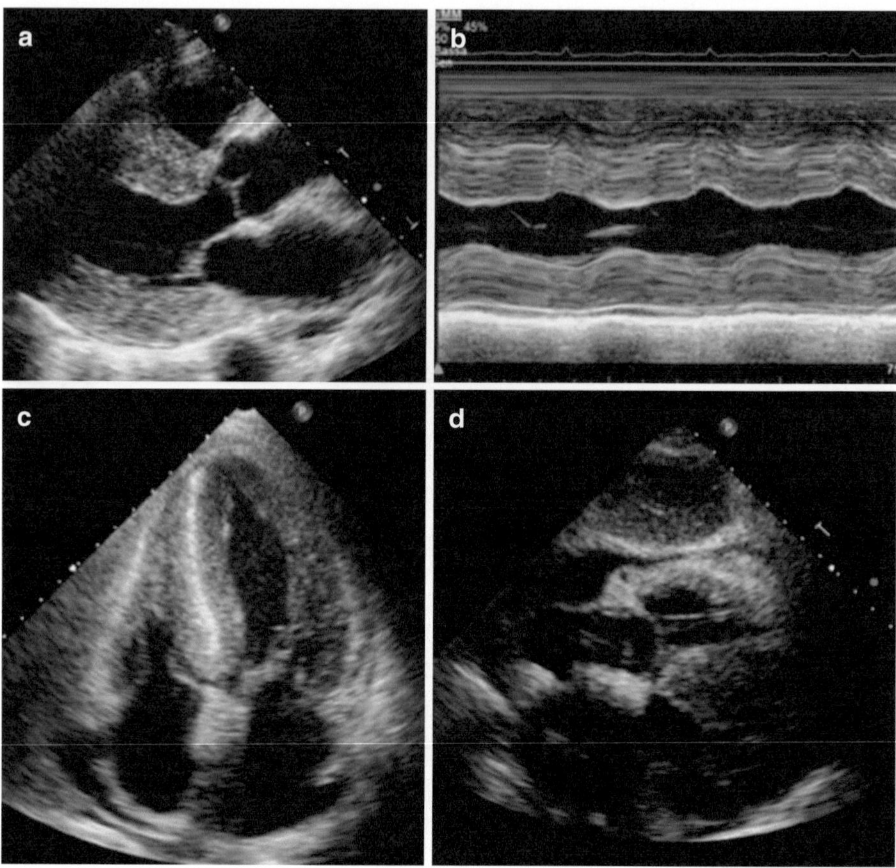

Fig. 20.3 Echocardiogram from a 72-year-old woman with cardiac amyloidosis. The left ventricle (LV) is severely hypertrophic (interventricular septum thickness 26 mm). Also, thickening of the right ventricle (RV) is evident. A granular sparkling appearance of the ventricular myocardium is evident. There is moderate thickening of valve leaflets and inter-atrial septum. Pericardial effusion is present. Parasternal long-axis view (**a**); M-mode echocardiogram of the left ventricle (**b**); apical four-chamber view (**c**); subcostal view (**d**)

diastolic dysfunction, which can involve both ventricles. The right ventricle (RV) can be involved in CA, frequently showing hypertrophy and dysfunction. Ghio et al. [21] studied 74 patients with AL amyloidosis and showed that 20 % of them had RV dysfunction [by tricuspid annular proximal systolic excursion (TAPSE)]. Diastolic dysfunction may be present in various degrees in CA. Doppler echocardiography has a main role in this setting. Advanced disease is frequently characterized by a restrictive filling pattern (RFP) (Fig. 20.4). In 1989, Klein et al. [22] were the first to describe the characteristics of LV filling pattern in patients with CA using Doppler echocardiography.

The above described echocardiographic abnormalities were reported and are seen in patients affected by symptomatic, clinically evident, CA and usually in an

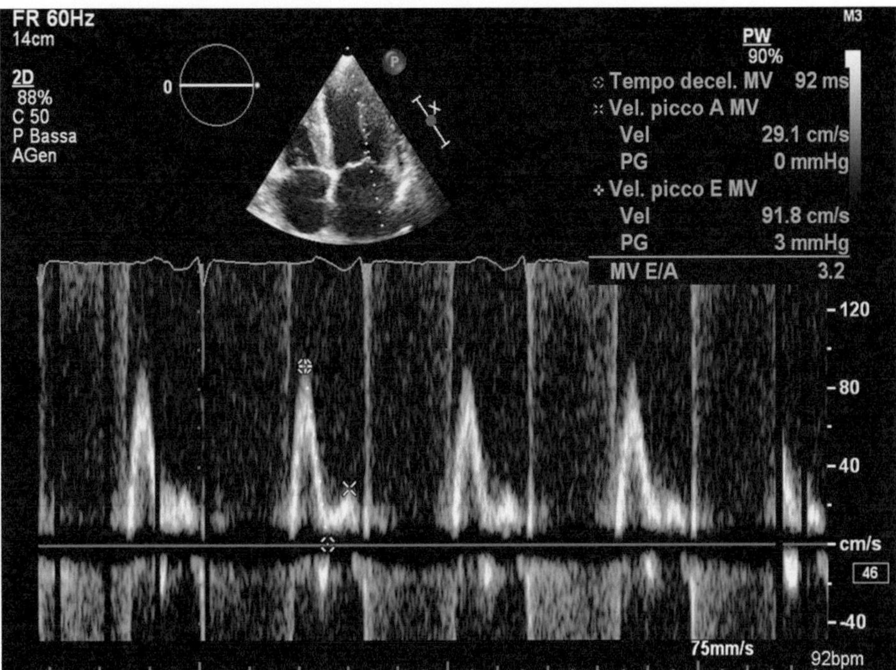

Fig. 20.4 Echocardiogram from a 50-year-old woman with cardiac amyloidosis. Transmitral pulsed Doppler shows severe diastolic dysfunction with restrictive filling pattern (E-wave velocity = 92 cm/s, A-wave velocity = 29 cm/s, E/A ratio = 3.2, E-wave deceleration time = 92 ms)

advanced stage. Efforts have been employed to identify cardiac involvement in the early stage of the disease in asymptomatic or mildly symptomatic patients.

Tissue-Doppler imaging (TDI) has shown reduced diastolic velocities in both early and late cardiac amyloid, so even early diastolic dysfunction could be identified, even in presence of minimal wall thickening [23]. As in healthy controls, in CA patients, there is a gradient of tissue velocities from the base to the apex, but peak systolic tissue velocities at the base and mid ventricle are significantly lower in CA patients with advanced disease and HF in comparison with early-stage asymptomatic patients [24].

Doppler myocardial imaging could have a role also in assessing RV dysfunction. Bellavia et al. [25] showed that E' velocity (at the RV free wall) measured using TDI, as well as TAPSE, are often reduced in patients with AL amyloidosis and normal echocardiogram and are independent predictors of death.

Furthermore, as mentioned in Chap. 19, TDI can have a role in distinguishing restrictive physiology due to amyloid from constrictive pericarditis (CP). Sometimes the differential diagnosis is not easy, because the two diseases share some clinical and morphologic features. Peak early diastolic velocity from the lateral mitral annulus by TDI are usually markedly reduced in patients with CA compared with CP and normal individuals, which suggests that this measurement can provide a clinically valuable distinction between these two conditions [26].

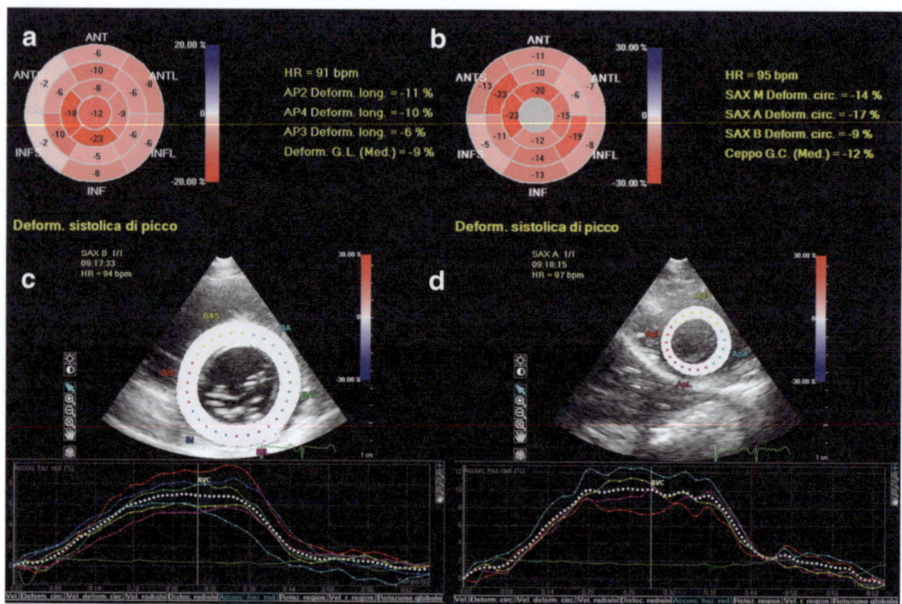

Fig. 20.5 Assessment of 2D speckle-tracking strain in a patient with amyloidosis. The left ventricle (LV) had a moderate hypertrophy (interventricular septum 14 mm, posterior wall 13 mm, mass 160 g/mq) and a moderate systolic dysfunction (ejection fraction 43 %). Strain imaging revealed global reduction of longitudinal (**a**), circumferential (**b**), and radial (**c, d**) strain, with a progressive increase in strain values from base to apex. Bull's eye plot showing results of longitudinal strain analysis (**a**): basal LV level −5.3 %, mid level −7.1 %, apical level −14.5 %, and global −9 %. Bull's eye plot with circumferential strain values (**b**): basal −9 %, mid −14 %, apical −17 %, and global −12 %. Radial strain assessed at basal LV (**c**) was 6.5 %, mid level 6.8 %, apical level 10 % (**d**), and global 7.8 %. *ANT* anterior, *ANTL* anterolateral, *ANTS* anteroseptal, *AP2* apical two-chamber view, *AP3* apical three-chamber view, *AP4* apical four-chamber view, *GC* global circumferential (strain), *GL* global longitudinal (strain), *HR* heart rate, *INF* inferior, *INFL* inferolateral, *INFS* inferoseptal, *SAX A* short-axis apical view, *SAX B* short-axis basal view, *SAX M* short-axis mid view

Advanced echocardiographic techniques also focus on segmental deformation and its role in the differential diagnosis between CA and other diseases that may have a similar appearance at 2D echocardiography. Such diseases comprise HCM, Fabry disease, and hypertensive heart disease. Sun et al. [27] reported that global longitudinal strain detected by 2D speckle-tracking analysis was significantly lower in patients with CA compared with healthy controls but also compared with individuals with LV hypertrophy caused by HCM or hypertensive heart disease. Interestingly, CA is characterized by typical regional variations in longitudinal strain from base to apex. A relative apical-sparing pattern (Fig. 20.5, Clip 20.3a, 20.3b, and 20.3c) of longitudinal strain is an easily recognizable, accurate, and reproducible method of differentiating CA from other causes of LV hypertrophy [28].

Finally, Baccouche et al. [29] studied 12 patients with CA and 12 with HCM using 3D speckle-tracking echocardiography. These authors found important

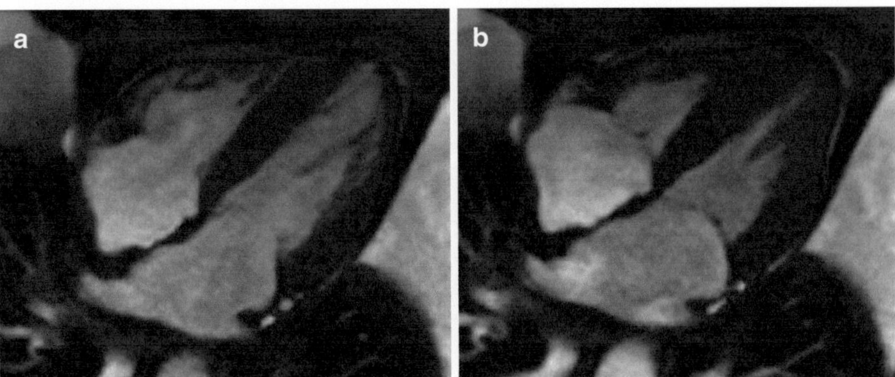

Fig. 20.6 Cardiac magnetic resonance (CMR) study in a 60-year-old patient affected by amyloid light-chain (AL) amyloidosis with cardiac involvement. End-diastolic (**a**) and end-systolic (**b**) frames. Note concentric LV thickening and severely impaired LV longitudinal function

differences between the two diseases. In particular, the basal–apical radial strain gradient displayed oppositional characteristics in CA and HCM. The increasing basoapical radial strain gradient contrasts the physiological, decreasing basoapical radial strain gradient observed in healthy hearts [30].

CMR is particularly useful in CA imaging assessment by its value in morphological assessment, wall thickness evaluation, and the differential with other CMP [8, 31–34]. CMR morphofunctional study confirms the classic appearance of the disease, characterized by a restrictive configuration of the heart, with small and thick ventricles and large atria, frequent presence of pericardial and pleural effusions and/or ascites, and sometimes hypertrophy of the atrial septum [8, 33] (Fig. 20.6).

In addition, CMR study can detect changes in myocardial tissue composition and architecture due to interstitial deposition of amyloid protein as changes in signal intensity on T1-weighted imaging. Furthermore, as myocardial intercellular amyloid deposition results in interstitial space expansion, late gadolinium-enhanced (LGE) CMR has main role in the diagnosis of CA. In fact, gadolinium chelates distribute in the extracellular space that is expanded by amyloid infiltration, leading to signal enhancement.

Syed et al. [34] performed LGE CMR in 120 patients referred to a tertiary center with histologically confirmed diagnosis of amyloidosis; 97 % of their CA patients had abnormal LGE, and 91 % had increased LV wall thickness on echocardiography. LGE pattern was global (transmural or subendocardial) in 83 % of cases (Fig. 20.7). Austin et al. [35] described a typical LGE pattern at CMR in CA patients, which is a diffuse circumferential LGE pattern involving the entire subendocardium and extending to adjacent myocardium. The diagnostic accuracy of this CMR pattern was superior to traditional noninvasive ECG and echocardiographic variables. However, LGE imaging has some limitations in CA, dealing in particular with contraindication in patients with severe renal impairment and by the fact that the above described patterns of LGE are often not uniform and are quite variable,

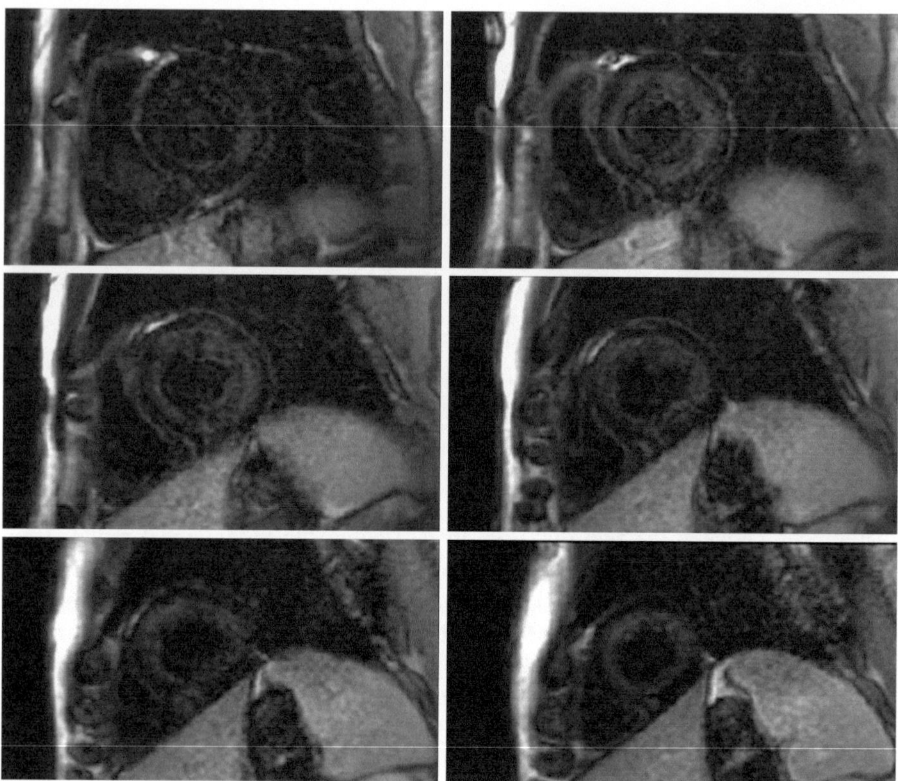

Fig. 20.7 Cardiac magnetic resonance (CMR) gadolinium-contrast-enhanced study in a patient with cardiac amyloidosis. The short-axis stack shows a global subendocardial late gadolinium enhancement (LGE) evident from the base to the apex of the left ventricle, corresponding to amyloid infiltration of myocardium

leading to confusion in interpretation [34]. An interesting development in CMR is the advent of techniques that provide quantitative information on diffuse myocardial fibrosis by measuring the intrinsic magnetic resonance relaxation parameter T1 of the myocardium and mapping its spatial distribution. Karamitsos et al. [36] described a cohort of AL amyloidosis showing how native T1 correlates with systolic and diastolic dysfunction and has the potential to be more sensitive in detecting early disease than is LGE imaging.

Another interesting new method that may play a future important role in assessing CA is extracellular volume measurement using CMR. Banypersad et al. [37] demonstrated the progressive increase of extracellular volume values from normals to patients with AL amyloidosis without cardiac involvement, and those with definite cardiac involvement. Thus, this measurement has potential to become the first noninvasive test able to quantify cardiac amyloid burden.

Amyloid deposits in the heart may be also detected by single-photon-emission computed tomography (SPECT) using technetium-99m (^{99m}Tc)-aprotinin, a protease inhibitor [38–40] and ^{99m}Tc-labelled phosphate derivatives, particularly in patients with hereditary transthyretin-related (TTR) amyloidosis [41–45]. The latter methods have important roles in differential diagnosis between TTR and AL amyloidoses and an improved capability in quantifying cardiac amyloid infiltration burden compared with LGE CMR [46].

An increased thallium-201 (^{201}Tl)—a perfusion tracer—washout rate at rest–redistribution myocardial scintigraphy was reported in patients with CA and may reflect the severity of amyloid deposits in the myocardium [47]. SPECT studies with [^{123}I]-metaiodobenzylguanidine (MIBG), an analog of norepinephrine, demonstrate myocardial dysinnervation (possibly due to the presence of amyloid deposits or a specific involvement of the autonomic system) both in patients with familial amyloidotic polyneuropathy [48, 49] and in those with AL amyloidosis and autonomic neuropathy [50]. Positron emission tomography (PET) with N-[methyl-11C]2-(4'-methylamino-phenyl)-6-hydroxybenzothiazole ([^{11}C]-PIB), a tracer used to evaluate brain amyloidosis, was suggested as a method for studying systemic amyloidosis types AL and ATTR affecting the heart [51]. Parasympathetic myocardial denervation was also found in patients with familial amyloidotic polyneuropathy with [^{11}C]-methylquinuclidinyl benzilate (MQNB) PET [49].

CA is historically considered a disease with poor short-term prognosis [3]. However, as demonstrated by Rapezzi et al. [8], it must not to be considered as a single entity, but the different underlying etiologies must be taken in account, especially when considering outcome, being that AL CA is the most aggressive form.

Echocardiography has a main role not only for determining cardiac involvement but in predicting outcome and monitoring cases over time. As shown by Klein et al. [22], Doppler-derived LV diastolic-filling variables and, in particular, the presence of RFP, are important predictors of survival in this disease. The same authors subsequently focused on the prognostic significance of a progression of LV-filling Doppler parameters during short-term follow-up that particularly affect patients with nonsevere thickening of LV walls [52]. Additional echocardiographic abnormalities, such as LA enlargement and RV dysfunction, were related with a worse prognosis in this disease [53]. Ghio et al. [21] found that RV dysfunction assessed by TAPSE was associated with a more severe LV involvement, higher plasma levels of N-terminal prohormone of brain natriuretic peptide (NT-proBNP) and poor prognosis. Speckle tracking showed that RV dysfunction seems to develop later than LV amyloid deposition, but, when it occurs, prognosis dramatically worsens [54]. In a large population of biopsy-proven AL CA patients, Buss et al. [55] showed that both TDI-derived longitudinal strain and speckle-tracking-derived global longitudinal strain were independent predictors of survival, with incremental power beyond standard clinical and serological parameters. The authors also demonstrated how NT-proBNP was strongly correlated with the parameters of longitudinal function considered above. Furthermore, Bellavia et al. [56], in a large cohort of patients with AL amyloidosis, identified peak longitudinal systolic strain of the basal anteroseptal segment as the main independent echocardiographic predictor of survival.

CMR, in addition to offering the clinician an excellent tool by which to attain a detailed view of morphological and functional abnormalities and to differentiate CA from other disease entities, may have a prognostic value [56]. First, this technique has an important role in early diagnosis of cardiac involvement, providing the opportunity to initiate early an adequate therapy [34, 57]. In addition, as reported by Austin et al. [35], the presence of typical diffuse circumferential LGE pattern at CMR is the only independent prognostic predictor on Cox proportional hazards analysis.

An additional clinical point must be considered in prognostic assessment of the disease. Although prognosis is generally poor in CA, long-term survival is rare but possible, and it is generally observed when the disease (and cardiac involvement) is detected at an early stage and adequate treatment is promptly implemented [58].

Finally, the underlying pathomechanisms of systolic and diastolic dysfunction associated with CA remain widely unknown. It has been hypothesized that a possible direct toxic effect of amyloid proteins could initially induce myocardial hypertrophy and then lead to systolic and/or diastolic dysfunction [59]. As the disease progresses, more amyloid deposits lead to atrophy and cardiomyocyte apoptosis and remodeling toward collagen formation and subsequent fibrosis [8]. Probably, this toxic effect is not equally present in all the types of amyloidosis. For example, Ng et al. [60] observed that patients with senile systemic amyloidosis (SSA) manifested a somewhat less aggressive disease course with respect to AL amyloidosis, despite the presence of more severe LV wall hypertrophy. A possible direct toxic effect related to the circulating monoclonal light chains in AL amyloidosis was hypothesized.

20.2.2 Sarcoidosis

Sarcoidosis is a chronic immune-mediated disease characterized by formation of granulomas in multiple organs (lungs, lymphatic system, liver, skin, eyes, nervous system, heart). Estimated prevalence is ~10.9 cases per 100,000 population [61]. The heart is involved in 20–30 % of cases, but only 5 % are clinically evident and symptomatic [62–64]. Every part of the heart can be involved in the disease. The predominant sites of myocardial involvement, in decreasing order of frequency, are LV free walls and papillary muscles, basal aspect of the interventricular septum (IVS), the RV wall, and atrial walls [63]. Clinical manifestations of cardiac sarcoidosis are variable and nonspecific; they range from asymptomatic conduction abnormalities to fatal ventricular arrhythmias, depending upon the location and extent of infiltration. Complete heart block is the most common finding (23–30 % of patients with clinically evident disease) [62–64]; first-degree heart block and bundle-branch blocks (BBB) also often occur due to involvement of the basal septum by scar tissue or granulomas or to that of the nodal artery, causing ischemia in the conduction system. Ventricular tachycardia is the most frequent arrhythmia in sarcoidosis (23 %), and sudden death (SD) secondary to ventricular arrhythmias has been described [63]; supraventricular arrhythmias are less common (15 % of cases). HF can be another manifestation and may be secondary to widespread infiltration of the myocardium, ventricular aneurysms, arrhythmias, cor pulmonale caused by pulmonary hypertension, valvular regurgitation, or a combination of these processes. End-stage HF is the cause of death in 25 % of patients affected by this disease, making it the second most frequent cause of death after SD (67 %). Other clinical manifestations include chest pain, pseudonecrosis Q waves at ECG, and pericardial abnormalities, such as pericardial effusion (3–19 % of cases), CP, and—rarely—cardiac tamponade [63].

The diagnosis of cardiac sarcoidosis can be very challenging from the clinical point of view. EMB, despite its specificity, has a low sensitivity as a result of patchy or focal infiltration [65]. The echocardiographic appearance of cardiac sarcoidosis varies among affected patients, ranging from normal to dilated ventricular chambers and normal to decreased regional and global systolic function. Ventricles may be globally hypokinetic, or the patchy nature of sarcoid infiltration of the heart may result in regional WMA [66]. Segmental WMA characteristically do not conform to any particular coronary distribution [66–68]. Two-dimensional echocardiographic morphologic abnormalities of cardiac sarcoid vary according to disease activity and include wall thickening due to granulomatous expansion and wall thinning due to fibrosis [66–68]. A typical site of these abnormalities, particularly wall thinning, is the basal anterior septum, the appearance of which in a young patient with dilated cardiomyopathy (DCM) is highly suggestive of sarcoidosis [67]. Scar retraction and aneurysms may develop, especially if the patient has been treated with corticosteroids. Sun et al. [69] assessed the prevalence of the above-described echocardiographic abnormalities in a large series of patients implanted with a pacemaker or an implanted cardiac defibrillator (ICD) and absence of coronary artery disease. Two abnormalities were analyzed: type 1, presenting with marked thinning and akinesis of the basal IVS; and type 2, presenting as localized aneurismal bulging of the posterolateral wall. Their prevalence was relatively low (15 and 6 cases, respectively, of 1,357 consecutive patients).

Pulmonary involvement occurs in 90 % of patients with sarcoidosis; thus Doppler echocardiographic examination should include assessment of pulmonary pressures and RV function to detect early signs of pulmonary hypertension [70]. In asymptomatic patients with extracardiac sarcoidosis, speckle-tracking echocardiography revealed alterations in strain and rotational indices [71]. Newly diagnosed sarcoid patients appear to have lower global longitudinal strain, despite having a well-preserved global systolic myocardial function. Moreover, LV twist appears to be increased in the patient population with respect to the control population. Therefore, deformation imaging could be a valuable adjunct for screening this patient group [71].

In suspected cardiac sarcoidosis, CMR can provide information when assessing myocardial edema and fibrosis leading to postinflammatory scarring [72]. Smedema et al. [73] studied 58 cases of biopsy-proven pulmonary sarcoidosis and report sensitivity and specificity of CMR as 100 and 78 %, respectively, and positive and negative predictive values as 55 and 100 %, respectively, with an overall accuracy of 83 %. The preferential involvement of LV basal septal and lateral segments was confirmed by this technique (Fig. 20.8).

Myocardial perfusion imaging with ^{201}Tl and ^{99m}Tc-sestamibi SPECT may show patterns of reverse distribution, in which perfusion defects at rest decrease under

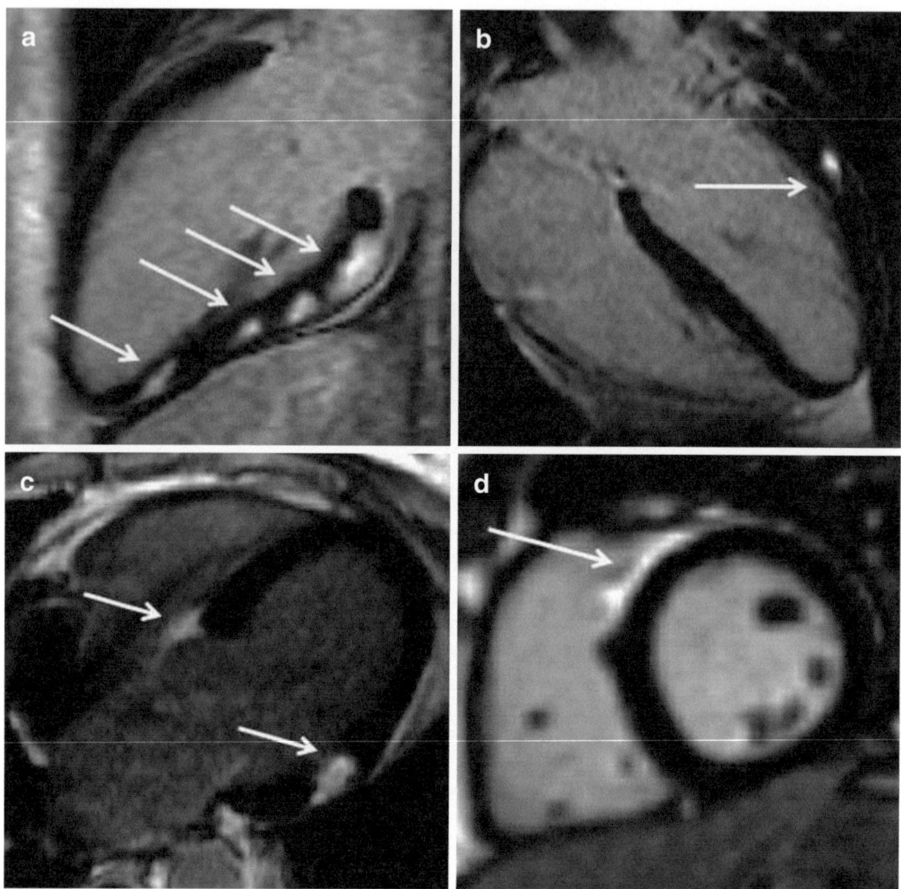

Fig. 20.8 Four examples of late gadolinium enhancement (LGE) distribution (*arrows*) in cardiac sarcoidosis. Patchy diffuse LGE at the inferior wall (**a**), focal LGE at the basal lateral wall (**b**), focal LGE at the basal septum and lateral wall (**c**), LGE scar at the anterior septum (**d**)

stress conditions, possibly due to focal reversible microvascular constriction in coronary arterioles around the granulomas. However, 67 gallium (^{67}Ga) scintigraphy can detect cardiac involvement in sarcoidosis during its inflammatory phase because of accumulation of this tracer in inflamed areas [74–76].

PET imaging with [^{18}F]-fluorodeoxyglucose ([^{18}F]-FDG) PET—a glucose analog preferentially taken up and retained in areas of inflammation—was demonstrated in cardiac sarcoidosis to provide functional imaging of inflammatory disease activity (typically seen as a patchy, focal uptake pattern) [72, 77–80]. In a meta-analysis of seven studies and 164 patients, [^{18}F]-FDG PET was reported to have 89 % sensitivity and 78 % specificity for detecting active sarcoidosis [80]. When using both [^{18}F]-FDG and [^{13}N]-ammonia (^{13}N-NH$_3$) or rubidium-82 (^{82}Rb) to assess myocardial perfusion, a characteristic pattern of perfusion defect and increased

[^{18}F]-FDG signal (perfusion–metabolism mismatch) is seen in active cardiac sarcoidosis [81–84].

In cardiac sarcoidosis, early diagnosis and effective treatment are absolutely necessary to improve long-term prognosis. Imaging—and in particular, CMR—and PET are important tools in prognostic stratification and treatment choice [82]. Cardiac PET identifies patients at higher risk of death and ventricular tachycardia due to the presence of focal perfusion defects and abnormal [^{18}F]-FDG uptake [83]. LGE at CMR can also be an important prognostic indicator. Patel et al. [85] described a cohort of 81 patients with biopsy-proven extracardiac sarcoidosis: LGE was present in 26 %, and these patients had a ninefold higher rate of adverse events (death, defibrillator shock, pacemaker requirement) and an 11.5-fold higher rate of cardiac death than patients without damage.

20.2.3 Wegener Granulomatosis

Wegener granulomatosis is characterized by necrotizing granulomatous inflammation involving vessels of multiple organs, particularly respiratory system and kidneys. Heart involvement is quite common (36–82 % of cases), but most frequently, it remains subclinical [86, 87]. Clinically evident HF is rare.

A high frequency of echocardiographic abnormalities is reported in Wegener granulomatosis. In a series of 85 patients [86], 86 % had echocardiographic abnormalities, and 36 % appeared directly related to Wegener granulomatosis. In particular, WMA, LV systolic dysfunction with decreased EF, and pericardial effusion were found, respectively, in 65, 50, and 19 % of patients with related abnormalities. Other findings include valvulitis, LV aneurysm, and a large intracardiac mass. The mass (16-mm tick at the LV OT), which was removed surgically, consisted of granulomatous tissue with negative culture results. Echocardiographic screening of patients with active Wegener granulomatosis may be of clinical value because cardiac involvement is often silent and associated with increased morbidity and worse prognosis [86].

The possible incremental value of 2D speckle-tracking echocardiography over standard echocardiography to detect myocardial abnormalities in Wegener granulomatosis shows that despite normal LV EF, global systolic LV abnormalities detected by speckle-tracking imaging are common in affected individuals, reflecting subclinical involvement of the myocardium, which is underdiagnosed using standard echocardiography. Among all global peak-systolic deformational parameters, longitudinal systolic strain/strain rate was the most commonly decreased, suggesting subendocardial and midwall involvement in this group of patients [88].

20.2.4 Primary Cardiac Lymphoma

Primary cardiac lymphoma is a rare neoplastic disease (1 % of primary cardiac tumors, 0.5 % of extra-nodal lymphomas) that involves myocardium and pericardium without extracardiac involvement [89, 90]. It is more frequent in immunocompromised patients and usually presents with myocardial thickening and intracardiac masses; nevertheless, forms undistinguishable from a restrictive/infiltrative CMP are described [90]. From the clinical point of view, patients usually present HF associated with diastolic and systolic dysfunction. ECG shows low voltages (despite LV hypertrophy at echo); mild pericardial effusion may be present. Diagnosis is challenging and always requires EMB [class IIa recommendation in "unexplained" forms of restrictive CMP, according to American College of Cardiology (ACC)/AHA (American Heart Association)/European Society of Cardiology (ESC) guidelines] [91].

20.3 Storage Cardiomyopathies

The majority of the storage CMP here described can be considered among the so-called lysosomal storage diseases, considering that they are caused by a deficiency of lysosomal enzymes, membrane transporters, or other proteins involved in lysosomal biology, and that the main accumulation of different substrates occurs within lysosomes [92].

20.3.1 Anderson-Fabry Disease

Anderson-Fabry disease is a progressive, multisystemic, lysosomal storage disease with an X-linked inheritance pattern [92, 93]. It is caused by a deficiency of alpha-galactosidase A, a lysosomal enzyme involved in the metabolism of glycosphingo-lipids. It results in accumulation of glycosphingolipids within the cells of multiple organs (primarily skin, kidneys, vessels, and heart), causing multisystem clinical manifestations. The incidence is reported to be ~1:100,000 live births, but this is probably underestimated [92–94]. Cardiac involvement is frequent (40–60 % of cases) and can mimic HCM [92, 95, 96], accounting for 0.5–6 % of cases initially diagnosed as HCM according to different case series [95–98].

ECG is characterized by high QRS voltages (signs of LV hypertrophy) with repolarization abnormalities; moreover, a short PR interval is present in 40 % of cases. With disease progression, many cases develop atrioventricular and/or intra-ventricular conduction defects, sick sinus syndrome, and supraventricular and ventricular arrhythmias [94]. Presentation is clinically heterogeneous; symptoms may be variable (angiokeratomas, acroparesthesias, pain crises, fever, chronic fatigue, hearing loss, etc.). Major renal or cardiac dysfunction is uncommon in early stages but frequently manifests in late stages [93, 98, 99]. The demonstration of deficient alpha-galactosidase activity in plasma or leukocytes by enzymatic assay provides a conclusive diagnosis in male patients; in female patients, diagnostic confirmation should be made by genetic analysis [93].

Progressive thickening of cardiac walls represents the main consequence of glycosphingolipid deposition and is the main echocardiographic feature of Fabry

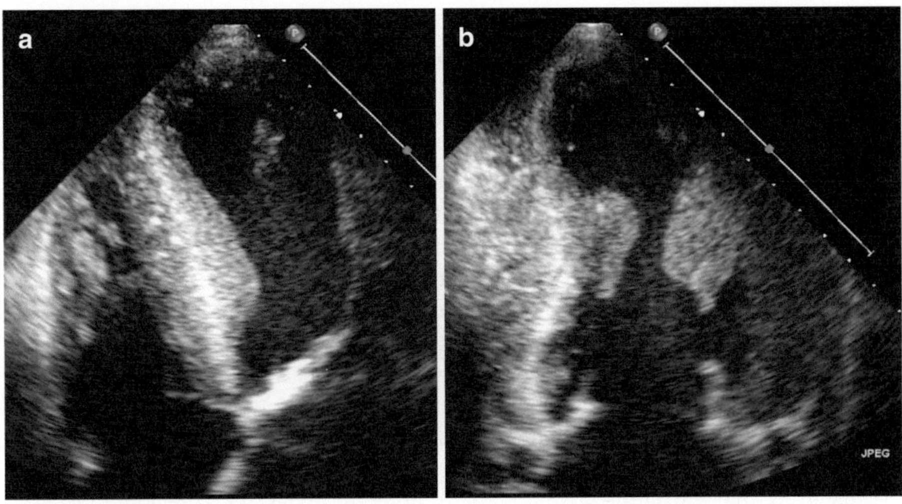

Fig. 20.9 Echocardiogram from a 52-year-old man with Fabry disease and cardiac involvement. The left ventricle is severely hypertrophic (interventricular septum thickness 29 mm) and moderately dilated (end-diastolic volume 175 ml). A granular sparkling appearance of ventricular myocardium is evident. There is moderate thickening of valve leaflets without significant stenosis. Apical four-chamber view (**a**); apical two-chamber view (**b**)

CMP (Fig. 20.9, Clips 20.4 and 20.5) [99, 100]. LV hypertrophy is reported in up to 50 % of male and one third of female Fabry patients [99, 100]. In most cases, LV hypertrophy is concentric; however, Fabry CMP may present with eccentric, apical, or asymmetric septal hypertrophy, so that it may mimic HCM [95–100]. LV obstruction is rare at rest but is reported in 43 % of patients during effort [101]. LV systolic function is usually preserved in most patients until advanced disease stage, but a few patients may progressively develop systolic dysfunction and refractory HF [102]. RV involvement largely parallels LV involvement. RV hypertrophy can be found in ~50–70 % of all patients with Fabry disease (dependent on gender and age) [103, 104]. Interestingly, there is no reduction in RV hypertrophy under enzyme replacement therapy, which is in contrast to LV response [104]. Valve abnormalities are observed frequently in Fabry patients, but although globotriaosylceramide storage is present in valve tissue, valve abnormalities are usually only mild. Mildly dilated aortic root is common in Fabry disease: increased aortic root diameter is reported in affected male compared with female patients and healthy controls [105].

On 2D echocardiography, a binary appearance of the endocardial border corresponding to endomyocardial sphingolipid compartmentalization, creating a two-layered appearance of the myocardium, was reported as a specific sign of the disease [106]; however, in a subsequent study [107], this sign was considered unreliable, being present also in some cases of HCM.

Finally, the Tei Index—a marker for combined diastolic and systolic dysfunction derived by dividing the sum of isovolumic contraction and relaxation times by ejection time—was assessed in a large cohort of genetically confirmed Fabry patients and was higher in those with evidence of LV hypertrophy and/or LGE on CMR with respect to patients without cardiac involvement [108].

According to recent studies, early cardiac involvement in Fabry disease could be detected using advanced echocardiographic techniques. A study with TDI in Fabry patients with EMB-proven cardiac involvement showed a reduction of both diastolic and systolic myocardial velocities recorded at septal and lateral corners of the mitral annulus [109]. Reduction of TDI velocities can, in fact, represent the sign of initial intrinsic myocardial impairment not yet manifesting with LV hypertrophy and conventional parameters of diastolic or even systolic dysfunction. According to those authors, TDI can also be useful in detecting cardiac involvement in female carriers with no systemic manifestations of disease.

Furthermore, Gruner et al. [110] showed that patients with Fabry disease lose the normal base-to-apex circumferential strain gradient. In another study on 51 patients affected by Fabry CMP and 25 controls [111], longitudinal strain rates in basal, mid, and apical segments of each wall and radial strain rates of the inferolateral wall were estimated by measuring the spatial velocity gradient using 2D color-Doppler myocardial imaging. Interestingly, in Fabry patients, functional abnormalities tend to occur more often in the LV lateral wall, LV longitudinal function appears to be impaired earlier than radial function, and—concerning regional ventricular dysfunction—only the LV but not the RV seems to be involved.

One additional advantage of deformation imaging is the possibility of indirectly assessing the presence of fibrosis. Weidemann et al. [112], using strain-rate imaging (by real-time 2D color-Doppler myocardial imaging), showed that all myocardial segments with LGE at CMR displayed a typical deformation pattern consisting of a first peak in early systole, followed by a rapid fall in strain rate close to zero and a second peak during isovolumic relaxation. This double-peak sign was never observed in segments of healthy controls but was present in ten segments without LGE. Interestingly, these false-positive segments were visualized in Fabry patients who often subsequently developed a fast, progressive fibrosis, as demonstrated by a follow-up CMR study.

In 101 consecutive Fabry patients, quantitative measurement of myocardial fibrosis at contrast CMR was compared with regional myocardial deformation assessed by speckle-tracking imaging [113]. Results suggest that the latter can be used as a tool for indirect evaluation of LGE in Fabry disease. Patients with LGE had lower global systolic longitudinal strain than those without. Loss of global deformation, quantified by speckle tracking, was predominantly affected by abnormalities of basal posterior and lateral segments, and global systolic strain correlated with the amount of LGE. Patients with severe LGE showed the lowest deformation values in basal posterolateral segments when compared with patients with mild or no LGE [113]. An improvement in regional myocardial function under enzyme replacement therapy and, in particular, of systolic radial strain rate using real-time 2D color-Doppler myocardial imaging, is reported in the early disease stage without LGE [114].

CMR study can be helpful in the diagnostic characterization of Fabry CMP and in the evaluation of disease progression [115, 116]. Moon et al. [117] reported LGE

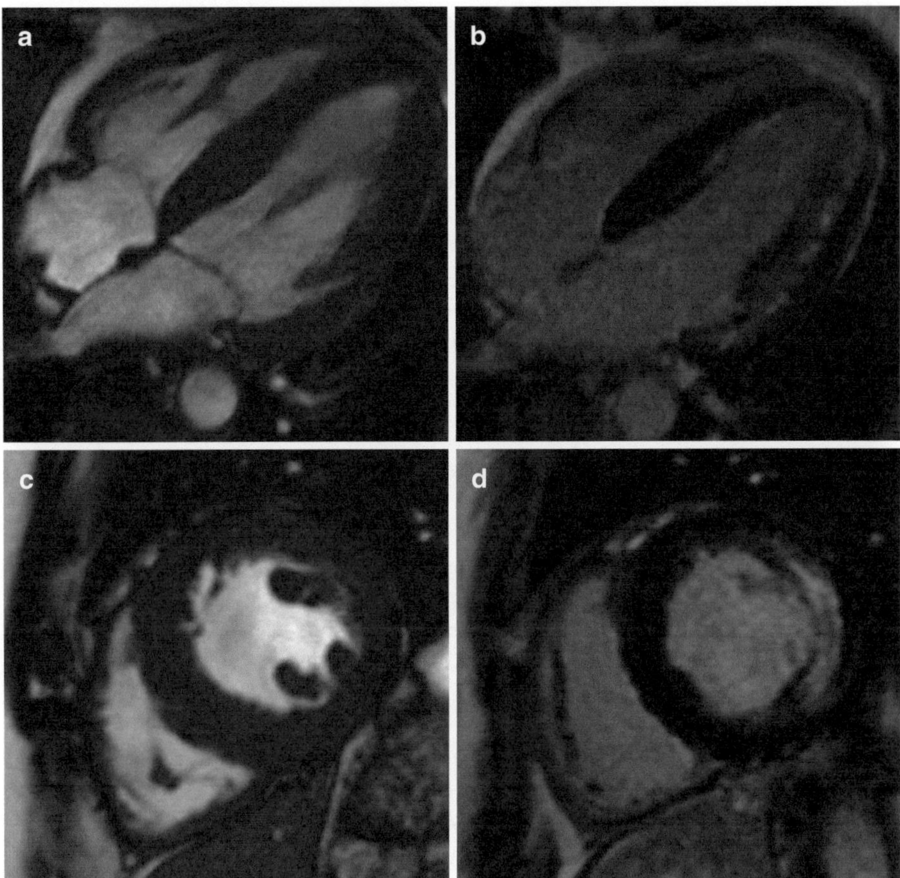

Fig. 20.10 CMR of a 46 years old man with Fabry disease. There is a concentric hypertrophy of the LV seen at the 4 chamber view (**a**) and short-axis view (**c**) with lateral late gadolinium enhancement (**b**, **d**)

patterns in a typical distribution involving the basal inferolateral wall, sparing the endocardium, in 50 % of affected patients (Fig. 20.10). Replacement fibrosis, detected as the presence of LGE at CMR, is considered a sign of disease progression [116] and is present also in affected female patients without LV hypertrophy, suggesting that hypertrophy and fibrosis are not necessarily associated [118]. Moreover, Sado et al. [119] demonstrated that native T1 values of the myocardium are lower in Fabry patients than healthy controls and patients affected by other diseases characterized by LV hypertrophy. This finding is probably related to the intracellular accumulation of glycosphingolipid in myocytes (presence of fat lowers T1 values). Other imaging techniques can be employed in selected cases. Myocardial perfusion reserve measured at rest and during dipyridamole-induced hyperemia by PET and ^{15}O-labeled water is reduced in patients with Fabry disease with cardiac involvement compared with controls [120]. Fibrotic myocardial changes on CT were observed in affected patients as hypointense areas at early phases and abnormal enhancement at late acquisition after iodinated contrast administration [121].

In Anderson-Fabry disease, there is evidence that early identification and initiation of enzyme replacement treatment is associated with significant reduction in myocardial mass and improved myocardial function and exercise capacity, whereas patients with advanced forms of myocardial involvement show no improvement [122]. Within this framework, CMR is a useful tool for assessing early cardiac involvement and LV wall thickening. As shown by Sado et al. [119], CMR and the use of native T1 mapping distinguishes Fabry disease from other common causes, showing no apparent overlap, and may be useful in identifying very early cardiac involvement (before the development of LV hypertrophy) and thus guide treatment preventing possible damage to cardiac tissues.

20.3.2 Glycogenoses, Danon Disease, *PRKAG2* Cardiomyopathy

Glycogen storage diseases are a group of genetic metabolic disorders caused by deficient activity of enzymes involved in glycogen metabolism [123]. They are usually clinically evident at birth or within the first year of life. Major clinical features include skeletal myopathy [hypotonia, generalized muscle weakness, calf pseudo-hypertrophy, elevated creatine kinase (CK) levels], hepatomegaly, and metabolic abnormalities (hypoglycemia and hyperlipemia). Inheritance is usually autosomal recessive.

More than ten different forms of glycogen storage diseases are described, and cardiac involvement is present in at least three of them (type II, or Pompe disease; type III, or Cori-Forbes disease; type IV, or Andersen disease). Usually, cardiomegaly and severe ventricular hypertrophy are identified at birth or at prenatal echocardiography. LV hypertrophy may be massive, with progressive LV OT obstruction. ECG usually shows very high QRS voltages, sometimes associated with ventricular pre-excitation; furthermore, during disease progression, deposition of glycogen results in conduction defects [124].

Diagnosis is made by measuring enzymatic activity and/or molecular genetic testing. Enzyme replacement therapy, started in the early phases, is effective in improving survival, ventilator-independent survival, motor-skills acquisition and in reducing cardiac mass [125].

Echocardiography in patients (generally infants/young children) affected by Pompe disease shows severe thickening of the IVS, free wall, and papillary muscles, sometimes with a tumour-like appearance, small LV cavity, and normal to poor LV function [126, 127]. Similar features can be present in Andersen disease. In Cori-Forbes disease, echocardiogram shows concentric LV thickening, increased myocardial refractile pattern and granular appearance, and decreased LV dimension.

Danon disease is a rare X-linked-dominant disorder caused by a mutation in the *LAMP2* gene, which encodes for a lysosomal membrane protein (LAMP). LAMP-2 deficiency results in lysosomal glycogen storage disease characterized in male patients by a triad of HCM with HF, skeletal myopathy, and mental retardation [128]. Retinal involvement is also frequent and can lead to a severe visual impairment. Affected female individuals usually show a later onset (30 vs 16 years) and a less-severe disease presentation, sometimes isolated to the heart. Symptoms are similar to those present in HCM (HF, arrhythmias, syncope, angina). ECG shows very high QRS voltages and, in some series, ventricular pre-excitation due to the presence of single or multiple accessory pathways [129]. Palpitations or syncope may be related to the ventricular myopathic process (ventricular tachycardia) or accessory pathways (orthodromic or antidromic precipitating tachycardia). Biological diagnosis involves the demonstration of normal or high acid maltase activity in combination with muscle biopsies showing large vacuoles (filled with glycogen and products of cytoplasmic degradation) and an absence of LAMP-2 protein on immunohistochemical analysis. The diagnosis can be confirmed by molecular analysis of the *LAMP2* gene.

Echocardiographic characteristics include a marked symmetrical increase in LV wall thickness (range 20–60 mm), significantly greater than that typically found in patients with HCM [129, 130]. LV systolic dysfunction is often severely impaired; LV OT obstruction is uncommon [130].

Some reports show additional advantage of advanced echocardiographic techniques in patients with Danon disease. In particular, real-time 3D echocardiography is useful for diagnosing and characterizing apical thrombus and LV noncompaction (NC) in young patients [131]. Entire trabecular projections and intertrabecular recesses are visualized simultaneously using this technique, and distinctions between compacted and NC LV myocardium and thrombus located within the NC LV myocardium are easily demarcated. Miani et al. [132] show a possible incremental value of 3D speckle-tracking strain imaging in Danon disease; 3D strain analysis could thus permit early recognition of cardiac involvement by detecting concealed myocardial abnormalities related to fibrosis and guide decision making around ICD implantation. In fact, in a young man followed because of being a carrier of *LAMP2* mutation, despite apparently normal 2D and 3D conventional echocardiography, 3D speckle-tracking imaging revealed impaired longitudinal strain of the inferior wall basal segment, the same area presenting myocardial fibrosis at contrast CMR.

There are few reports in the literature on CMR in Danon disease. Usually, severe hypertrophy is associated with various pattern of LGE (from subendocardial, to transmural, to subepicardial). Rest-perfusion deficits and poor LV function can also be observed [133, 134].

Danon disease carries a poor prognosis, with uncommon survival beyond 25 years of age and the need to consider heart transplantation early [129, 135]. Echocardiography and CMR are also important in prognostic assessment, as they identify a severe phenotype at a very young age and in close follow-up. Transition from severe concentric hypertrophy with preserved LV systolic function to wall thinning and severe systolic impairment may be observed. Within this framework, echocardiography has a primary role in patient monitoring and treatment choice [136].

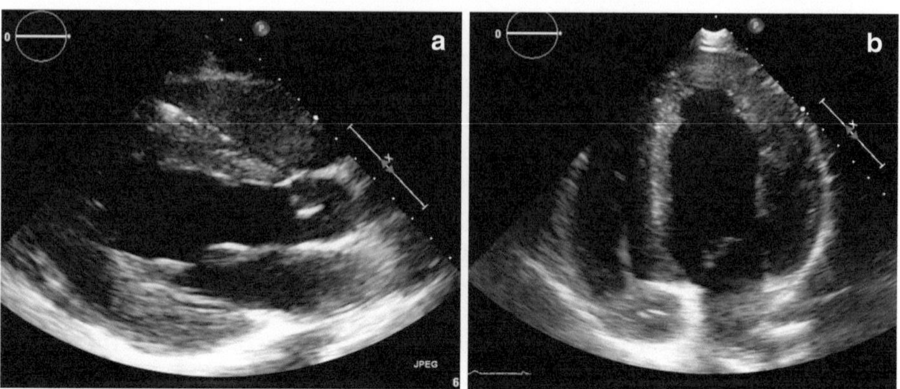

Fig. 20.11 Echocardiogram from a 20-year-old man with *PRKAG2* gene cardiac syndrome. The left ventricle is moderately hypertrophic (interventricular septum thickness 15 mm). Papillary muscles are also thickened. Note the presence of pace maker (early implanted) in right chambers (**a**). Parasternal long-axis view (**a**); apical four-chamber view (**b**)

The *PRKAG2* gene encodes for an enzyme called adenosine monophosphate (AMP)-activated protein kinase (AMPK). AMPK deficiency leads to extralysosomal glycogen storage disorder, which can express with isolated adult-onset HCM or familial Wolff-Parkinson-White syndrome [129]. An association between HCM, conduction abnormalities, and skeletal muscle glycogenosis are described [137].

Diagnosis requires molecular genetic analysis. Severe LV hypertrophy mimicking HCM (Fig. 20.11, Clips 20.6 and 20.7), in association with electrophysiologic abnormalities (including Wolff-Parkinson-White syndrome) and atrioventricular block are the main features of the syndrome [138, 139]. In a population of 41 patients, LV hypertrophy was present in 32 (78 %) >18 years, with a mean of 21 mm (median 18 mm, range 13–45 mm). The pattern of hypertrophy varied within families, ranging between asymmetric septal hypertrophy, concentric hypertrophy, and distal hypertrophy. RFP was present in 37 % of patients [138].

20.3.3 Mucopolysaccharidoses, Mucolipidoses, Gangliosidoses, Sphingolipidoses

20.3.3.1 Mucopolysaccharidoses

Mucopolysaccharidoses are metabolic lysosomal storage disorders [92, 123] caused by absent or defective activity of lysosomal enzymes involved in the catabolism of complex carbohydrates (mucopolysaccharides or glycosaminoglycans). This enzymatic deficiency limits the breakdown of mucopolysaccharides into simpler molecules, leading to accumulation of partially degraded mucopolysaccharides within the cells of different organs. Seven disease types and numerous subtypes are described; all are inherited in an autosomic recessive manner and affect both sexes equally.

The clinical phenotype is highly variable. The disease usually becomes clinically evident within the first decade of life and has a rapid progression, although milder forms with later onset are described. Affected patients may have normal intellect or may be severely retarded, with developmental delay and/or behavioral problems. Other clinical features include coarse facies, bone abnormalities, macrocephaly and hydrocephalus, upper airway complications (narrowed trachea, thickened vocal cords, enlarged tongue), hypertrichosis, massive hepatosplenomegaly, progressive skeletal dysplasia, short stature, progressive corneal clouding with visual impairment, and hearing loss.

Cardiac involvement is common in all subtypes of mucopolysaccharidoses. The most severe form is seen in type 1 (Hurler-Scheie syndrome) [140]. Prominent valvular thickening, diffuse coronary artery disease, myocardial hypertrophy, and secondary pulmonary hypertension are common. In patients with cardiac involvement, SD due to arrhythmias and/or coronary artery disease may occur [141]. In the later stages of the disease, valvular defects (mitral and/or aortic valve stenosis or insufficiency) may become hemodynamically important [141], and cases of successful treatment with valve replacement are described [142]. Severe forms of endomyocardial fibroelastosis are also described [140]. LV hypertrophy at ECG is uncommon; low QRS voltages may be due to poor conductance of mucopolysaccharides.

Diagnosis is made through clinical examination, mucopolysaccharides levels in urine, and various enzyme assays. Prognosis is usually poor; death occurs early and usually due to cardiorespiratory complications or end-stage neurodegenerative disorders.

20.3.3.2 Mucolipidoses

Mucolipidoses are a group of inherited inborn errors of metabolism characterized by deficiency in lysosomal enzymes involved in degradation of lipids and carbohydrates, with consequent accumulation of these molecules within cells; the pattern of inheritance is autosomal recessive. Clinical features and cardiovascular involvement are similar to those observed in mucopolysaccharidoses. Aortic and mitral valve (MV) prolapse may coexist. Moreover, cases of DCM, HCM, endocardial fibroelastosis, and accumulation of foam cells in the myocardium are described [143].

20.3.3.3 Gangliosidoses

Gangliosidoses are a group of autosomal-recessive metabolic disorders characterized by accumulation of gangliosides within cells. Clinical features are similar to those observed in mucopolysaccharidoses. Cardiac involvement is common and includes HCM, DCM, endocardial fibroelastosis, conduction delay, and valves defects.

20.3.3.4 Sphingolipidoses

Sphingolipidoses are another group of storage diseases inherited by an autosomal-recessive modality and characterized by lysosomal accumulation of sphingolipids. Gaucher disease is caused by a deficiency in beta-glucocerebrosidase and

Niemann-Pick disease by a deficiency in acid sphingomyelinase [92]. In both diseases, cardiac involvement is rare and is characterized by a variety of reported abnormalities, such as myocardial involvement with hypertrophic, restrictive, or dilated phenotypes; valvular fibrosis and calcifications with possible regurgitation and/or stenosis; pericardial calcification; effusion and sometimes constriction; and aortic calcifications. Cardiac consequences of pulmonary hypertension with cor pulmonale are also reported [92, 123].

20.3.4 Hemochromatosis

Hemochromatosis is an iron-overload disorder characterized by excessive accumulation of iron within the cells of multiple organs. It may result from a genetic defect (hereditary hemochromatosis; *HFE* gene) with an autosomal-recessive inheritance pattern, or it can be secondary to other causes (chronic blood transfusions). From the clinical point of view, hemochromatosis is characterized by liver cirrhosis, diabetes mellitus, hypogonadotropic hypogonadism, and arthritis. Heart involvement is most frequently characterized by HF with LV systolic dysfunction [144]. ECG usually shows normal QRS complexes, even if, in advanced forms, voltages can be reduced and repolarization abnormalities can become evident. Cessation of blood transfusions, phlebotomy, and chelation therapy proved effective in reversing cardiac abnormalities. Some patients may require combined liver and heart transplantation [145].

Diastolic dysfunction is the predominant early finding both in patients with primary hemochromatosis [146] and secondary iron overload [147]. Elevation in the peak transmitral early-filling velocity (E wave), increased E deceleration time, and increased LA size are consistently abnormal diastolic parameters [148]. Iron-overload CMP, regardless of origin, is characterized by RCM, which invariably progresses to an end-stage DCM that is often not distinguishable from idiopathic DCM [67, 149].

CMR is the best noninvasive imaging technique for identifying iron-overload CMP. Assessing cardiac and hepatic involvement in hemochromatosis using T2* is a very useful diagnostic tool [150]. T2* is a measure of magnetic relaxation and is typically shortened when particulate hemosiderin storage iron disturbs the magnetic microenvironment. Myocardial T2* correlates well with cardiac iron concentration measured from biopsy specimens, in contrast to liver iron concentration and serum ferritin. In patients with myocardial iron overload, T2* values are typically <20 ms, with a range of clinical interest between 5 and 20 ms. Moreover, declining myocardial T2* is associated with increasing risk of LV dysfunction and increasing likelihood of cardiac events in transfusion-dependent thalassanemia [150, 151]. Myocardial T2* <10 ms significantly increases HF risk within the first year, and the risk rises steeply with further reduction in T2* [152].

Myocardial iron load evaluation is also possible with dual-energy cardiac CT. In particular, Hounsfield unit values of septal muscle correlate strongly with T2* values at CMR [153]. The diagnostic capabilities of these imaging techniques in hemochromatosis have important consequences in patient management. In fact, echocardiography has a limited value in screening patients for myocardial iron deposition, whereas CMR has the potential to identify the presence of iron in the heart and quantify myocardial iron load [154]. In patients with myocardial iron overload, T2* can diagnose the disease early and guide the physician toward adequate treatment [153, 155]. Recognition and intervention in an early stage of the disease is important because chelation therapy may delay or prevent the occurrence of iron-overload DCM [154].

20.3.5 Wilson Disease

Wilson disease is a rare autosomal-recessive disorder characterized by multiorgan copper accumulation. The disease particularly affects the liver and central nervous system. Cardiac involvement is uncommon; nevertheless, cardiac hypertrophy and increased cardiac copper concentration are described [156]. Cardiologic manifestations of the disease are HCM, DCM, arrhythmias (AF, sinoatrial block, atrioventricular blocks), and autonomic dysfunction.

20.3.6 Friedreich Ataxia

Friedreich ataxia is an autosomal recessive neurodegenerative disease caused by a mutation in the frataxin gene on chromosome 9 [157]. Frataxin deficiency results in abnormal accumulation of intramitochondrial iron, defective mitochondrial respiration, and overproduction of oxygen free radicals, with evidence of oxidant-induced intracellular damage. Mean age at onset is 10–15 years. Patients present with progressive ataxia, dysarthria, muscle weakness, and optic nerve atrophy. Patients usually become wheelchair-dependent around 20–25 years of age.

Cardiac involvement is frequent (>90 % in neurologically symptomatic patients) and usually becomes clinically evident 4–5 years after disease onset. The disease is characterized by LV hypertrophy, usually concentric and without LV OT [158]. Sometimes, evolution toward DCM may be seen. Cardiac symptoms include arrhythmias (ventricular tachycardia) and HF, which may be severe. However, noncardiac dyspnea secondary to severe scoliosis and neuromuscular impairment of respiratory muscles is usually associated. QRS voltage at ECG may not correspond to the extent of LV hypertrophy present at imaging, probably because of extensive myocardial fibrosis. Prognosis and quality of life are poor; the average time from symptom onset to death is 36 years; therapy thus far is supportive only [159].

Concentric LV hypertrophy is the most commonly reported echocardiographic finding [160] (Fig. 20.12, Clips 20.8, 20.9, and 20.10). Different patterns of LV hypertrophy, unrelated to disease duration, are described [161]. All ventricular structures, including papillary muscles, may be thickened, but asymmetric septal hypertrophy and LV OT obstruction are rare [161, 162]. LV diastolic relaxation is reduced, but LV cavity size and EF are usually normal [160, 162]. The prognosis is

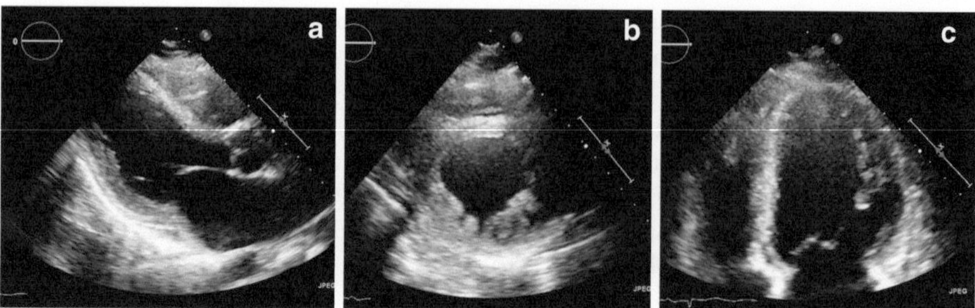

Fig. 20.12 Echocardiogram from a 31-year-old man with Friedreich ataxia with cardiac involvement. Normal chamber dimension; left ventricle is moderately hypertrophic (interventricular septum 16 mm). Parasternal long-axis view (**a**); parasternal short-axis view (**b**); apical four-chamber view (**c**)

particularly poor, with progressive cardiac deterioration when a DCM pattern is involved [161]. Valvular insufficiency, if present, is usually mild.

20.3.7 Cardiac Oxalosis

Primary hyperoxaluria is a rare autosomal recessive disease caused by a mutation in genes encoding for hepatic enzymes involved in glyoxylate metabolism (*AGXT* gene in type 1 and *GRHPR* gene in type 2). As a result, substrate glyoxylate accumulates and is converted to oxalate, which forms insoluble calcium oxalate salts that accumulate in renal and extrarenal tissues. Primary hyperoxaluria type 1 has an incidence of 1:100,000 live births in Europe; type 2 is rarer. The higher prevalence is observed in specific populations, especially if a high rate of consanguinity is present [163].

Clinical presentation and onset are variable. The severe infantile form is characterized by failure to thrive, nephrocalcinosis, and early end-stage renal failure. Forms with later onset are usually less severe in presentation (from recurrent urolithiasis with nephrocalcinosis and progressive renal failure during adolescence to occasional renal stones in adulthood). Other manifestations include urinary tract infections, dysuria and hematuria, vascular calcification with distal gangrene, visual defects with brown-colored retinal deposits, skin nodules, and joint and bone involvement leading to fractures in long-term dialysis-dependent patients. Diagnosis relies on measuring levels of urine oxalate. Confirmation is made by measuring specific enzymatic activity at liver biopsy and/or from molecular genetic testing.

Cardiac involvement is described in both types of primary hyperoxaluria and is characterized by myocardial hypertrophy and severe diastolic dysfunction [164]. HF may be severe and can be associated with conduction abnormalities secondary to extensive conduction-tissue infiltration by calcium oxalate [164–167]. Associated severe mitral regurgitation (MR) necessitating MV repair is described [166]. Treatment (hemodialysis, combined liver and kidney transplantation) demonstrates inconsistent effects on cardiac symptoms and echocardiographic features [166, 167].

Biventricular diffuse hypertrophy is the echocardiographic pattern usually observed in primary oxalosis with cardiac involvement [168]. EF may be normal in the early stage of this disease, but mild to moderate biventricular dilation and dysfunction are observed in advanced cases [168]. The myocardium can be characterized by patchy, echo-dense, speckled reflection most prominent in the papillary muscles [166, 168]. Diastolic dysfunction with signs of elevated filling pressures and RFP is common [164, 165, 168].

20.3.8 Mitochondrial Diseases

Mitochondrial diseases comprise several disorders secondary to dysfunction in oxidative phosphorylation. They can be included among the group of metabolic CMP [123]. Their causes are genetic defects, which are localized either in nuclear or mitochondrial DNA (matrilinear hereditary transmission; Chap. 2). Mitochondrial diseases are characterized by high clinical heterogeneity ranging from oligosymptomatic states to complex syndromes [169]. Furthermore, identical DNA mutations may produce different diseases, and different mutations can lead to undistinguishable clinical syndromes. Cardiac involvement can present with HCM, DCM phenotypes, or rarer forms of CMP (LV NC, restrictive, histiocytoid) or arrhythmias (ventricular pre-excitation, conduction diseases). The most frequent morphologic pattern is the association of LV hypertrophy and systolic dysfunction, mimicking HCM with hypokinetic end-stage evolution [170, 171]. Pathogenetic mechanisms are still poorly understood, but a marked induction of mitochondrial biogenesis is recognized as a prominent feature of end-stage mitochondrial DNA (mtDNA)-related CMP [172]. Proliferation of intermyofibrillar mitochondria, which can represent a biological response to deficient oxidative phosphorylation, can have a detrimental effect on cardiac muscle, interfering with sarcomeric function and contributing to adverse cardiac remodeling [169, 172]. Bioptic and pathological studies revealed cardiomyocyte enlargement with lipid vacuoles, interstitial fibrosis, and proliferation of polymorphic mitochondria at ultrastructural analysis. Typical extracardiac manifestations involve skeletal myopathy, neurological disorders, and ophthalmologic, gastroenterologic, and endocrine features [169]. Cardiac involvement in these diseases is usually an important predictor of morbidity and mortality. Specific therapies are not yet available.

In mitochondrial CMP, reported echocardiographic abnormalities include ventricular hypertrophy, dilatation, and systolic dysfunction [170]. In a study of 101 children with mitochondrial disease, 20 % of patients had CMP diagnosed by echo-Doppler investigations, all characterized by hypertrophic, nonobstructive phenotype [171]. In the majority of patients with hypertrophy, both the LV posterior wall and IVS in diastole are increased. The majority of patients with CMP had normal LV inner diameter in diastole and fractional shortening at the time of diagnosis [171]. In the late stage of disease, the LV is dilated and poorly contracting, and the diagnosis can be confused with DCM. At this stage, hypertrophy of the myocardium in terms of increased wall thickness is diminished in a dilated ventricle, whereas hypertrophy in terms of LV mass is preserved or even exaggerated [171]. Thus, the typical echocardiographic pattern of mitochondrial CMP can mimic HCM with hypokinetic end-stage evolution (Table 20.1).

References

1. Rapezzi C, Arbustini E, Caforio AL et al (2013) Diagnostic work-up in cardiomyopathies: bridging the gap between clinical phenotypes and final diagnosis. A position statement from the ESC Working Group on Myocardial and Pericardial Diseases. Eur Heart J 34:1448–1458
2. Klein AL, Oh JK, Miller FA, Seward JB, Tajik AJ (1988) Two-dimensional and Doppler echocardiographic assessment of infiltrative cardiomyopathy. J Am Coll Cardiol 1:48–59
3. Falk RH (2005) Diagnosis and management of the cardiac amyloidoses. Circulation 112:2047–2060
4. Shah KB, Inoue Y, Mehra MR (2006) Amyloidosis and the heart. A comprehensive review. Arch Intern Med 166:1805–1813
5. Kyle RA, Linos A, Beard CM et al (1992) Incidence and natural history of primary systemic amyloidosis in Olmsted County, Minnesota, 1950 through 1989. Blood 79:1817
6. Jaccard A, Moreau P, Leblond V et al (2007) High-dose melphalan versus melphalan plus dexamethasone for AL amyloidosis. N Engl J Med 357:1083–1093
7. Finocchiaro G, Pinamonti B, Merlo M et al (2013) Focus on cardiac amyloidosis: a single-center experience with a long-term follow-up. J Cardiovasc Med (Hagerstown) 14:281–288
8. Rapezzi C, Merlini G, Quarta CC, Riva L, Longhi S, Leone O, Salvi F, Ciliberti P, Pastorelli F, Biagini E, Coccolo F, Cooke RM, Bacchi-Reggiani L, Sangiorgi D, Ferlini A, Cavo M, Zamagni E, Fonte ML, Palladini G, Salinaro F, Musca F, Obici L, Branzi A, Perlini S (2009) Systemic cardiac amyloidoses: disease profiles and clinical courses of the 3 main types. Circulation 120:1203–1212
9. Rahman JE, Heleou EF, Gelzer-Bell R et al (2004) Noninvasive diagnosis of biopsy-proven cardiac amyloidosis. J Am Coll Cardiol 43:410
10. Merlini G, Wechalekar AD, Palladini G (2013) Systemic light chain amyloidosis: an update for treating physicians. Blood 121(26):5124–5130. doi:10.1182/blood-2013-01-453001
11. Kyle RA, Greipp PR (1983) Amyloidosis (AL). Clinical and laboratory features in 229 cases. Mayo Clin Proc 58(10):665–683
12. Picano E, Pinamonti B, Ferdeghini EM et al (1991) Two-dimensional echocardiography in myocardial amyloidosis. Echocardiography 8:253–258
13. Hongo M, Kono J, Yamada H et al (1991) doppler echocardiographic assessment of left ventricular diastolic filling in patients with amyloid heart disease. J Cardiol 21:391–401
14. Liu D, Niemann M, Hu K, Herrmann S, Stork S, Knop S, Ertl G, Weidemann F (2011) Echocardiographic evaluation of systolic and diastolic function in patients with cardiac amyloidosis. Am J Cardiol 108(4):591–598. doi:10.1016/j.amjcard.2011.03.092
15. Falk RH, Plehn JF, Deering T, Schick EC Jr, Boinay P, Rubinow A, Skinner M, Cohen AS (1987) Sensitivity and specificity of the echocardiographic features of cardiac amyloidosis. Am J Cardiol 59(5):418–422
16. Murtagh B, Hammill SC, Gertz MA et al (2005) Electrocardiographic findings in primary systemic amyloidosis and biopsy-proven cardiac involvement. Am J Cardiol 95:535–537
17. Carroll JD, Gaasch WH, McAdam KP (1982) Amyloid cardiomyopathy: characterization by a distinctive voltage/mass relation. Am J Cardiol 49:9–13
18. Tsai SB, Seldin DC, Wu H, O'Hara C, Ruberg FL, Sanchorawala V (2011) Myocardial infarction with "clean coronaries" caused by amyloid light-chain AL amyloidosis: a case report and literature review. Amyloid 18(3):160–164. doi:10.3109/13506129.2011.571319

19. Selvanayagam JB, Hawkins PN, Paul B, Myerson SG, Neubauer S (2007) Evaluation and management of the cardiac amyloidosis. J Am Coll Cardiol 50(22):2101–2110. doi:10.1016/j.jacc.2007.08.028

20. Dubrey SW, Hawkins PN, Falk RH (2011) Amyloid diseases of the heart: assessment, diagnosis, and referral. Heart 97(1):75–84. doi:10.1136/hrt.2009.190405

21. Ghio S, Perlini S, Palladini G, Marsan NA, Faggiano G, Vezzoli M, Klersy C, Campana C, Merlini G, Tavazzi L (2007) Importance of the echocardiographic evaluation of right ventricular function in patients with AL amyloidosis. Eur J Heart Fail 9(8):808–813. doi:10.1016/j.ejheart.2007.05.006

22. Klein AL, Hatle LK, Burstow DJ, Seward JB, Kyle RA, Bailey KR, Luscher TF, Gertz MA, Tajik AJ (1989) Doppler characterization of left ventricular diastolic function in cardiac amyloidosis. J Am Coll Cardiol 13(5):1017–1026

23. Koyama J, Ray-Sequin PA, Davidoff R, Falk RH (2002) Usefulness of pulsed tissue Doppler imaging for evaluating systolic and diastolic left ventricular function in patients with AL (primary) amyloidosis. Am J Cardiol 89(9):1067–1071

24. Koyama J, Ray-Sequin PA, Falk RH (2003) Longitudinal myocardial function assessed by tissue velocity, strain, and strain rate tissue Doppler echocardiography in patients with AL (primary) cardiac amyloidosis. Circulation 107(19):2446–2452. doi:10.1161/01.CIR.0000068313.67758.4F

25. Bellavia D, Pellikka PA, Dispenzieri A, Scott CG, Al-Zahrani GB, Grogan M, Pitrolo F, Oh JK, Miller FA Jr (2012) Comparison of right ventricular longitudinal strain imaging, tricuspid annular plane systolic excursion, and cardiac biomarkers for early diagnosis of cardiac involvement and risk stratification in primary systematic (AL) amyloidosis: a 5-year cohort study. Eur Heart J Cardiovasc Imaging 13(8):680–689. doi:10.1093/ehjci/jes009

26. Garcia MJ, Rodriguez L, Ares M, Griffin BP, Thomas JD, Klein AL (1996) Differentiation of constrictive pericarditis from restrictive cardiomyopathy: assessment of left ventricular diastolic velocities in longitudinal axis by Doppler tissue imaging. J Am Coll Cardiol 27(1):108–114. doi:10.1016/0735-1097(95)00434-3

27. Sun JP, Stewart WJ, Yang XS, Donnell RO, Leon AR, Felner JM, Thomas JD, Merlino JD (2009) Differentiation of hypertrophic cardiomyopathy and cardiac amyloidosis from other causes of ventricular wall thickening by two-dimensional strain imaging echocardiography. Am J Cardiol 103(3):411–415. doi:10.1016/j.amjcard.2008.09.102

28. Phelan D, Collier P, Thavendiranathan P, Popovic ZB, Hanna M, Plana JC, Marwick TH, Thomas JD (2012) Relative apical sparing of longitudinal strain using two-dimensional speckle-tracking echocardiography is both sensitive and specific for the diagnosis of cardiac amyloidosis. Heart 98(19):1442–1448. doi:10.1136/heartjnl-2012-302353

29. Baccouche H, Maunz M, Beck T, Gaa E, Banzhaf M, Knayer U, Fogarassy P, Beyer M (2012) Differentiating cardiac amyloidosis and hypertrophic cardiomyopathy by use of three-dimensional speckle tracking echocardiography. Echocardiography 29(6):668–677. doi:10.1111/j.1540-8175.2012.01680.x

30. Saito K, Okura H, Watanabe N, Hayashida A, Obase K, Imai K, Maehama T, Kawamoto T, Neishi Y, Yoshida K (2009) Comprehensive evaluation of left ventricular strain using speckle tracking echocardiography in normal adults: comparison of three-dimensional and two-dimensional approaches. J Am Soc Echocardiogr 22(9):1025–1030. doi:10.1016/j.echo.2009.05.021

31. Sharma N, Howlett J (2013) Current state of cardiac amyloidosis. Curr Opin Cardiol 28:242–248

32. Quarta CC, Kruger JL, Falk RH (2012) Cardiac amyloidosis. Circulation 126:e178–e182

33. Fattori R, Rocchi G, Celletti F, Bertaccini P, Rapezzi C, Gavelli G (1998) Contribution of magnetic resonance imaging in the differential diagnosis of cardiac amyloidosis and symmetric hypertrophic cardiomyopathy. Am Heart J 136:824–830

34. Syed IS, Glockner JF, Feng D, Araoz PA, Martinez MW, Edwards WD, Gertz MA, Dispenzieri A, Oh JK, Bellavia D, Tajik AJ, Grogan M (2010) Role of cardiac magnetic resonance imaging in the detection of cardiac amyloidosis. JACC Cardiovasc Imaging 3:155–164

35. Austin BA, Tang WH, Rodriguez ER, Tan C, Flamm SD, Taylor DO, Starling RC, Desai MY (2009) Delayed hyper-enhancement magnetic resonance imaging provides incremental diagnostic and prognostic utility in suspected cardiac amyloidosis. JACC Cardiovasc Imaging 2:1369–1377

36. Karamitsos TD, Piechnik SK, Banypersad SM, Fontana M, Ntusi NB, Ferreira VM, Whelan CJ, Myerson SG, Robson MD, Hawkins PN, Neubauer S, Moon JC (2013) Noncontrast T1 mapping for the diagnosis of cardiac amyloidosis. JACC Cardiovasc Imaging 6:488–497

37. Banypersad SM, Sado DM, Flett AS, Gibbs SD, Pinney JH, Maestrini V, Cox AT, Fontana M, Whelan CJ, Wechalekar AD, Hawkins PN, Moon JC (2013) Quantification of myocardial extracellular volume fraction in systemic al amyloidosis: an equilibrium contrast cardiovascular magnetic resonance study. Circ Cardiovasc Imaging 6:34–39

38. Aprile C, Marinone G, Saponaro R, Bonino C, Merlini G (1995) Cardiac and pleuropulmonary AL amyloid imaging with technetium-99m labelled aprotinin. Eur J Nucl Med 22:1393–1401

39. Han S, Chong V, Murray T, McDonagh T, Hunter J, Poon FW, Gray HW, Neilly JB (2007) Preliminary experience of 99mtc-aprotinin scintigraphy in amyloidosis. Eur J Haematol 79:494–500

40. Schaadt BK, Hendel HW, Gimsing P, Jonsson V, Pedersen H, Hesse B (2003) 99mtc-aprotinin scintigraphy in amyloidosis. J Nucl Med 44:177–183

41. Karp K, Naslund U, Backman C, Eriksson P (1987) Technetium-99m pyrophosphate single-photon emission computed tomography of the heart in familial amyloid polyneuropathy. Int J Cardiol 14:365–369

42. Puille M, Altland K, Linke RP, Steen-Muller MK, Kiett R, Steiner D, Bauer R (2002) 99mtc-dpd scintigraphy in transthyretin-related familial amyloidotic polyneuropathy. Eur J Nucl Med Mol Imaging 29:376–379

43. Perugini E, Guidalotti PL, Salvi F, Cooke RM, Pettinato C, Riva L, Leone O, Farsad M, Ciliberti P, Bacchi-Reggiani L, Fallani F, Branzi A, Rapezzi C (2005) Noninvasive etiologic diagnosis of cardiac amyloidosis using 99mtc-3,3-diphosphono-1,2-propanodicarboxylic acid scintigraphy. J Am Coll Cardiol 46:1076–1084

44. Rapezzi C, Guidalotti P, Salvi F, Riva L, Perugini E (2008) Usefulness of 99mtc-dpd scintigraphy in cardiac amyloidosis. J Am Coll Cardiol 51:1509–1510; author reply 1510

45. Bokhari S, Castano A, Pozniakoff T, Deslisle S, Latif F, Maurer MS (2013) (99m)tc-pyrophosphate scintigraphy for differentiating light-chain cardiac amyloidosis from the transthyretin-related familial and senile cardiac amyloidoses. Circ Cardiovasc Imaging 6:195–201

46. Minutoli F, Di Bella G, Mazzeo A, Donato R, Russo M, Scribano E, Baldari S (2013) Comparison between (99m)tc-diphosphonate imaging and mri with late gadolinium enhancement in evaluating cardiac involvement in patients with transthyretin familial amyloid polyneuropathy. AJR Am J Roentgenol 200:W256–W265

47. Kodama K, Hamada M, Kuwahara T, Nakamura M, Shigematsu Y, Hiwada K, Iwata T, Hoshii Y, Ishihara T (1999) Rest-redistribution thallium-201 myocardial scintigraphic study in cardiac amyloidosis. Int J Card Imaging 15:371–378

48. Tanaka M, Hongo M, Kinoshita O, Takabayashi Y, Fujii T, Yazaki Y, Isobe M, Sekiguchi M (1997) Iodine-123 metaiodobenzylguanidine scintigraphic assessment of myocardial sympathetic innervation in patients with familial amyloid polyneuropathy. J Am Coll Cardiol 29:168–174

49. Delahaye N, Dinanian S, Slama MS, Mzabi H, Samuel D, Adams D, Merlet P, Le Guludec D (1999) Cardiac sympathetic denervation in familial amyloid polyneuropathy assessed by iodine-123 metaiodobenzylguanidine scintigraphy and heart rate variability. Eur J Nucl Med 26:416–424

50. Hongo M, Urushibata K, Kai R, Takahashi W, Koizumi T, Uchikawa S, Imamura H, Kinoshita O, Owa M, Fujii T (2002) Iodine-123 metaiodobenzylguanidine scintigraphic analysis of myocardial sympathetic innervation in patients with al (primary) amyloidosis. Am Heart J 144:122–129

51. Antoni G, Lubberink M, Estrada S, Axelsson J, Carlson K, Lindsjo L, Kero T, Langstrom B, Granstam SO, Rosengren S, Vedin O, Wassberg C, Wikstrom G, Westermark P, Sorensen J (2013)

In vivo visualization of amyloid deposits in the heart with 11c-pib and pet. J Nucl Med 54:213–220

52. Klein AL, Hatle LK, Taliercio CP, Oh JK, Kyle RA, Gertz MA, Bailey KR, Seward JB, Tajik AJ (1991) Prognostic significance of Doppler measures of diastolic function in cardiac amyloidosis. A Doppler echocardiography study. Circulation 83(3):808–816

53. Mohty D, Pibarot P, Dumesnil JG, Darodes N, Lavergne D, Echahidi N, Virot P, Bordessoule D, Jaccard A (2011) Left atrial size is an independent predictor of overall survival in patients with primary systemic amyloidosis. Arch Cardiovasc Dis 104(12):611–618. doi:10.1016/j.acvd.2011.10.004

54. Cappelli F, Porciani MC, Bergesio F, Perlini S, Attana P, Moggi Pignone A, Salinaro F, Musca F, Padeletti L, Perfetto F (2012) Right ventricular function in AL amyloidosis: characteristics and prognostic implication. Eur Heart J Cardiovasc Imaging 13(5):416–422. doi:10.1093/ejechocard/jer289

55. Buss SJ, Emami M, Mereles D, Korosoglou G, Kristen AV, Voss A, Schellberg D, Zugck C, Galuschky C, Giannitsis E, Hegenbart U, Ho AD, Katus HA, Schonland SO, Hardt SE (2012) Longitudinal left ventricular function for prediction of survival in systemic light-chain amyloidosis: incremental value compared with clinical and biochemical markers. J Am Coll Cardiol 60(12):1067–1076. doi:10.1016/j.jacc.2012.04.043

56. Bellavia D, Pellikka PA, Al-Zahrani GB, Abraham TP, Dispenzieri A, Miyazaki C, Lacy M, Scott CG, Oh JK, Miller FA Jr (2010) Independent predictors of survival in primary systemic (Al) amyloidosis, including cardiac biomarkers and left ventricular strain imaging: an observational cohort study. J Am Soc Echocardiogr 23(6):643–652. doi:10.1016/j.echo.2010.03.027

57. Ruberg FL, Appelbaum E, Davidoff R, Ozonoff A, Kissinger KV, Harrigan C, Skinner M, Manning WJ (2009) Diagnostic and prognostic utility of cardiovascular magnetic resonance imaging in light-chain cardiac amyloidosis. Am J Cardiol 103(4):544–549. doi:10.1016/j.amjcard.2008.09.105

58. Finocchiaro G, Merlo M, Pinamonti B, Barbati G, Santarossa E, Doimo S, Bussani R, Sinagra G (2013) Long term survival in patients with cardiac amyloidosis. Prevalence and characterisation during follow-up. Heart Lung Circ 22(8):647–654. doi:10.1016/j.hlc.2013.01.010

59. Brenner DA, Jain M, Pimentel DR, Wang B, Connors LH, Skinner M, Apstein CS, Liao R (2004) Human amyloidogenic light chains directly impair cardiomyocyte function through an increase in cellular oxidant stress. Circ Res 94(8):1008–1010. doi:10.1161/01.RES.0000126569.75419.74

60. Ng B, Connors LH, Davidoff R, Skinner M, Falk RH (2005) Senile systemic amyloidosis presenting with heart failure: a comparison with light chain-associated amyloidosis. Arch Intern Med 165(12):1425–1429. doi:10.1001/archinte.165.12.1425

61. Chapelon-Abric C, de Zuttere D, Duhaut P et al (2004) Cardiac sarcoidosis: a retrospective study of 41 cases. Medicine (Baltimore) 83:315–334

62. Silverman KJ, Hutchins GM, Bulkley BH (1978) Cardiac sarcoid: a clinicopathologic study of 84 unselected patients with systemic sarcoidosis. Circulation 58:1204–1211

63. Roberts WC, McAllister HA Jr, Ferrans VJ (1977) Sarcoidosis of the heart. A clinicopathologic study of 35 necropsy patients (group 1) and review of 78 previously described necropsy patients (group 11). Am J Med 63:86–108

64. Kim JS, Jusdson MA, Donnino R et al (2009) Cardiac sarcoidosis. Am Heart J 157:9–21

65. Bargout R, Kelly RF (2004) Sarcoid heart disease: clinical course and treatment. Int J Cardiol 97:173–182

66. Dubrey SW, Falk RH (2010) Diagnosis and management of cardiac sarcoidosis. Prog Cardiovasc Dis 52(4):336–346. doi:10.1016/j.pcad.2009.11.010

67. Seward JB, Casaclang-Verzosa G (2010) Infiltrative cardiovascular diseases: cardiomyopathies that look alike. J Am Coll Cardiol 55(17):1769–1779. doi:10.1016/j.jacc.2009.12.040

68. Uemura A, Morimoto S, Kato Y, Hiramitsu S, Ohtsuki M, Kato S, Sugiura A, Miyagishima K, Iwase M, Hishida H (2005) Relationship between basal thinning of the interventricular septum and atrioventricular block in patients with cardiac sarcoidosis. Sarcoidosis Vasc Diffuse Lung Dis 22(1):63–65

69. Sun BJ, Lee PH, Choi HO et al (2011) Prevalence of echocardiographic features suggesting cardiac sarcoidosis in patients with pacemaker or implantable cardiac defibrillators. Korean Circ J 41:313–320

70. Baughman RP (2007) Pulmonary hypertension associated with sarcoidosis. Arthritis Res Ther 9(Suppl 2):S8. doi:10.1186/ar2192

71. Aggeli C, Felekos I, Tousoulis D, Gialafos E, Rapti A, Stefanadis C (2013) Myocardial mechanics for the early detection of cardiac sarcoidosis. Int J Cardiol. doi:10.1016/j. ijcard.2013.07.010

72. Galati G, Leone O, Rapezzi C (2014) The difficult diagnosis of isolated cardiac sarcoidosis: usefulness of an integrated MRI and PET approach. Heart 100:89–90

73. Smedema JP, Snoep G, van Kroonenburgh MP, van Geuns RJ, Dassen WR, Gorgels AP, Crijns HJ (2005) Evaluation of the accuracy of gadolinium-enhanced cardiovascular magnetic resonance in the diagnosis of cardiac sarcoidosis. J Am Coll Cardiol 45:1683–1690

74. Le Guludec D, Menad F, Faraggi M, Weinmann P, Battesti JP, Valeyre D (1994) Myocardial sarcoidosis. Clinical value of technetium-99m sestamibi tomoscintigraphy. Chest 106:1675–1682

75. Okayama K, Kurata C, Tawarahara K, Wakabayashi Y, Chida K, Sato A (1995) Diagnostic and prognostic value of myocardial scintigraphy with thallium-201 and gallium-67 in cardiac sarcoidosis. Chest 107:330–334

76. Eguchi M, Tsuchihashi K, Hotta D, Hashimoto A, Sasao H, Yuda S, Nakata T, Shijubou N, Abe S, Shimamoto K (2000) Technetium-99m sestamibi/tetrofosmin myocardial perfusion scanning in cardiac and noncardiac sarcoidosis. Cardiology 94:193–199

77. Yamagishi H, Shirai N, Takagi M, Yoshiyama M, Akioka K, Takeuchi K, Yoshikawa J (2003) Identification of cardiac sarcoidosis with (13)n-nh(3)/(18)f-fdg pet. J Nucl Med 44:1030–1036

78. Ishimaru S, Tsujino I, Takei T, Tsukamoto E, Sakaue S, Kamigaki M, Ito N, Ohira H, Ikeda D, Tamaki N, Nishimura M (2005) Focal uptake on 18f-fluoro-2-deoxyglucose positron emission tomography images indicates cardiac involvement of sarcoidosis. Eur Heart J 26:1538–1543

79. Tahara N, Tahara A, Nitta Y, Kodama N, Mizoguchi M, Kaida H, Baba K, Ishibashi M, Hayabuchi N, Narula J, Imaizumi T (2010) Heterogeneous myocardial fdg uptake and the disease activity in cardiac sarcoidosis. JACC Cardiovasc Imaging 3:1219–1228

80. Youssef G, Leung E, Mylonas I, Nery P, Williams K, Wisenberg G, Gulenchyn KY, Dekemp RA, Dasilva J, Birnie D, Wells GA, Beanlands RS (2012) The use of 18f-fdg pet in the diagnosis of cardiac sarcoidosis: a systematic review and metaanalysis including the Ontario experience. J Nucl Med 53:241–248

81. Chen S, Bokhari S (2011) Diagnosis of cardiac sarcoidosis through mismatched defects seen on n-13 nh3/f-18 fdg cardiac pet. Clin Nucl Med 36:1156–1157

82. Radulescu B, Imperiale A, Germain P, Ohlmann P (2010) Severe ventricular arrhythmias in a patient with cardiac sarcoidosis: Insights from mri and pet imaging and importance of early corticosteroid therapy. Eur Heart J 31:400

83. Blankstein R, Osborne M, Naya M, Waller A, Kim CK, Murthy VL, Kazemian P, Kwong RY, Tokuda M, Skali H, Padera R, Hainer J, Stevenson WG, Dorbala S, Di Carli MF (2013) Cardiac positron emission tomography enhances prognostic assessments of patients with suspected cardiac sarcoidosis. J Am Coll Cardiol 63:329–336

84. Mc Ardle BA, Birnie DH, Klein R, de Kemp RA, Leung E, Renaud J, DaSilva J, Wells GA, Beanlands RS, Nery PB (2013) Is there an association between clinical presentation and the location and extent of myocardial involvement of cardiac sarcoidosis as assessed by (1)(8)f-fluorodoexyglucose positron emission tomography? Circ Cardiovasc Imaging 6:617–626

85. Patel MR, Cawley PJ, Heitner JF, Klem I, Parker MA, Jaroudi WA, Meine TJ, White JB, Elliott MD, Kim HW, Judd RM, Kim RJ (2009) Detection of myocardial damage in patients with sarcoidosis. Circulation 120(20):1969–1977. doi:10.1161/CIRCULATIONAHA.109.851352

86. Oliveira GH, Seward JB, Tsang TS et al (2005) Echocardiographic findings in patients with Wegener granulomatosis. Mayo Clin Proc 80:1435–1440

87. Miszalski-Jamka T, Szczeklik W, Sokołowska B et al (2011) Cardiac involvement in Wegener's granulomatosis resistant to induction therapy. Eur Radiol 21:2297–2304

88. Miszalski-Jamka T, Szczeklik W, Nycz K, Sokolowska B, Gorka J, Bury K, Musial J (2012) Two-dimensional speckle-tracking echocardiography reveals systolic abnormalities in granulomatosis with polyangiitis (Wegener's). Echocardiography 29(7):803–809. doi:10.1111/j.1540-8175.2012.01699.x

89. Miguel CE, Bestetti RB (2011) Primary cardiac lymphoma. Int J Cardiol 149:358–363

90. Lee GY, Kim WS, Ko YK et al (2013) Primary cardiac lymphoma mimicking infiltrative cardiomyopathy. Eur J Heart Fail 15:589–591

91. Cooper LT, Baughman KL, Feldman AM et al (2007) The role of endomyocardial biopsy in the management of cardiovascular disease: a scientific statement from the American Heart Association, the American College of Cardiology, and the European Society of Cardiology. Circulation 116:2216–2233

92. Linhart A, Elliott PM (2007) The heart in Anderson-Fabry disease and other lysosomal storage disorders. Heart 93:528–535. doi:10.1136/hrt.2005.063818

93. Zarate YA, Hopkin RJ (2008) Lysosomal storage disease 3. Fabry's disease. Lancet 372:1427–1435

94. Schiffmann R, Warnock DG, Banikazemi M et al (2009) Fabry disease: progression of nephropathy, and prevalence of cardiac and cerebrovascular events before enzyme replacement therapy. Nephrol Dial Transplant 24:2102–2111

95. Colucci WS, Lorell BH, Schoen FJ et al (1982) Hypertrophic obstructive cardiomyopathy due to Fabry's disease. N Engl J Med 307:926–928

96. Sachdev B, Takenaka T, Teraguchi H et al (2002) Prevalence of Anderson-Fabry disease in male patients with late onset hypertrophic cardiomyopathy. Circulation 105:1407–1411

97. Monserrat L, Gimeno-Blanes JR, Marin F et al (2007) Prevalence of Fabry disease in a cohort of 508 unrelated patients with hypertrophic cardiomyopathy. J Am Coll Cardiol 50:2399–2403

98. Elliott P, Baker R, Pasquale F et al (2011) Prevalence of Anderson-Fabry disease in patients with hypertrophic cardiomyopathy: the European Anderson-Fabry disease survey. Heart 97:1957–1960

99. Linhart A, Palecek T, Bultas J et al (2000) New insights in cardiac structural changes in patients with Fabry's disease. Am Heart J 139:1101–1108

100. Kampmann C, Linhart A, Baehner F, Palecek T, Wiethoff CM, Miebach E, Whybra C, Gal A, Bultas J, Beck M (2008) Onset and progression of the Anderson-Fabry disease related cardiomyopathy. Int J Cardiol 130(3):367–373. doi:10.1016/j.ijcard.2008.03.007

101. Calcagnino M, O'Mahony C, Coats C et al (2011) Exercise-induced left ventricular outflow tract obstruction in symptomatic patients with Anderson-Fabry disease. J Am Coll Cardiol 58:88–89

102. Shah JS, Lee P, Hughes D et al (2005) The natural history of left ventricular systolic function in Anderson-Fabry disease. Heart 91:533–534

103. Palecek T, Dostalova G, Kuchynka P, Karetova D, Bultas J, Elleder M, Linhart A (2008) Right ventricular involvement in Fabry disease. J Am Soc Echocardiogr 21(11):1265–1268. doi:10.1016/j.echo.2008.09.002

104. Niemann M, Breunig F, Beer M, Herrmann S, Strotmann J, Hu K, Emmert A, Voelker W, Ertl G, Wanner C, Weidemann F (2010) The right ventricle in Fabry disease: natural history and impact of enzyme replacement therapy. Heart 96(23):1915–1919. doi:10.1136/hrt.2010.204586

105. Barbey F, Qanadli SD, Juli C, Brakch N, Palecek T, Rizzo E, Jeanrenaud X, Eckhardt B, Linhart A (2010) Aortic remodelling in Fabry disease. Eur Heart J 31(3):347–353. doi:10.1093/eurheartj/ehp426

106. Pieroni M, Chimenti C, De Cobelli F et al (2006) Fabry's disease cardiomyopathy: echocardiographic detection of endomyocardial glycosphingolipid compartmentalization. J Am Coll Cardiol 47:1663–1671

107. Mundigler G, Gaggi M, Heinze G et al (2011) The endocardial binary appearance ('binary sign') is un unreliable marker for echocardiographic detection of Fabry disease in patients with left ventricular hypertrophy. Eur J Echocardiogr 12:744–749

108. Niemann M, Breunig F, Beer M, Hu K, Liu D, Emmert A, Herrmann S, Ertl G, Wanner C, Takenaka T, Tei C, Weidemann F (2011) Tei index in fabry disease. J Am Soc Echocardiogr 24(9):1026–1032. doi:10.1016/j.echo.2011.05.021

109. Pieroni M, Chimenti C, Ricci R, Sale P, Russo MA, Frustaci A (2003) Early detection of Fabry cardiomyopathy by tissue Doppler imaging. Circulation 107(15):1978–1984. doi:10.1161/01.CIR.0000061952.27445.A0

110. Gruner C, Verocai F, Carasso S, Vannan MA, Jamorski M, Clarke JT, Care M, Iwanochko RM, Rakowski H (2012) Systolic myocardial mechanics in patients with Anderson-Fabry disease with and without left ventricular hypertrophy and in comparison to nonobstructive hypertrophic cardiomyopathy. Echocardiography 29(7):810–817. doi:10.1111/j.1540-8175.2012.01704.x

111. Weidemann F, Breunig F, Beer M, Sandstede J, Stork S, Voelker W, Ertl G, Knoll A, Wanner C, Strotmann JM (2005) The variation of morphological and functional cardiac manifestation in Fabry disease: potential implications for the time course of the disease. Eur Heart J 26(12):1221–1227. doi:10.1093/eurheartj/ehi143

112. Weidemann F, Niemann M, Herrmann S, Kung M, Stork S, Waller C, Beer M, Breunig F, Wanner C, Voelker W, Ertl G, Bijnens B, Strotmann JM (2007) A new echocardiographic approach for the detection of non-ischaemic fibrosis in hypertrophic myocardium. Eur Heart J 28(24):3020–3026. doi:10.1093/eurheartj/ehm454

113. Kramer J, Niemann M, Liu D, Hu K, Machann W, Beer M, Wanner C, Ertl G, Weidemann F (2013) Two-dimensional speckle tracking as a non-invasive tool for identification of myocardial fibrosis in Fabry disease. Eur Heart J 34(21):1587–1596. doi:10.1093/eurheartj/eht098

114. Weidemann F, Niemann M, Breunig F, Herrmann S, Beer M, Stork S, Voelker W, Ertl G, Wanner C, Strotmann J (2009) Long-term effects of enzyme replacement therapy on fabry cardiomyopathy: evidence for a better outcome with early treatment. Circulation 119(4):524–529. doi:10.1161/CIRCULATIONAHA.108.794529

115. Yousef Z, Elliott PM, Cecchi F, Escoubet B, Linhart A, Monserrat L, Namdar M, Weidemann F (2013) Left ventricular hypertrophy in fabry disease: a practical approach to diagnosis. Eur Heart J 34:802–808

116. Koeppe S, Neubauer H, Breunig F et al (2012) MR-based analysis of regional cardiac function in relation to cellular integrity in Fabry disease. Int J Cardiol 160:53–58

117. Moon JC, Sachdev B, Elkington AG, McKenna WJ, Mehta A, Pennell DJ, Leed PJ, Elliott PM (2003) Gadolinium enhanced cardiovascular magnetic resonance in anderson-fabry disease. Evidence for a disease specific abnormality of the myocardial interstitium. Eur Heart J 24:2151–2155

118. Niemann M, Herrmann S, Hu K et al (2011) Differences in Fabry cardiomyopathy between female and male patients: consequences for diagnostic assessment. JACC Cardiovasc Imaging 4:592–601

119. Sado DM, White SK, Piechnik SK, Banypersad SM, Treibel T, Captur G, Fontana M, Maestrini V, Flett AS, Robson MD, Lachmann RH, Murphy E, Mehta A, Hughes D, Neubauer S, Elliott PM, Moon JC (2013) Identification and assessment of anderson-fabry disease by cardiovascular magnetic resonance noncontrast myocardial t1 mapping. Circ Cardiovasc Imaging 6:392–398

120. Kalliokoski RJ, Kalliokoski KK, Sundell J, Engblom E, Penttinen M, Kantola I, Raitakari OT, Knuuti J, Nuutila P (2005) Impaired myocardial perfusion reserve but preserved peripheral endothelial function in patients with fabry disease. J Inherit Metab Dis 28:563–573

121. Funabashi N, Toyozaki T, Matsumoto Y, Yonezawa M, Yanagawa N, Yoshida K, Komuro I (2003) Images in cardiovascular medicine. Myocardial fibrosis in fabry disease demonstrated by multislice computed tomography: comparison with biopsy findings. Circulation 107:2519–2520

122. Beer M, Weidemann F, Breunig F, Knoll A, Koeppe S, Machann W, Hahn D, Wanner C, Strotmann J, Sandstede J (2006) Impact of enzyme replacement therapy on cardiac morphology and function and late enhancement in Fabry's cardiomyopathy. Am J Cardiol 97(10):1515–1518. doi:10.1016/j.amjcard.2005.11.087

123. Guertl B, Noehammer C, Hoefler G (2000) Metabolic cardiomyopathies. Int J Exp Pathol 81:349–372

124. van der Ploeg AT, Reuser AJJ (2008) Lysosomal storage disease 2. Pompe's disease. Lancet 372:1342–1353

125. Chien YH, Hwu WL, Lee NC (2013) Pompe disease: early diagnosis and early treatment make a difference. Pediatr Neonatol 54:219–227

126. Lorber A, Luder AS (1987) Very early presentation of Pompe's disease and its cross-sectional echocardiographic features. Int J Cardiol 16(3):311–314

127. Shapir Y, Roguin N (1985) Echocardiographic findings in Pompe's disease with left ventricular obstruction. Clin Cardiol 8(3):181–185

128. Danon MJ, Oh SJ, Di Mauro S et al (1981) Lysosomal glycogen storage disease with normal acid maltase. Neurology 31:51–57

129. Arad M, Maron BJ, Gorham JM et al (2005) Glycogen storage diseases presenting as hypertrophic cardiomyopathy. N Engl J Med 352:362–372

130. Charron P, Villard E, Sebillon P, Laforet P, Maisonobe T, Duboscq-Bidot L, Romero N, Drouin-Garraud V, Frebourg T, Richard P, Eymard B, Komajda M (2004) Danon's disease as a cause of hypertrophic cardiomyopathy: a systematic survey. Heart 90(8):842–846. doi:10.1136/hrt.2003.029504

131. Tada H, Harimura Y, Yamasaki H, Sekiguchi Y, Ishizu T, Seo Y, Kawano S, Aonuma K (2010) Utility of real-time 3-dimensional echocardiography and magnetic resonance imaging for evaluation of Danon disease. Circulation 121(17):e390–e392. doi:10.1161/CIR.0b013e3181de7097

132. Miani D, Nucifora G, Piccoli G, Proclemer A, Badano LP (2012) Incremental value of three-dimensional strain imaging in Danon disease. Eur Heart J Cardiovasc Imaging 13(10):804. doi:10.1093/ehjci/jes099

133. Nucifora G, Miani D, Piccoli G, Proclemer A (2012) Cardiac magnetic resonance imaging in Danon disease. Cardiology 121:27–30

134. Piotrowska-Kownacka D, Kownacki L, Kuch M, Walczak E, Kosieradzka A, Fidzianska A, Krolicki L (2009) Cardiovascular magnetic resonance findings in a case of danon disease. J Cardiovasc Magn Reson 11:12

135. Maron BJ, Roberts WC, Arad M, Haas TS, Spirito P, Wright GB, Almquist AK, Baffa JM, Saul JP, Ho CY, Seidman J, Seidman CE (2009) Clinical outcome and phenotypic expression in LAMP2 cardiomyopathy. JAMA 301(12):1253–1259. doi:10.1001/jama.2009.371

136. Maron BJ, Roberts WC, Ho CY, Kitner C, Haas TS, Wright GB, Moazami N, Feldman DS (2010) Profound left ventricular remodeling associated with LAMP2 cardiomyopathy. Am J Cardiol 106(8):1194–1196. doi:10.1016/j.amjcard.2010.06.035

137. Laforêt P, Richard P, Said MA et al (2006) A new mutation in PRKAG2 gene causing hypertrophic cardiomyopathy with conduction system disease and muscular glycogenosis. Neuromuscul Disord 16:178–182

138. Murphy RT, Mogensen J, McGarry K, Bahl A, Evans A, Osman E, Syrris P, Gorman G, Farrell M, Holton JL, Hanna MG, Hughes S, Elliott PM, Macrae CA, McKenna WJ (2005) Adenosine monophosphate-activated protein kinase disease mimicks hypertrophic cardiomyopathy and Wolff-Parkinson-White syndrome: natural history. J Am Coll Cardiol 45(6):922–930. doi:10.1016/j.jacc.2004.11.053

139. Fabris E, Brun F, Porto AG, Losurdo P, Vitali Serdoz L, Zecchin M, Severini GM, Mestroni L, Di Chiara A, Sinagra G (2013) Cardiac hypertrophy, accessory pathway, and conduction system disease in an adolescent: the PRKAG2 cardiac syndrome. J Am Coll Cardiol 62(9):e17. doi:10.1016/j.jacc.2013.02.099

140. Rigante D, Segni G (2002) Cardiac structural involvement in mucopolysaccharidoses. Cardiology 98:18–20

141. Dangel JH (1998) Cardiovascular changes in children with mucopolysaccharide storage diseases and related disorders: clinical and echocardiographic findings in 64 patients. Eur J Pediatr 157:534–538

142. Butman SM, Karl L, Copeland JG (1989) Combined aortic and mitral valve replacement in an adult with Scheie's disease. Chest 96:209–210

143. Satoh Y, Sakamoto K, Fujibayashi Y et al (1983) Cardiac involvement in mucolipidosis. Importance of non-invasive studies for detection of cardiac abnormalities. Jpn Heart J 24:149–159

144. Hoffbrand AV (2001) Diagnosing myocardial iron overload. Eur Heart J 22:2140–2141

145. Alexander J, Kowdley KV (2005) Hereditary hemochromatosis: genetics, pathogenesis, and clinical management. Ann Hepatol 4:240–247

146. Palka P, Macdonald G, Lange A, Burstow DJ (2002) The role of Doppler left ventricular filling indexes and Doppler tissue echocardiography in the assessment of cardiac involvement in hereditary hemochromatosis. J Am Soc Echocardiogr 15(9):884–890

147. Kremastinos DT, Tsiapras DP, Tsetsos GA, Rentoukas EI, Vretou HP, Toutouzas PK (1993) Left ventricular diastolic Doppler characteristics in beta-thalassemia major. Circulation 88(3):1127–1135

148. Seliem MA, Al-Saad HI, Bou-Holaigah IH, Khan MN, Palileo MR (2002) Left ventricular diastolic dysfunction in congenital chronic anaemias during childhood as determined by comprehensive echocardiographic imaging including acoustic quantification. Eur J Echocardiogr 3(2):103–110

149. Olson LJ, Baldus WP, Tajik JA (1987) Echocardiographic features of idiopathic hemochromatosis. Am J Cardiol 60:885–889

150. Anderson LJ, Holden S, Davis B, Prescott E, Charrier CC, Bunce NH, Firmin DN, Wonke B, Porter J, Walker JM, Pennell DJ (2001) Cardiovascular t2-star (t2*) magnetic resonance for the early diagnosis of myocardial iron overload. Eur Heart J 22:2171–2179

151. Wood JC, Tyszka JM, Carson S, Nelson MD, Coates TD (2004) Myocardial iron loading in transfusion-dependent thalassemia and sickle cell disease. Blood 103:1934–1936

152. Suksaranjit P, Prasidthrathsint K (2013) Clinical implication of T2* cardiac magnetic resonance imaging in cardiac siderosis. Am J Med 126:e9–e10

153. Hazirolan T, Akpinar B, Unal S, Gumruk F, Haliloglu M, Alibek S (2008) Value of dual energy computed tomography for detection of myocardial iron deposition in thalassaemia patients: initial experience. Eur J Radiol 68:442–445

154. Jensen PD, Jensen FT, Christensen T, Eiskjaer H, Baandrup U, Nielsen JL (2003) Evaluation of myocardial iron by magnetic resonance imaging during iron chelation therapy with deferrioxamine: indication of close relation between myocardial iron content and chelatable iron pool. Blood 101(11):4632–4639. doi:10.1182/blood-2002-09-2754

155. Anderson LJ, Westwood MA, Holden S, Davis B, Prescott E, Wonke B, Porter JB, Walker JM, Pennell DJ (2004) Myocardial iron clearance during reversal of siderotic cardiomyopathy with intravenous desferrioxamine: a prospective study using T2* cardiovascular magnetic resonance. Br J Haematol 127(3):348–355. doi:10.1111/j.1365-2141.2004.05202.x

156. Kuan P (1987) Cardiac Wilson's disease. Chest 91:579–583

157. Dürr A, Cossee M, Agid Y et al (1996) Clinical and genetic abnormalities in patients with Friedreich's ataxia. N Engl J Med 335:1169–1175

158. Child JS, Perloff JK, Bach PM et al (1986) Cardiac involvement in Friedreich's ataxia: a clinical study of 75 patients. J Am Coll Cardiol 7:1370–1378

159. Leone M, Rocca WA, Rosso MG et al (1988) Friedreich's disease: survival analysis in an Italian population. Neurology 38:1433–1438

160. Alboliras ET, Shub C, Gomez MR, Edwards WD, Hagler DJ, Reeder GS, Seward JB, Tajik AJ (1986) Spectrum of cardiac involvement in Friedreich's ataxia: clinical, electrocardiographic and echocardiographic observations. Am J Cardiol 58(6):518–524

161. Dutka DP, Donnelly JE, Nihoyannopoulos P, Oakley CM, Nunez DJ (1999) Marked variation in the cardiomyopathy associated with Friedreich's ataxia. Heart 81(2):141–147
162. Morvan D, Komajda M, Doan LD, Brice A, Isnard R, Seck A, Lechat P, Agid Y, Grosgogeat Y (1992) Cardiomyopathy in Friedreich's ataxia: a Doppler-echocardiographic study. Eur Heart J 13(10):1393–1398
163. Cochat P, Hulton SA, Acquaviva C et al (2012) Primary hyperoxaluria Type 1: indications for screening and guidance for diagnosis and treatment. Nephrol Dial Transplant 27:1729–1736
164. Schulze MR, Wachter R, Schmeisser A et al (2006) Restrictive cardiomyopathy in a patient with primary hyperoxaluria type II. Clin Res Cardiol 95:235–240
165. Vélez-Roa S, Depierreux M, Nortier J et al (2006) Cardiac oxalosis: a rare cause of diastolic dysfunction. Eur Heart J 27:2496
166. Van Driessche L, Dhondt A, De Sutter J (2007) Heart failure with mitral valve regurgitation due to primary hyperoxaluria type 1: case report with review of the literature. Acta Cardiol 62:202–206
167. Detry O, Honoré P, DeRoover A et al (2002) Reversal of oxalosis cardiomyopathy after combined liver and kidney transplantation. Transpl Int 15:50–52
168. Palka P, Duhig E, Carey L, Galbraith A (2001) Primary oxalosis with cardiac involvement: echocardiographic features of an unusual form of cardiomyopathy. Circulation 103(24): E122–E123
169. Bates MGD, Bourke JP, Giordano C et al (2012) Cardiac involvement in mitochondrial DNA disease: clinical spectrum, diagnosis, and management. Eur Heart J 33:3023–3033
170. Sebastiani M, Giordano C, Nediani C et al (2007) Induction of mitochondrial biogenesis is a maladaptive mechanism in mitochondrial cardiomyopathies. J Am Coll Cardiol 50:1362–1369
171. Anan R (1991) Cardiac involvement in mitochondrial disease: a clinical study of 38 patients. Igaku Kenkyu 61(2):49–61
172. Holmgren D, Wahlander H, Eriksson BO, Oldfors A, Holme E, Tulinius M (2003) Cardiomyopathy in children with mitochondrial disease; clinical course and cardiological findings. Eur Heart J 24(3):280–288

Other Cardiomyopathies: Clinical Assessment and Imaging in Diagnosis and Patient Management

21

Marco Merlo, Davide Stolfo, Giancarlo Vitrella, Elena Abate, Bruno Pinamonti, Francesco Negri, Anita Spezzacatene, Marco Anzini, Enrico Fabris, Francesca Brun, Lorenzo Pagnan, Manuel Belgrano, Giorgio Faganello, and Gianfranco Sinagra

Electronic supplementary material The online version of this chapter (doi: 10.1007/978-3-319-06019-4_21) contains supplementary material, which is available to authorized users. Videos can also be accessed at http://www.springerimages.com/videos/978-3-319-06018-7.

M. Merlo (✉) • D. Stolfo • G. Vitrella • E. Abate • B. Pinamonti, MD • F. Negri
A. Spezzacatene • M. Anzini • E. Fabris • G. Sinagra, MD, FESC
Department of Cardiology, University Hospital of Trieste,
via P. Valdoni 7, Trieste 34139, Italy
e-mail: supermerloo@libero.it; davide.stolfo@gmail.com;
giancarlo.vitrella@gmail.com; abate.elena@gmail.com;
bruno.pinamonti@gmail.com; francesco_negri@yahoo.it;
anita.spe@gmail.com; marcoanzini@gmail.com;
enrico.fabris@hotmail.it; gianfranco.sinagra@aots.sanita.fvg.it

F. Brun
Department of Cardiology, University Hospital of Trieste,
via P. Valdoni 7, Trieste 34100, Italy
e-mail: frabrun77@gmail.com

L. Pagnan, MD • M. Belgrano, MD
Radiology Unit, University Hospital of Trieste,
via P. Valdoni 7, Trieste 34139, Italy
e-mail: pagny@inwind.it; belgranom@gmail.com

G. Faganello, MD
Cardiovascular Center, Azienda per i Servizi Sanitari n° 1,
via Slataper, 9, Trieste 34125, Italy
e-mail: giorgio.faganello@libero.it

B. Pinamonti, G. Sinagra (eds.), *Clinical Echocardiography and Other Imaging Techniques in Cardiomyopathies*, DOI 10.1007/978-3-319-06019-4_21,
© Springer International Publishing Switzerland 2014

21.1 Introduction

The nonspecific nature of the term cardiomyopathy (CMP) allows a number of diseases directly or indirectly affecting myocardial function to be included under this heading. In fact, in the classification of CMP, some myocardial diseases cannot properly be defined: dilated (DCM), hypertrophic (HCM), right arrhythmogenic (ARVC), restrictive (RCM), and infiltrative/storage CMP. These myocardial diseases are generally defined unclassified or other CMP. They are not extremely rare in clinical practice and are characterized by pathophysiologic processes that are not completely understood. Therefore, their management represents a challenge for clinical cardiologists. Interestingly, some of these CMP are characterized by partial to complete reversibility when etiologic factors are removed (reversible CMP) [1]. Finally, a peculiar form of CMP is left ventricular noncompaction (LV NC), with typical clinical–instrumental characteristics that are not yet widely known.

21.2 Peripartum Cardiomyopathy

The definition of peripartum CMP was first established according to the following four criteria adapted from the study by Demakis et al. [2]:

- Development of heart failure (HF) in the last month of pregnancy or within 5 months of delivery
- Absence of an identifiable cause for HF other than pregnancy
- Absence of recognizable heart disease before the last month of pregnancy (requiring imaging data)
- Left ventricular systolic dysfunction demonstrated by classic echocardiographic criteria, such as depressed shortening fraction or ejection fraction in the last month of pregnancy or within 5 months of delivery [3]

Peripartum CMP remains an exclusion diagnosis (all other causes of HF must be ruled out), and it seems to be linked with several risk factors, such as one or more prior pregnancies, multifetal pregnancy, older maternal age, and high blood pressure [4]. Many etiological processes occurring during pregnancy have been suggested as being causative, such as viral myocarditis, coronary artery spasm, small-vessel disease, abnormal immune response to pregnancy, and excessive prolactin excretion [4].

Common echocardiographic findings of peripartum CMP include globally decreased LV systolic function and LV enlargement, usually without LV hypertrophy (Clips 21.1a, 21.1b, 21.1c, and 21.1d). The primary echocardiographic diagnostic criteria are LV systolic dysfunction [LV ejection fraction (EF) <0.45 and/or M-mode fractional shortening <30 %) and LV dilatation (LV end-diastolic diameter >2.7 cm/m^2) between the last month of pregnancy and the first 5 months postpartum in the absence of other known causes of systolic HF [3]. Additionally, LV thrombus is not rare in patients with LV EF <35 % [5]. Peripartum CMP is frequently associated with preeclampsia (22 % vs 3–5 % in the general population) [6]. In this context marked LV hypertrophy can be exceptionally observed (Fig. 21.1, Clips 21.2a, 21.2b, 21.2c, 21.2d, 21.2e, 21.2f, 21.2g, 21.2h, and 21.2i), which is usually reversible, such as impaired LV contractility.

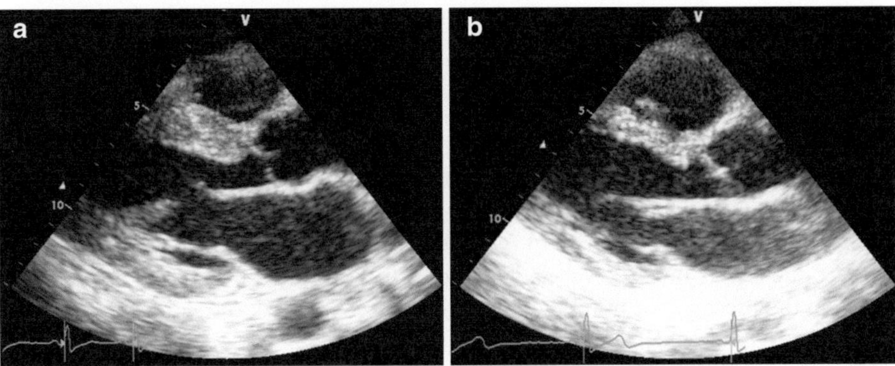

Fig. 21.1 (**a**, **b**) Echocardiographic study in a 42-year-old woman with peripartum cardiomyopathy associated with preeclampsia. Parasternal long-axis view (**a**), diastolic frame, of the first echocardiogram postdelivery documenting severe left ventricular (LV) hypertrophy (septal wall thickness 17 mm, posterior wall thickness 14 mm), with diffuse hypokinesis and severe systolic dysfunction [fractional shortening 15 %, ejection fraction (EF) 32 %]. After 6 months of therapy with beta-blocker and angiotensin-converting-enzyme inhibitor, echocardiography in the parasternal long-axis view, diastolic frame (**b**) shows normal LV wall thickness (septal wall thickness 9 mm, posterior wall thickness 9 mm), with normal regional wall motion and systolic function (fractional shortening 39 %, EF 64 %)

There are few data about the use of advanced echocardiographic technologies in this disease. A similar counterclockwise rotation during systole of both the base and the apex at speckle-tracking analysis was reported in one case of peripartum CMP associated with LV NC [7]. This subtle deformation abnormality has been interpreted as secondary to dysfunction of basal and midwall subepicardial fibers, with resultant predominant effect exerted by the subendocardial fibers in this region. These abnormalities were reversible after optimal medical therapy. However, further investigation is required.

Studies on cardiac magnetic resonance (CMR) in the acute phases of peripartum CMP show the presence of edema at T2 sequences and on early gadolinium enhancement, suggesting an inflammatory etiology for this condition. In addition, late gadolinium enhancement (LGE) seems to identify cases with unfavorable prognosis [8, 9].

Although peripartum CMP shares many features with other forms of nonischemic CMP, women affected by this disease have a higher rate of spontaneous recovery of LV function [5]. Monitoring patients after diagnosis should include serial echocardiograms to identify improvement in systolic function in response to conventional HF medical treatment. Less severely impaired LV EF and lower LV dimensions at the time of diagnosis are predictors of complete LV function recovery and good outcome [10].

Previous studies assessed prognostic implications of LV contractile reserve at initial diagnosis and demonstrated that improved LV EF during dobutamine stress echocardiography accurately correlates with subsequent recovery of LV function and confers a benign prognosis to this CMP [11].

The existing literature indicates that many patients with peripartum CMP actually have myocarditis. The diagnosis of myocarditis is more suspicious in the presence of progressive worsening of LV dilation and systolic dysfunction at serial echocardiographic evaluations. In these cases, endomyocardial biopsy (EMB) can be useful to modify therapeutic strategies.

Finally, one important question asked by women with a history of this disease is whether they can safely get pregnant again. For women with persistently reduced LV EF, there is a substantial risk of recurrent HF. On the other hand, for women who recover, the risk is much lower and can be further stratified by a stress echocardiogram: in the presence of normal contractile reserve, the risk of recurrent disease or HF seems to be low [4].

21.3 Tako-Tsubo Cardiomyopathy

Tako-tsubo, or stress-induced CMP, is an acute, usually reversible, disorder of the heart characterized by transient LV dysfunction [12–15]. Clinical presentation is usually similar to an acute coronary syndrome, with precordial pain and dyspnea. Other symptoms may include palpitations, syncope, or even cardiac arrest or sudden death (SD). A trigger, such as a stressful physical or psychological event, can usually be detected in 27–100 % of cases. Many diagnostic criteria have been formulated, but the most widely accepted are those of the Mayo Clinic in the United States [13], which require normality of the epicardial coronary arteries. Tako-tsubo syndrome may be confused with stress syndrome caused by underlying pheochromocytoma, and attention should be paid to this clinically important differential diagnosis. The etiology and pathogenesis are presently unknown. One possibility is stress-induced catecholamine release, producing cardiac stunning through direct toxic damage to myocytes and/or vasoconstriction with ischemia [16]. The apical region is the most vulnerable area, probably due to the large number of adrenergic receptors [14]. Treatment is symptomatic and is determined by the complications occurring during the acute phase. Complications are estimated to occur in 19 % of cases, mortality varies between 0 and 12 % [15], and recurrence is rare.

Echocardiography plays a major role in achieving this diagnosis. In fact, the most salient feature of this disease is the unusual LV contractile pattern noted at the time of admission. Typically, it is characterized by a transient hypokinesis, akinesis, or dyskinesis of the LV apical and mid segments, usually with compensatory hyperkinesia of the basal portions (Fig. 21.2, Clip 21.3a) [17]. Moreover, regional wall motion abnormalities (WMA) extend beyond a single epicardial vascular distribution [18]. Global contractile LV function is usually significantly impaired. The time course for cardiac function improvement is variable, from a few days to several weeks; however, LV function typically recovers completely (Fig. 21.2, Clip 21.3b).

Atypical forms of stress-induced CMP have been increasingly reported. Transient midventricular ballooning with preserved basal and apical contractility (inverted tako-tsubo CMP) has been described [19]. Additionally, LV apical thrombosis may occur during the early stage of the disease due to transient apical akinesis and

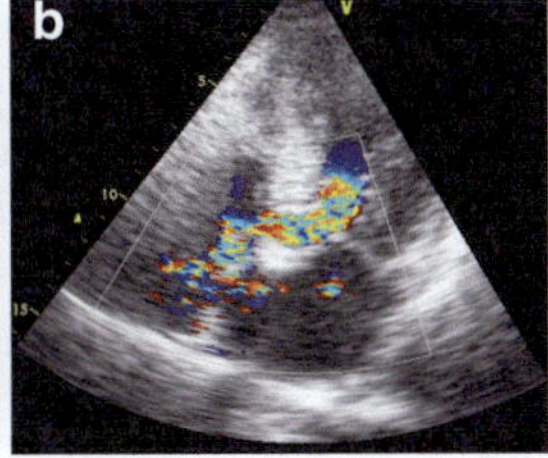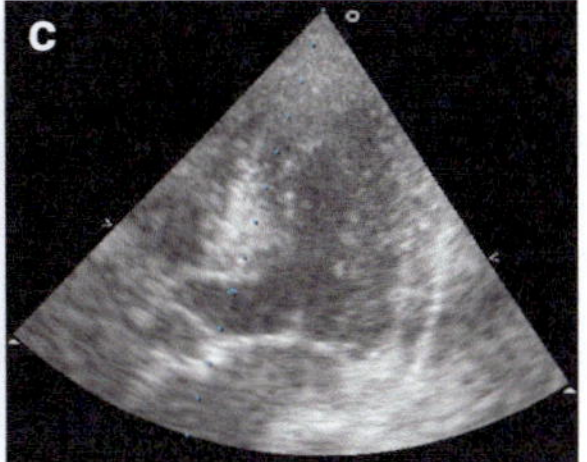

Fig. 21.2 (**a–c**) A 79-year-old woman with tako-tsubo-like cardiomyopathy. Echocardiography at the time of admission shows left ventricular (LV) apical akinesis, hypokinesis of the mid segments with compensatory hyperkinesis of the basal portions, and moderate systolic dysfunction (**a**) in the apical four chamber view, systolic frame. Apical long-axis view (**b**) recorded with color-Doppler imaging demonstrates marked turbulence in the LV outflow tract (OT), consistent with dynamic LV OT obstruction in the presence of a sigmoid interventricular septum. An echocardiogram performed 4 months later shows complete recovery of LV wall motion and systolic function (**c**) in the apical long-axis view, systolic frame

aneurysm formation [20]. The use of contrast agents can be particularly helpful to highlight apical thrombosis and if there is a difficult acoustic window.

Dynamic LV outflow tract (OT) obstruction is a relatively common complication of stress-induced CMP, with a reported incidence of >10 % (Fig. 21.2, Clip 21.3c) [21]. There are probably some predisposing factors to LV OT obstruction, i.e., sigmoid interventricular septum or a small LV or LV OT; more importantly, this complication is frequently precipitated by certain conditions, such as hypovolemia, ionotropic drugs, and counterpulsation.

Stress-induced CMP is also frequently complicated by acute mitral regurgitation (MR). Systolic anterior motion (SAM) of the mitral valve (MV) is typically associated with LV OT gradient and accounts for one half of acute MR. MV tethering with increased valve tenting area the in presence of LV systolic dysfunction and LV enlargement has been proposed as an alternative mechanism responsible for MR in this disease [22].

Right ventricular (RV) involvement and dysfunction is relatively common and is associated with lower LV EF [23]. Conversely, ventricular rupture is an extremely rare life-threatening complication of stress-induced CMP. There are a few cases reported in literature, principally in elderly female patients [24].

Myocardial viability and contractile reserve could be evaluated with low-dose dobutamine stress echocardiography in suspected stress-induced CMP. However, particular caution must be taken considering that increasing doses of dobutamine can worsen LV OT gradient. Furthermore, the possible occurrence of tako-tsubo CMP as a complication of dobutamine stress echocardiography has been reported [25].

Finally, if transthoracic echocardiography (TTE) is limited by poor acoustic windows, transesophageal echocardiography (TEE) can provide clearer image quality and allows careful evaluation of MV anatomy and full definition of the MR [17].

Advanced echocardiographic techniques could be useful in diagnosis and prognostic stratification of tako-tsubo CMP. Both 2D and 3D imaging allows recognition of the contractile pattern, mainly when the apex is involved; 3D imaging may allow better visualization of contracting and noncontracting segments when medial segments are involved. Myocardial contrast echocardiography seems to be a useful tool by which to clarify the mechanisms involved the myocardial injury and to distinguish stress-induced CMP from acute coronary syndrome. In one study, myocardial perfusion was relatively preserved in patients with tako-tsubo CMP compared with those with myocardial infarction. The authors of that study concluded that myocardial contrast echocardiography had a high sensitivity, specificity, and positive and negative predictive values for detecting stress-induced CMP (91, 86.2, 83, and 93 %, respectively) [26]. In addition, transient impairment of coronary flow reserve, assessed by Doppler coronary flow analysis during dipyridamole test, has also been reported in this disease [27]. Finally, at 2D strain by speckle-tracking analysis, a progressive decrease of longitudinal strain values from base to apex was reported in patients with classical stress-induced CMP [17].

CMR in this CMP exhibits the characteristic finding of transmural high T2 signal in the midanterior wall and apical segments, matching the distribution of WMA [28, 29]. This abnormality can persist after 3 months from the acute event although is substantially decreased compared with the acute phase [30]. Myocardial inflammation may also be found at global relative enhancement and quantitative T1 mapping sequences [31, 32].

Patients with tako-tsubo CMP usually do not exhibit hypoenhancement at first-pass perfusion [33], or by LGE [34, 35], thus helping differentiate this condition from acute myocardial infarction with spontaneous coronary recanalization or acute myocarditis [35]. When LGE is found, it is focal or patchy and has decreased signal intensity compared with ischemic LGE [36, 37]. This finding is usually indicative of a more severe acute condition, which tends to resolve within 6 months [38].

CMR data from a large multicenter registry of patients with tako-tsubo CMP revealed four distinct patterns of regional ventricular ballooning [36]:
- Apical (82 %)
- Biventricular (34 %)
- Midventricular (17 %)
- Basal (1 %)

Single-photon-emission CT (SPECT) findings include reduced apical perfusion assessed with technetium-99 m (^{99m}Tc)-tetrofosmin in the acute phase, which recedes during follow-up [39–41]. Severely impaired myocardial fatty-acid metabolism assessed with ^{123}I-beta-methyl-p-iodophenyl pentadecanoic acid (^{123}I-BMIPP) [42–44], and apical sympathetic dysinnervation in the acute phase assessed by ^{123}I-metaiodobenzylguanidine (MIBG) uptake [43, 45–47] were also found, mismatched from perfusion defects.

Positron emission tomography (PET) studies also report perfusion/metabolism mismatch involving the apical akinetic area assessed by [^{18}F]-fluorodeoxyglucose (FDG) and [^{13}N]-ammonia or by thallium-201 radiochemical thallium chloride (^{201}Tl) SPECT [48–50]. Glucose metabolism assessed by [^{18}F]-FDG PET and sympathetic function assessed by [^{123}I]-MIBG SPECT seem to be strictly correlated in affected segments [46].

In tako-tsubo CMP, LV apical WMA is typically transient and resolves over a period of days to weeks. Therefore, follow-up echocardiographic reevaluation is essential to monitor its resolution and recovery of LV systolic function. The prognosis is generally favorable; reported in-hospital mortality rates range from 0 to 8 % [18]. As it is difficult to predict subsequent occurrence of complications immediately after the onset of the disease, serial echocardiographic evaluations should be performed during the in-hospital period. There is no established consensus on how to manage stress- induced CMP, but early detection of complications, such as the occurrence of LV OT gradient or apical thrombosis, can protect against a poor outcome and may lead to some changes in therapeutic strategies.

In this disease, RV involvement is relatively common, and RV dysfunction is associated with lower LV EF, longer hospitalization, more complications, such as severe HF, and need for intra-aortic balloon pump and cardiopulmonary resuscitation [23]. LV EF at admission is one of the independent predictors of mortality [51]. Moreover, absence of LV function recovery within 1 week was an independent factor associated with mortality [52]. Other prognostic indicators of worse outcome are intraventricular thrombus formation and LV OT gradient occurrence [17]. Recurrence of stress-induced CMP occurs in approximately 10 % of patients [53] and is unpredictable from imaging data at first manifestation.

21.4 Tachycardia-Induced Cardiomyopathy

Tachycardia-induced CMP (TIC) is a frequent cause of reversible HF secondary to persistent supraventricular or ventricular arrhythmias and in the absence of pre-existing structural heart disease [54]. Early diagnosis is crucial for prompt re-establishment of sinus rhythm and normal heart rate, with consequent improvement or even normalization of myocardial function. The pathogenesis is still controversial: Elevated heart rate causes structural alterations of myocytes, mitochondrial abnormalities, oxidative stress, and loss of contractile tissue due to necrosis or apoptosis. Moreover, tachycardia reduces myocardial perfusion, leading to myocardial stunning, interstitial fibrosis, and neurohumoral variations with elevations in natriuretic peptide, endothelin, catecholamines, and the renin-angiotensin-aldosterone system (RAAS).

Strict clinical and echocardiographic follow-up is very important in order to recognize relapses, which tend to be more severe and life threatening. Furthermore, due to the fact that LV remodeling can occur despite EF and heart rate normalization, long-term treatment with beta-blockers and angiotensin-converting enzyme (ACE) inhibitors is recommended.

In TIC, imaging techniques are essential to exclude other causes of ventricular dysfunction and to assess its reversibility after normalization of atrial or ventricular rate; echocardiography, being widely available and inexpensive, is the cornerstone in establishing the presence of LV dysfunction and narrowing the list of differential diagnoses. LV systolic dysfunction is the typical model of presentation. However, other aspects can sustain the diagnostic hypothesis. Usually, myocardial thickness

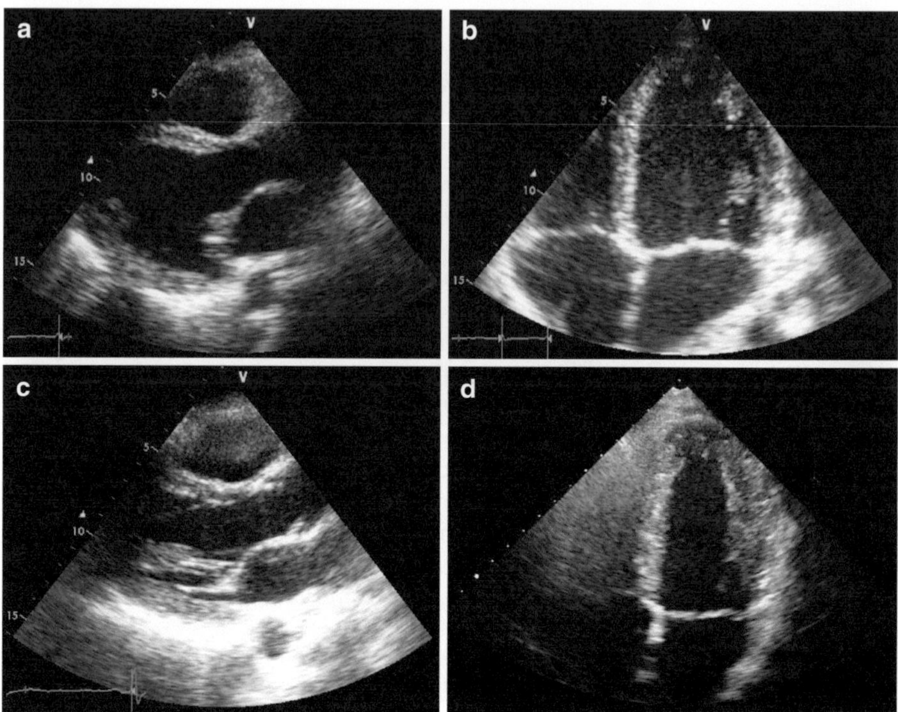

Fig. 21.3 (**a–d**) Echocardiographic study in a 32-year-old patient with atrial fibrillation (AF) and tachycardia-induced cardiomyopathy. Echocardiogram shows mild left ventricular (LV) dilation [end-diastolic diameter corrected for body surface area (BSA) 32 mm/mq), with normal wall thickness, diffuse hypo-akinesis, and severe systolic dysfunction [ejection fraction (EF) 22 %] in the parasternal long-axis (**a**) and apical four-chamber views (**b**), systolic frames. The echocardiogram performed 5 months after successful radiofrequency catheter ablation of AF shows normal LV dimensions (end-diastolic diameter corrected for BSA 26 mm/mq), wall motion, and systolic function (EF 60 %) in the parasternal long-axis (**c**) and apical four-chamber (**d**) views, systolic frames

is preserved, indicating the absence of scar tissue. Moreover, some studies suggest that the absence of severe LV dilation may support the diagnosis of TIC rather than DCM accompanied by supraventricular tachycardia (Fig. 21.3, Clips 21.4a, 21.4b, 21.4c, and 21.4d) [55, 56]. In fact, Jeong et al. [55] reported that LV end-diastolic dimension ≤61 mm could predict TIC with a sensitivity of 100 % and a specificity of 71 % in patients with HF and tachyarrhythmia.

LV diastolic dysfunction should be considered a component of TIC and is indeed sometimes the first expression of the disease [57]. However, it is particularly difficult to assess at Doppler in the presence of tachyarrhythmias. Contractile reserve at low-dose dobutamine stress echocardiography has been reported as a predictor of LV function recovery after catheter ablation of AF in TIC [58].

TEE can provide better image quality in patients with a poor acoustic window. Moreover, it is essential to identify left atrial appendage clots when restoring sinus rhythm is the chosen treatment. Finally, TEE and intracardiac echocardiography may be helpful during catheter ablation of arrhythmias, even without fluoroscopy [59]. There are a few data regarding the application of new and advanced echocardiographic technologies in the setting of TIC. Alterations in LV torsion have been reported in an experimental model [60]. Strain and strain-rate imaging can provide detailed regional and global LA functional assessment [61]. In patients who have undergone catheter ablation for atrial fibrillation, LA strain and strain rate during atrial filling (parameters of LA reservoir function) are known to be better predictors of sinus rhythm maintenance [62]. Real-time 3D TEE has been demonstrated to be feasible during ablation procedures, allowing fluoroscopy-free navigation and precise anatomical delineation of atrial structure [63]. CMR with LGE may differentiate TIC, which seldom shows LGE from primary CMP, in which LGE is frequent [64]. Myocardial glucose metabolism assessed by [^{18}F]-FDG PET was found to be impaired in TIC [65].

The improvement of LV function after normalization of the heart rate is a hallmark of TIC. Therefore, multiple evaluations are necessary to identify changes in LV EF. Echocardiography is probably the most feasible and less expensive technique allowing close follow-up of these patients. The time course of improvement in biventricular systolic function has not been fully established; generally it can be observed soon after heart rate normalization [66]. If LV systolic dysfunction does not improve, other causes of impaired LV function must be reconsidered, justifying an "impure" form of TIC (possible association with dilated CMP, myocarditis, or ischemic heart disease).

It should be noted that patients with a history of successfully treated TIC are susceptible to a more severe CMP if the offending tachyarrhythmia recurs [67]. For this reason, patients should be periodically evaluated after complete LV function restoration.

21.5 Myocarditis

Myocarditis is an inflammatory disease of the myocardium and is diagnosed by established histological [68] (Fig. 21.4), immunological, and immunohistochemical criteria [69]. Most cases of myocarditis observed in clinical practice in the Western world are ascribable to viral infections and to the related reaction of the immune system. On the other hand, myocarditis can also be triggered by many specific causes, such as bacterial or parasitic infections, autoimmune diseases, hypersensitivity processes, hypercatecholaminergic states, drugs, toxic substances, and physical agents [69]. Clinical presentation of myocarditis is polymorphic, ranging from subclinical or benign forms to major clinical syndromes, such as severe HF or life-threatening ventricular arrhythmias. However, for simplification purposes, it can be categorized into three main patterns according to disease onset: HF, arrhythmias (hypokinetic or hyperkinetic, supraventricular or ventricular), and chest pain [70]. Moreover, myocarditis is characterized by great variability in its natural history evolution, ranging from resolution, to relapse, to development of DCM, or to unexpected SD. Patients presenting with chest pain and preserved LV function are

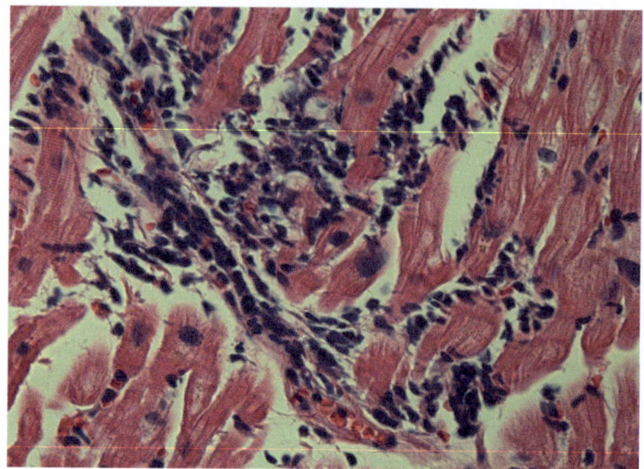

Fig. 21.4 Endomyocardial biopsy, histologic pattern, in a case of myocarditis (hematoxylin and eosin ×40). Severe lymphocytic infiltrates are present and are associated with "fraying" of myocytes (Dallas criteria)

projected through a favorable natural history, whereas those presenting with HF and significant LV dysfunction are generally characterized by a worse prognosis. On the other hand, it is important to emphasize that spontaneous (or therapeutically induced) improvement of ventricular function within a few months of symptom onset is described for 40–50 % of patients and identifies a subgroup with a fair long-term prognosis [70]. Advanced analysis of myocardial tissue samples collected with endomyocardial biopsy is thus far the only way to diagnose the disease definitively and to guide eventual treatment using immunomodulating drugs.

In clinical practice, myocarditis and pericarditis may coexist. This clinical condition is known as perimyocarditis (or myopericarditis) [71]. A precise definition of perimyocarditis is still lacking. Consequently, the true incidence and prevalence of this disease remain unknown. The diagnosis is usually based on the combination of chest pain, pericardial rubs, increased inflammation indexes, electrocardiographic (ECG) and echocardiographic abnormalities (most frequently, pericardial effusion), with troponin release [71]. Clinical presentation is variable and may affect any or all cardiac chambers. Usually, chest pain is the main symptom and is associated with concomitant or recent flu-like syndrome, whereas ventricular/supraventricular arrhythmias and HF with LV dysfunction are rarely observed. Natural history is excellent (survival rate 100 %) during long-term follow-up, regardless of specific etiology and the presence of myocardial involvement (troponin release and WMA at echocardiography) at admission; relapses are relatively infrequent (<10 %) [72].

Typically, patients with myocarditis who present with recent onset of HF demonstrate at echocardiographic study a global impairment of ventricular function without significant remodeling of ventricular chambers, which often maintain a normal or augmented wall thickness and an ellipsoidal shape. Moreover, patchy WMA not corresponding to coronary distribution or ECG changes are often observed (Fig. 21.5, Clips 21.5a and 21.5b) [73, 74]. Additional elements, such as the presence of pericardial effusion, diastolic dysfunction, transient pseudohypertrophy of the ventricular wall, intraventricular thrombi [sometimes multiple and mobile (Fig. 21.6, Clips 21.6a, 21.6b, and 21.6c)] and alteration of the

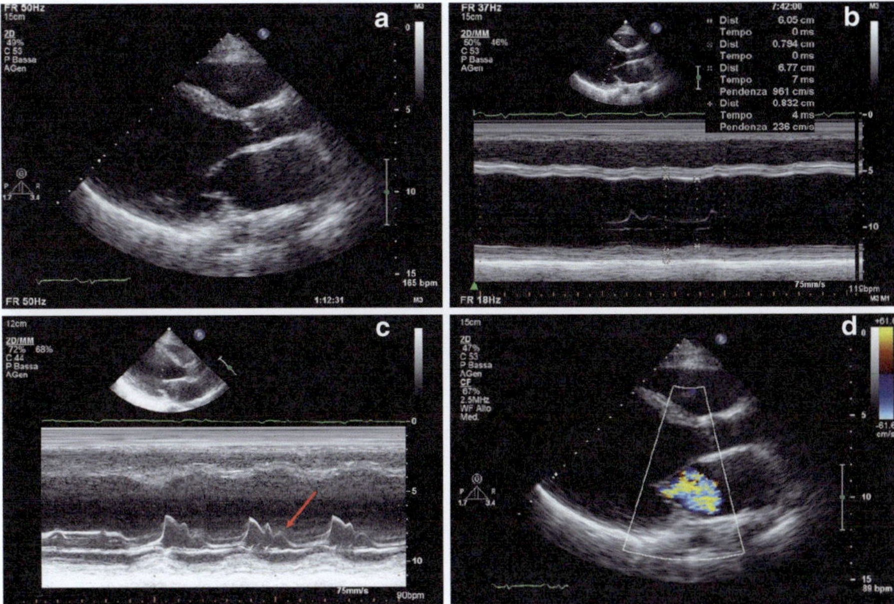

Fig. 21.5 (**a–d**) Echocardiographic study in a 33-year-old patient with myocarditis and severe heart failure. Parasternal long-axis view (**a**) and M-mode (**b**) show severe left ventricular (LV) dilation (end-diastolic diameter corrected for body surface area 39 mm/m^2), normal wall thickness, and severe systolic dysfunction (fractional shortening 12 %, ejection fraction 15 %). M-mode recorded at the level of the mitral valve (**c**) shows a B bump (*arrow*), a sign of elevated LV diastolic pressure. Color-Doppler imaging reveals severe functional mitral regurgitation (**d**)

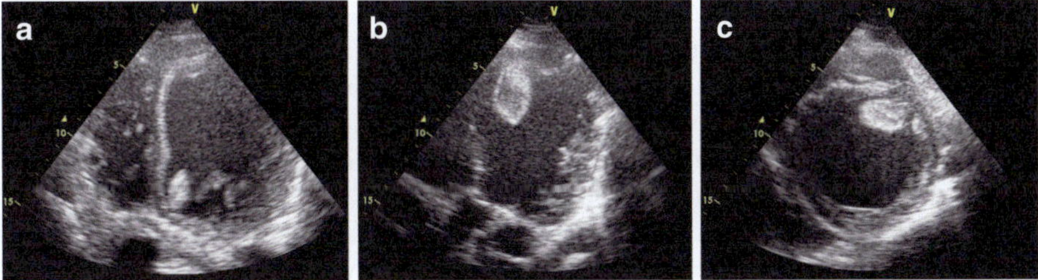

Fig. 21.6 (**a–c**) Echocardiogram in a patient with acute myocarditis and severe left ventricular (LV) dysfunction showing multiple pedunculated and mobile thrombi in the LV cavity. Apical four-chamber view (**a**) demonstrating thrombus in the LV attached to the anterior mitral annulus. Apical long-axis view (**b**) showing another pedunculated mobile thrombus attached to the septal apex. Parasternal short-axis view (**c**) in which the apical thrombus is clearly visible

echocardiographic myocardial texture, may further strengthen, if correctly contextualized, the suspicion of myocarditis [73, 75–77]. On the other hand, patients who present with arrhythmias or chest pain and those with perimyocarditis usually exhibit ventricular chambers characterized by normal dimensions, regional wall motion, and global function, even if WMA or transient mild ventricular dysfunction may be observed [72, 78]. In such cases, careful re-evaluation of those

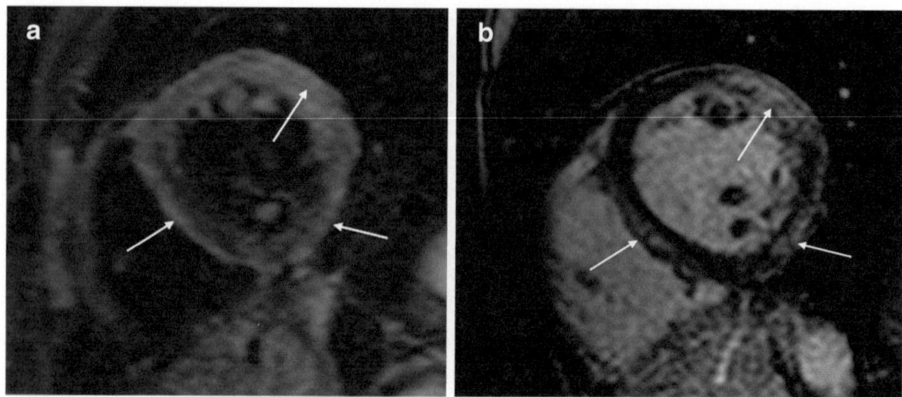

Fig. 21.7 (**a, b**) Cardiac magnetic resonance study in acute myocarditis. Midventricular short-axis T2-weighed image (**a**) showing multiple foci of myocardial edema (*arrows*). Midventricular short-axis T1-weighted image after gadolinium contrast administration (**b**) showing late gadolinium enhancement (transmural or subepicardial) in regions corresponding to hyperintensity seen at T2 imaging (*arrows*)

abnormalities with a short-term follow-up is recommended in order to track disease evolution and promptly recognize potentially extensive myocardial involvement.

Recent studies show that LV strain and strain rate may be promising diagnostic parameters in acute myocarditis, even in the presence of normal standard indices, such as LV EF and wall motion. Di Bella et al. [79] demonstrated that strain Doppler echocardiography could detect longitudinal segmental myocardial dysfunction subsequent to myocardial edema in the acute phase of myocarditis.

Further studies using 2D speckle-tracking strain imaging demonstrate that, among all deformation parameters, longitudinal strain appears to be the most powerful index for diagnostic purposes [80, 81]. Furthermore, Escher et al. [82] demonstrated reduced 2D speckle-tracking global systolic longitudinal strain and strain rate in all their patients with biopsy-proven myocarditis (even in those who had preserved LV systolic function); in addition, at follow-up, deformation parameters were significantly lower in patients with than in those without inflammation and correlated significantly with lymphocytic infiltrates. Finally, in a preliminary report, myocardial contrast echocardiography enabled detection of regional perfusion defects that did not conform to a coronary distribution and were not apparent with conventional echocardiography, suggesting the diagnosis of myocarditis later confirmed by CMR [83].

CMR is extensively assessed in scientific literature and is frequently used in clinical practice to evaluate suspected myocarditis [84]. Acute myocarditis, particularly if presenting as acute chest pain and positive markers of myocardial damage without coronary artery disease, frequently has a characteristic pattern at LGE imaging of subepicardial enhancement involving the basal and mid segments of the LV free wall [85] (Fig. 21.7). T2- and T1-weighed early enhancement sequences may, respectively, demonstrate localized myocardial edema and global hyperemia in the inflamed myocardium [86, 87] (Fig. 21.7). The diagnostic accuracy of CMR compared with the gold-standard of EMB is very high when using a combination of two of the three aforementioned criteria [88].

The same diagnostic criteria were initially reported to have high diagnostic accuracy in cases of myocarditis with clinical presentation such as HF [89]. However, more recent data report limited accuracy when evaluating a single criterion or any combination thereof [90, 91]. These cases are usually characterized by lower-grade diffuse inflammation—which is often impossible to identify with early-enhancement T1- or T2-weighted sequences—and by diffuse interstitial fibrosis, which is missed by LGE sequences [92]. Delayed multidetector CT performed 5 min after contrast injection may be able to identify hyperenhancement similarly to LGE in CMR [93]. This may be a useful alternative in patients with contraindications to CMR.

Echocardiographic recognition of severe myocardial structural derangement with LV enlargement and systolic dysfunction permits identification of patients at risk of major clinical events (death, heart transplantation) in the long-term follow-up. More importantly, data published by our group show that improvement or normalization of LV function at 6 months echocardiographic re-evaluation are associated with a benign long-term prognosis, independently of the pattern of clinical presentation and LV function at presentation [70].

Promising data have been published in recent years on the prognostic role of CMR in the context of myocarditis. The presence of LGE is associated with increased global and arrhythmic cardiac mortality [94]. A pattern of LGE involving the septum, usually from human herpesvirus 6 (HHV6) or combined HHV6 parvovirus B-19 (PVB19) infections, may be predictive of persisting LV dilatation and dysfunction [95].

21.6 Chagas Disease

One peculiar form of myocarditis is Chagas disease, which is caused by *Trypanosoma cruzi*, a flagellated protozoan. This disease continues to represent a health threat for an estimated 28 million people, mostly those living in Latin America [96, 97]. Chagas disease classically presents in an acute or initial phase, which is followed by a chronic phase that can be categorized into indeterminate, cardiac, or digestive forms, each with different clinical manifestations [97]. Severe acute disease is rare (<1 %) and characterized by acute myocarditis, pericardial effusion, and/or meningoencephalitis. After the acute phase, an indeterminate phase usually lasting several years precedes the chronic phase of the disease. The most common and serious problems are cardiac and are caused by an inflammatory CMP as a result of immune reaction and/or the persistence of parasites in the heart. They manifest clinically with progressive HF, life-threatening arrhythmias, and/or thromboembolic events. According to severity of clinical, ECG, chest X-ray, and imaging abnormalities, chronic Chagas CMP is classified into four stages (A, B, C, D) with different mortality and morbidity rates [98]:

- Stage A, or indeterminate, characterized by the absence of symptoms and ECG and structural cardiac abnormalities

- Stage B, with ECG abnormalities (conduction defects and/or arrhythmias) in the absence of symptoms; mild/moderate LV WMA and systolic dysfunction may be present
- Stage C, LV dysfunction at imaging, and prior or current symptoms of HF
- Stage D: symptoms/signs of HF at rest, refractory to medical therapy [New York Heart Association (NYHA) IV]

Most patients affected by Chagas disease have no symptoms for decades after becoming infected with *T. cruzi*. In rare cases, acute myopericarditis can manifest at echocardiography as pericardial effusion, sometimes massive and with tamponade, and/or WMA [97, 99]. In chronic Chagas disease, echocardiographic abnormalities increase in frequency and severity according to the clinical stage of the disease [97, 99, 100]. The typical, although not pathognomonic, pattern is the presence of apical LV aneurysm, with or without global chamber dilatation and depressed systolic function (Clips 21.7a, 21.7b, 21.7c, and 21.7d) [99, 100]. Diastolic dysfunction is an important hallmark of Chagas disease and usually precedes systolic dysfunction [97]. Also, RV involvement is a typical feature of the disease and is usually associated with LV dysfunction; occasionally a RV apical aneurysm is observed [97]. Patients with LV aneurysms, similarly to those with this complication of myocardial infarction, are at risk of thrombosis and systemic embolism.

Few data are available regarding the usefulness of new echocardiographic techniques in Chagas disease. Tissue-Doppler-imaging (TDI) derived myocardial strain can demonstrate lower radial and longitudinal values compared with normal individuals and could quantify subtle segmental contractile dysfunction not detected visually [99]. Speckle-tracking technology is used to quantify global and segmental LV deformation (radial, circumferential, and longitudinal strain) and twist and untwisting velocities [101]. In that study, global strains showed a significant decreasing trend across groups of disease severity. Interestingly, patients in the indeterminate form had significantly lower radial strains in both the global and midinferior segment and lower twist and untwisting velocities compared with normal individuals. CMR may help in diagnosing Chagas CMP by demonstrating aneurysm formation with preferential sites at the apex and inferolateral walls. Aneurysms are easily detected with SSFP cine imaging. The pattern of LGE is variable and may involve any or all layers of the myocardial wall [102, 103].

Prognosis in Chagas disease mainly depends on the clinical stage of the disease [97]. No mortality is reported for patients in the indeterminate phase. In one series of 843 initially asymptomatic patients with Chagas disease [100], during long-term follow-up (mean 9.9 ± 5.3 years), a change in clinical stage, LV systolic dimension at M-mode echocardiography, and EF were the only independent predictors of mortality. The frequency and severity of echocardiographic abnormalities increases with increasing severity of disease stage. In that series, mortality and event rates were, respectively, 0 and 8 % of 505 patients in group 0; 1 and 26 % of 257 patients of group 1; and 14 and 52 % of 87 patients of group 2.

Nunes et al. [104] reported on the prognostic value of LA volume assessed by 2D echocardiography, adding incremental prognostic value to clinical factors (NYHA class), LV EF, RV function, and Doppler parameters of diastolic function [Ratio of transmitral E velocity to mitral annular E' velocity (E/E')]. In that series, an LA-indexed end-systolic volume >51 ml/m² was associated with significant excess mortality. The prognostic impact of TDI index on LV diastolic dysfunction (E/E') was subsequently analyzed by Nunes et al. [105], who showed a different and opposite prognostic significance of E/E' according to LV systolic dysfunction severity. In fact, a high E/E' (>15) was a strong adverse prognostic factor only for patients with mild to moderate LV EF depression (>30 %), whereas it was "protective" in the subset patients with severe LV systolic dysfunction. An interaction between RV dysfunction, frequent in the most severe cases with advanced congestive HF, was hypothesized.

21.7   Chemotherapy-Induced Cardiomyopathy

The incidence of complications after antineoplastic therapy is increasing in relation to the incidence of cancer and prolonged survival rate. Cardiotoxicity is one of the major complications. The Cardiac Review and Evaluation Committee established some criteria for diagnosing chemotherapy-related cardiac dysfunction [106], which consider clinical history, LV EF reduction, and presence of HF symptoms and signs. Echocardiography is recommended before the start of treatment and periodically during and after chemotherapy cycles. Anthracyclines (doxorubicin, daunomycin, idarubicin) are the most frequent chemotherapeutic agents involved in cardiotoxicity; however, adverse cardiotoxic effects are reported also for other drugs (mitoxantrone, 5-fluorouracil, cyclophosphamide, trastuzumab). Anthracycline may exhibit two different types of cardiac toxicity over time: early-onset cardiotoxicity (often expressed with ventricular or supraventricular arrhythmias), or late-onset chronic cardiotoxicity that emerges many years after chemotherapy has been completed. The risk and severity of anthracycline CMP is typically dose related. Clinical manifestations are those of severe biventricular HF with decreased EF and frequently severe diastolic dysfunction. Because of the progressive morphologic changes and the persistence of changes over a long period, symptoms are reported to occur any time up to months after stopping the drug. Although HF is reported to have a high mortality rate, successful treatment is possible [107].

Traditional therapies, such as anthracyclines, have been recognized for years as causing cardiovascular complications. Less expected were the cardiovascular effects of targeted cancer therapies, which were initially thought to be specific to cancer cells and would spare any adverse effects on the heart. In patients with breast cancer treated with anthracyclines, taxanes, and trastuzumab, systolic longitudinal myocardial strain and ultrasensitive troponin I measured at the completion of anthracycline therapy are useful for predicting subsequent cardiotoxicity and may help guide treatment [108].

Echocardiographic characteristics of anthracyclines-induced CMP are indistinguishable from other causes of LV dysfunction [109]. A typical pattern is a mildly dilated but severely dysfunctioning LV with severe diastolic dysfunction [restrictive

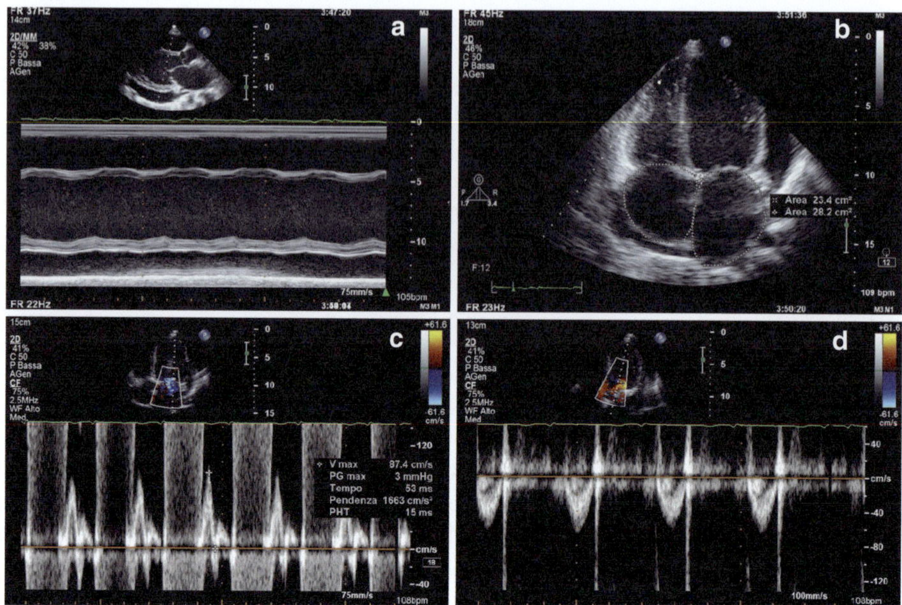

Fig. 21.8 (**a–d**) A 19-year-old patient with cardiomyopathy that developed after chemiotherapy (including anthracyclines) and radiotherapy for acute lymphatic leukemia. M-mode echocardiography (**a**), parasternal long-axis view, shows moderate left ventricular (LV) dilation (end-diastolic diameter corrected for body surface area 36 mm/mq), with severe systolic dysfunction (fractional shortening 11 %). There is also pericardial effusion posteriorly to the LV (21-mm thick), around the right atrium (12 mm), and laterally to the LV (14 mm), as shown in the apical four-chamber view (**b**), which also shows mild biatrial dilation. Pulsed-wave-Doppler interrogation of transmitral flow reveals a restrictive filling pattern (**c**). Pulsed-wave Doppler of the aortic valve (**d**) shows a low velocity (0.5 m/s), a sign of low cardiac output

filling pattern (RFP)}. RV dysfunction, MR, tricuspid regurgitation (TR), and pulmonary hypertension are frequently present (Fig. 21.8, Clips 21.8a, 21.8b, 21.8c, and 21.8d). Other antineoplastic drugs, such as the monoclonal antibody trastuzumab, can induce reversible forms of cardiac dysfunction [110].

Furthermore, several forms of cancer treatment, such as 5-fluorouracil, are associated with an increased risk of coronary artery disease and/or acute coronary syndrome, with transient regional hypokinesia at echocardiographic evaluation.

Strain and strain-rate imaging is used to detect subtle early impairment in cardiac contractility due to chemotherapeutic agents. Reduced strain and strain-rate parameters can, in fact, precede any appreciable change in LV EF and might therefore help in identifying patients who develop chemotherapy-related cardiotoxicity in an early subclinical stage (Fig. 21.9) [111]. Early subclinical abnormalities occur after low to moderate dosages of anthracycline-based chemotherapy and persist after 6 months, although without evidence of myocardial fibrosis by LGE [112].

CMR is able to detect significantly reduced LV EF and cardiac mass in survivors of childhood cancer previously undiagnosed with cardiotoxicity by 2D

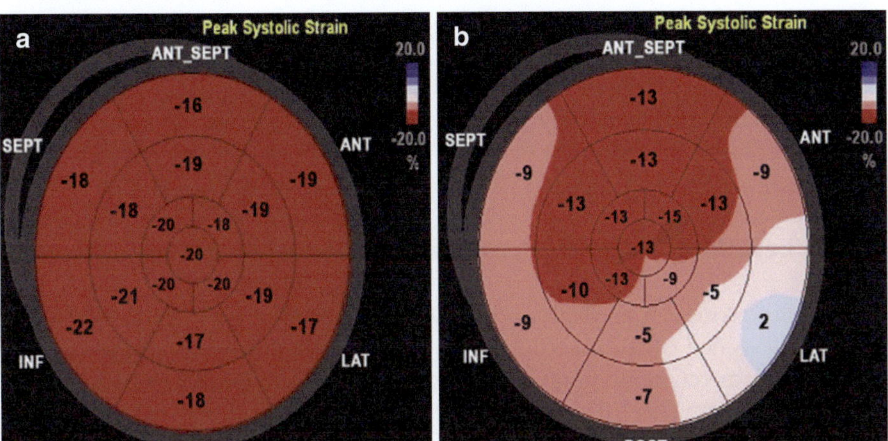

Fig. 21.9 (**a**, **b**) Normal 2D global longitudinal strain (−19.5 %) (**a**) measured in a 22-year-old woman before chemotherapy treatment. After 6 months of chemotherapy (**b**), a significant reduction in global longitudinal strain is observed (−10.1 %) despite persistence of normal left ventricular ejection fraction. *ANT* anterior, *ANT_SEPT* anteroseptal, *INF* inferior, *LAT* lateral, *POST* posterior, *SEPT* septal (From Oreto et al. [111], with permission)

echocardiography [113, 114]. Indexed LV mass by CMR is inversely associated with cumulative anthracycline dose and predictive of events at follow-up [115]; LGE is rare [114, 115]. Diffuse myocardial fibrosis seen at T1 mapping may represent an early marker of anthracycline cardiotoxicity [116, 117].

Conversely, when trastuzumab is combined with anthracyclines for human epidermal growth factor receptor-2 (HER-2)-positive breast cancer, subepicardial lateral wall LGE is often found in patients who develop drug-induced CMP [118]. Serial LV EF determination may be performed using ^{99m}Tc radionuclide ventriculography and has long been regarded as the gold standard for measuring anthracycline cardiotoxicity in adult patients [119]. Imaging with [^{123}I]-MIBG or ^{123}I-labelled antimyosin may detect subclinical changes before LV function is impaired in patients treated with anthracyclines [120].

Regular heart-function monitoring during treatment is important to detect cardiac involvement in neoplastic patients treated with chemotherapy. A baseline, LV EF evaluation is usually necessary. It is recommended that the same methodology be used for comparing serial studies [109]. Decreased longitudinal strain, together with troponin I, increases early after treatment with anthracyclines and trastuzumab, can predict cardiotoxicity development [108]. CMR imaging is also emerging as a promising tool in the oncology setting [113].

A clinically important deterioration in LV function can be variously defined (i.e., 10 % absolute decrease in LV fractional shortening, 10 % decrease in LV EF, or absolute LV EF value <55 %). Guidelines recommend discontinuing anthracycline therapy if LV deterioration is found and, preferably, is confirmed on two successive tests [110].

Treating anthracycline-induced LV dysfunction is the same as for treating other causes of myocardial dysfunction according to international HF guidelines. Echocardiography continues to be the mainstay of monitoring therapeutic efficacy, given that it is portable, widely available, noninvasive, causes minimal pain, and provides real-time data [110].

21.8 Left Ventricular Noncompaction

A position statement from the European Society of Cardiology categorized LV NC as an "unclassified CMP," asserting: "it is not clear whether it is a separate cardiomyopathy or merely a morphological trait shared by many phenotypically distinct cardiomyopathies" [121]. There is no gold-standard criteria for making this diagnosis, so that it can even be difficult to assess the real incidence of the disease. In 1990, Chin et al. [122] proposed echocardiographic criteria for diagnosing this entity. LV NC can be present from birth or it can develop later in life. It is difficult to identify strong predictors of outcome to select effective management strategies in this CMP due to the rarity of the disease and to different studies that are not comparable for type and number of patients included [123]. The standard therapy HF management should be applied to patients with LV NC and LV dysfunction.

Systemic thromboembolic events are commonly associated with LV NC. However, there is no agreement in the cardiology community regarding the use warfarin and/or antiplatelet therapy, particularly in patients with preserved LV EF, and the risk/benefit ratio must be individualized. Also the practice to use anticoagulation in patients with LV NC and significantly impaired LVEF is not based on robust data [124].

The typical echocardiographic features of LV NC are the presence of multiple, prominent LV endocardial trabeculations separated by multiple, deep intertrabecular recesses filled with blood from the ventricular cavity, with a predominant involvement of the apex, the lateral, and the inferior wall. Wall thickness of spared segments is normal [123]. Dimensions and shape of cardiac chambers are usually preserved [122], but, in the late stages of HF, the LV can also be significantly dilated. Noncompacted segments are usually hypokinetic, such as the noninvolved walls; therefore, the LV systolic function is commonly depressed (~60 % of patients). Maximal end-systolic ratio of the noncompacted endocardial layer to the compacted myocardium and the number of affected segments are independent predictors of LV systolic dysfunction [125].

RV involvement is reported in 20–30 % of cases [126], but it is very difficult to demonstrate due to the normal trabeculated pattern of the RV walls. Myocardial thickness is apparently increased, but with a patchy structure and deep intertrabecular recesses, which are radially oriented. Usually, these aspects are better appreciated in childhood (Fig. 21.10, Clips 21.9a and 21.9b). Considering its predominant direction, anomalous trabeculation should be assessed by multiple views. Oblique of-axis images or images in the parasternal short-axis view, which are not perpendicular to the LV long axis, can produce the morphological appearance of prominent

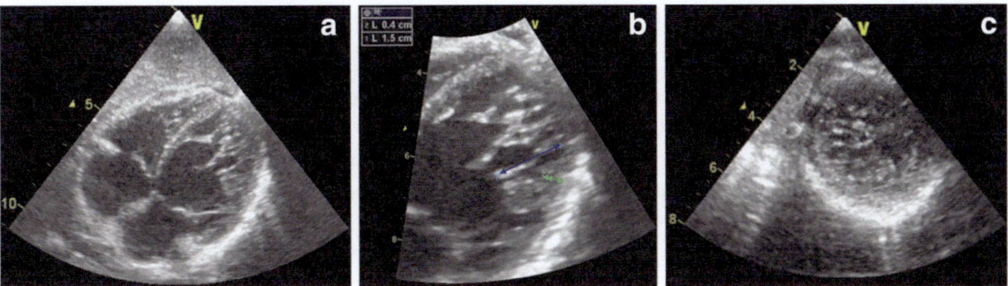

Fig. 21.10 (**a–c**) Echocardiographic study in a 6-year-old patient with left ventricular (LV) non-compaction. Subcostal four-chamber view (**a**) showing multiple endocardial trabeculations in the LV lateral wall, with normal wall thickness of the spared segments. Compacted myocardium thickness is 4 mm (*green arrow*); compacted+noncompacted myocardial thickness is 15 mm at end-diastole (*blue arrow*) (**b**). Subcostal short-axis view (**c**) showing the typical honeycomb appearance

trabeculations and thus mimic LV NC. It is therefore crucial to obtain images that are not foreshortened and are perpendicular to the ventricular long axis [124]. Color-Doppler flow imaging can be useful to detect intertrabecular recesses filled with blood in the LV cavity. In adults, prominent trabeculations are less evident; more frequently, there are echo-free spaces interrupting the homogeneous myocardial echogenic pattern [127]. Moreover, typically, progressive increase in the noncompacted/compacted segment ratio from base to apex is seen, showing the typical honeycomb appearance [128]. The presence of thrombi, which are hidden in the sponge-like myocardium, can be detected by 2D echocardiography, but the accuracy of CMR is certainly superior. Diastolic function is usually affected, and an restrictive pattern is present in 20–40 % of patients [126]. Atrial cavities are typically dilated [127]. Differential diagnosis can be challenging and includes apical form of HCM, a combination of apical HCM and LV NC, hypertensive CMP, endocardial fibroelastosis, abnormal chords, apical thrombus, or tumors [129]. Differential diagnosis between DCM and LV NC can be a challenge, especially in dilated ventricles. Furthermore, the degree of trabeculated LV myocardium is far more frequent than previously thought; this supports the concept of a continuous trait between the normal and pathological appearance of the myocardium [130]. Given the high interobserver variability, it is not sufficient to limit the diagnostic approach to a simple qualitative morphologic assessment. Therefore, three different quantitative diagnostic criteria exist (Table 21.1). All criteria are based on morphological findings and require the presence of prominent trabeculations, with deep intertrabecular recesses communicating with the ventricular cavity, as well as a two-layered appearance of the myocardium (trabecular myocardium as one layer, compacted myocardium as the second layer) [122, 131–134]. Chin et al. [122] calculated the ratio between the depth of the intertrabecular recesses and posterior wall thickness by comparing the distance between the epicardial surface trough of intertrabecular recesses (*X*) with the distance between the epicardial surface and peak trabeculations (*Y*) in end-diastole. A decade later, Jenni et al. [131] published their criteria for LV NC consisting of four components and validated with anatomical heart preparations. In contrast to

Table 21.1 Echocardiographic diagnostic criteria for left ventricular noncompaction (LV NC)

Study	Criteria
Chin et al. [122]	Two-layered structure of the myocardium (epicardial compacted, endocardial noncompacted layer)
	Determination of X to Y ratio (≤ 0.5). X: distance between epicardial surface and through intertrabecular recess; Y: distance between epicardial surface and peak of trabeculation
	Image acquisition. Parasternal short-axis view, measurements of X to Y ratio at end-diastole
Jenni et al. [127, 131]	Image acquisition. Short-axis views, measurement of noncompacted (N)/compacted (C) ratio at end-systole
	Thickened myocardium, with a two-layered structure consisting of a thin, compacted, epicardial layer/band (C) and a much thicker, noncompacted, endocardial layer (N) or trabecular meshwork with deep endomyocardial spaces; N/C ratio >2.0
	Predominant location of the pathology. Midlateral, midinferior, and apex
	Color-Doppler evidence of deep intertrabecular recesses filled with blood from the left ventricular cavity
	Absence of coexisting cardiac abnormalities (in the presence of isolated LV NC)
Stollberger et al. [132, 133]	More than three trabeculations protruding from the LV wall, located apically to the papillary muscles and visible in one image plane
	Trabeculations with the same echogenicity as the myocardium and synchronous movement with ventricular contractions. Perfusion of intertrabecular spaces from the LV cavity
	Ratio of noncompacted to compacted segment >2.0 at end-diastole (this criterion was introduced later)
	Image acquisition. Apical four-chamber view; transducer angulation, and image acquisition in atypical views to obtain the best technical picture quality for differentiation between false chords/aberrant bands and trabeculations
	Diagnostic criteria have changed in recent years

Chin et al., the Zurich group relied on measurements at end-systole because the thickness of the two layers is best visualized in that phase. The combination of these criteria was very specific [135]. The third criteria, by Stollberger et al. [132], required the presence of more than three trabeculations located apical to insertion of the papillary muscles, as visible in one apical image plane. These authors were the first to clearly define trabeculations as structures with the same echogenicity as the myocardium, moving synchronously with the ventricle.

Belanger et al. [136] also assessed the utility of the LV trabecular area as measured by echocardiography using a four-chamber view to identify LV NC.

Several limitations are reported regarding these criteria. Kohli et al. [137] demonstrated an unexpectedly high percentage (23.6 %) of patients with HF fulfilling one or more of the diagnostic criteria for LV NC, in addition to 8.3 % of healthy controls. Furthermore, the reproducibility of the measurement of noncompacted/compacted segment ratio, such as the quantification of trabeculations, has been shown to be poor [138]. Interestingly, a high proportion of young athletes (8.1 %) fulfilled conventional criteria for LV NC [139].

When noncompaction is subtle or incomplete, differential diagnosis with other disorders is uncertain. Contrast echocardiography can be helpful in such cases or when conventional echocardiographic images are poor, improving visualization of trabeculations and the compacted myocardium, and illustrating intertrabecular perfusion [140]. Moreover, TEE can support the diagnosis of LV NC, thus highlighting the spongy appearance of the LV walls and showing the peculiar morphology of the papillary muscles [141]. Finally, it can be helpful when intraventricular thrombi cannot be excluded by TTE.

A functional evaluation, in addition to morphological assessment, can be useful in LV NC diagnosis. Myocardial strain values are abnormal in patients with LV NC, even in the context of preserved systolic function [142]. In addition, an abnormal pattern of LV twist/rotation was observed on speckle-tracking echocardiography in patients with LV NC. In one study [143], rotation was clockwise at the base and counterclockwise at the apex in all controls as well as in patients with DCM. In contrast, LV base and apex rotated in the same direction (LV solid-body rotation) in all LV NC patients. Thus, LV solid-body rotation/twist may be a new objective, functional, and quantitative diagnostic criterion for this CMP. However, this feature might not be entirely specific [144] and was not present in all LV NC patients in another study [145]. In that study, the presence of rigid-body rotation was not associated with worse LV remodelling compared with LV NC individuals with normal twist.

Furthermore, Nieman et al. [146] found no difference in standard echocardiographic parameters between LV NC and DCM but observed a unique regional deformation pattern in LV NC characterized by preserved deformation in basal segments with decreased myocardial deformation in more apical segments. Conversely, in DCM, strain and strain rate were homogeneously reduced in all LV segments. Thus, the authors proposed this special regional deformation pattern as an additional diagnostic tool to differentiate LV NC from DCM (Fig. 21.11).

In LV NC, 3D echocardiography allows a more comprehensive LV assessment, including trabecular volume measurement, which may further aid in diagnosis (Fig. 21.12) [147]. Moreover, Bodiwala et al. [148] suggested the use of 3D echocardiography to visualize the trabecular meshwork, referred to as a honeycomb appearance, as an useful feature for differentiating LV NC from other diseases.

CMR has an important diagnostic contribution in suspected LV NC, particularly in patients with poor echocardiographic quality. A ratio between noncompacted and compacted myocardium >2.3:1 seen at steady-state free-precession (SSFP) CMR sequences was demonstrated to have high sensitivity and specificity and is the accepted diagnostic criterion for diagnosing this disease [149] (Fig. 21.13). However, when using this criterion, an unexpectedly high rate of LV NC is found [150]. Other proposed diagnostic criteria are the percentage of LV trabeculated mass >20 % [151, 152] or >25 %, or >15 g/m^2 indexed noncompacted myocardial mass [153]. Operators must be aware of the potential pitfalls in CMR, which have frequently led to overdiagnosis of LV NC, such as assessing long-axis instead of short-axis views [150], possibly due to incorrect piloting of long-axis planes [154].

LGE correlates with the extent of WMA and severity of clinical status [155–157]. However, these relations were not confirmed in other series [153, 158].

Multidetector CT (MDCT) of the heart may be a valuable diagnostic option. A noncompacted to compacted ratio of 2.2 or 2.3 measured in end-diastole, and involvement of two or more segments, is suggested to distinguish LV NC from other CMP and healthy individuals [159, 160].

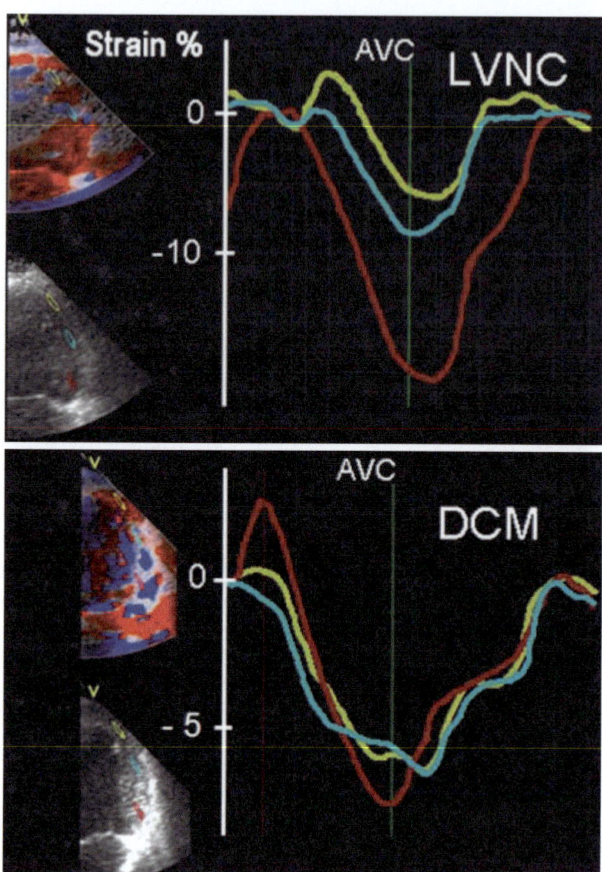

Fig. 21.11 Tissue-Doppler strain imaging performed in three lateral wall segments in a patient with left ventriculare noncompaction (*LV NC*) (*upper*) and dilated cardiomyopathy (*DCM*) (*lower*). *Yellow, blue,* and *red curves* show strain curves in apical, mid, and basal segments, respectively. There is an increasing gradient in end-systolic strain from the apex to the base in the patient with LV NC, whereas strain in the patient with DCM is homogeneously reduced. *AVC* aortic valve closure (From Niemann et al. [146], with permission)

Regional myocardial perfusion defects assessed by [^{13}N]-ammonia PET are described in most noncompacted segments and in a minority of normal segments. Coronary flow reserve is significantly decreased in most segments with WMA and not confined to noncompacted segments only [161].

Considering the possible prognostic implications of imaging, the presence of LV systolic dysfunction in LV NC is related with the number of affected segments and the thickness of the noncompacted layer [125]. LV dysfunction by itself places patients at a higher risk for morbidity and mortality [162]. Other echocardiographic predictors of adverse outcome are reported in previous studies, specifically the ratio of noncompacted to compacted layers, the number of affected segments, the LV end-diastolic diameter, and an a decreased E′ velocity of the LV lateral wall on TDI [123, 125, 163–165].

Patients with systolic dysfunction, even if asymptomatic, should be treated with evidenced-based HF therapy and need careful follow-up. Insertion of an implantable cardioverter defibrillator (ICD) for primary prevention should be considered, according to guidelines, for nonischemic CMP [166].

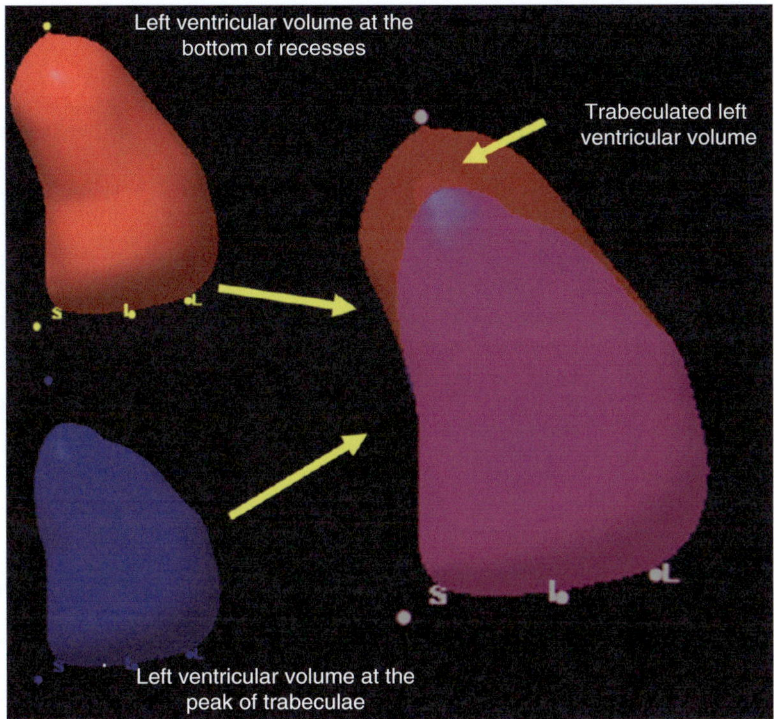

Fig. 21.12 Result of the 3Dechocardiographic analysis for trabeculated left ventricular (LV) volume estimation in a patient with LV noncompaction. After tracing the endocardial border at the bottom of the trabeculae and at the peak of the recesses, end-diastolic volumes including (*red*) and excluding (*blue*) trabeculae are obtained. Yellow arrows indicate that the difference between volumes (*blue* and *red*) corresponds to the trabeculated LV volume (indicated by the other yellow arrow), which is normalized by LV end-diastolic volume including trabeculae and represents the proportion of the LV cavity occupied by trabeculae (From Caselli et al. [147], with permission)

Fig. 21.13 Patient with left ventricular noncompaction (LV NC). Steady-state free-precession cardiac magnetic resonance, three-chamber image, taken at end-diastole showing a thick layer of noncompacted myocardium (*dotted arrows*) over compacted myocardium (*solid arrows*) in LV posterior wall

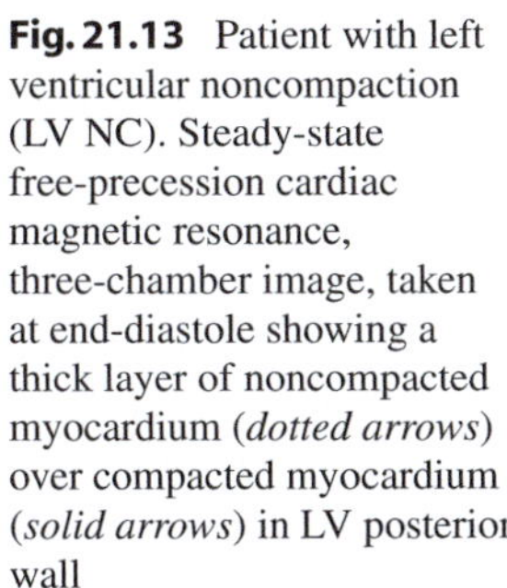

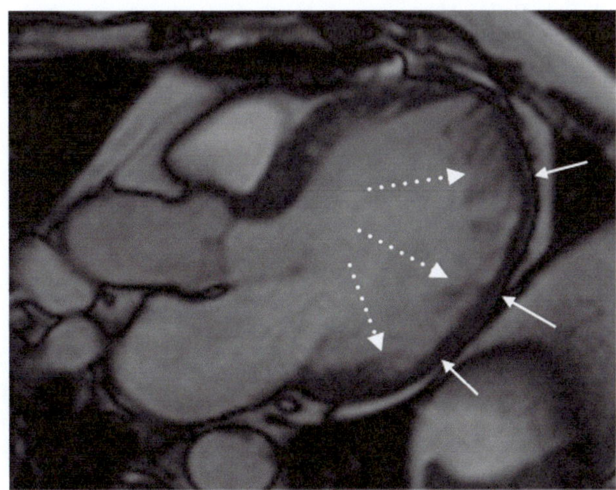

References

1. Huffman C, Wagman G, Fudim M et al (2010) Reversible cardiomyopathies – a review. Transplant Proc 42:3673–3678
2. Demakis JG, Rahimtoola SH, Sutton GC et al (1971) Natural course of peripartum cardiomyopathy. Circulation 44:1053–1061
3. Pearson GD, Veille JC, Rahimtoola S et al (2000) Peripartum cardiomyopathy: National Heart, Lung, and Blood Institute and Office of Rare Diseases (National Institutes of Health) workshop recommendations and review. JAMA 283:1183–1188
4. Givertz MM (2013) Cardiology patient page: peripartum cardiomyopathy. Circulation 127:e622–e626
5. Sliwa K, Skudicky D, Bergemann A et al (2000) Peripartum cardiomyopathy: analysis of clinical outcome, left ventricular function, plasma levels of cytokines and Fas/APO-1. J Am Coll Cardiol 35:701–705
6. Bello N, Rendon IS, Arany Z (2013) The relationship between pre-eclampsia and peripartum cardiomyopathy: a systematic review and meta-analysis. J Am Coll Cardiol 62:1715–1723
7. Peters F, Khandheria BK, dos Santos C et al (2013) Peripartum cardiomyopathy associated with left ventricular noncompaction phenotype and reversible rigid body rotation. Circ Heart Fail 6:e62–e63
8. Renz DM, Rottgen R, Habedank D et al (2011) New insights into peripartum cardiomyopathy using cardiac magnetic resonance imaging. Röfo 183:834–841
9. Arora NP, Mohamad T, Mahajan N et al (2014) Cardiac magnetic resonance imaging in peripartum cardiomyopathy: a new tool to evaluate an old enigma. Am J Med 347:112–7.
10. Blauwet LA, Libhaber E, Forster O et al (2013) Predictors of outcome in 176 South African patients with peripartum cardiomyopathy. Heart 99:308–313
11. Dorbala S, Brozena S, Zeb S et al (2005) Risk stratification of women with peripartum cardiomyopathy at initial presentation: a dobutamine stress echocardiography study. J Am Soc Echocardiogr 18:45–48
12. Maron BJ, Towbin JA, Thiene G et al (2006) Contemporary definitions and classification of the cardiomyopathies: an American Heart Association Scientific Statement from the Council on Clinical Cardiology, Heart Failure and Transplantation Committee; Quality of Care and Outcomes Research and Functional Genomics and Translational Biology Interdisciplinary Working Groups; and Council on Epidemiology and Prevention. Circulation 113:1807–1816
13. Bybee KA, Kara T, Prasad A et al (2004) Systematic review: transient left ventricular apical ballooning: a syndrome that mimics ST-segment elevation myocardial infarction. Ann Intern Med 141:858–865
14. Ruiz Bailen M, Aguayo de Hoyos E, Lopez Martnez A et al (2003) Reversible myocardial dysfunction, a possible complication in critically ill patients without heart disease. J Crit Care 18:245–252
15. Kawai S, Kitabatake A, Tomoike H et al (2007) Guidelines for diagnosis of takotsubo (ampulla) cardiomyopathy. Circ J 71:990–992
16. Lyon AR, Rees PS, Prasad S et al (2008) Stress (Takotsubo) cardiomyopathy – a novel pathophysiological hypothesis to explain catecholamine-induced acute myocardial stunning. Nat Clin Pract Cardiovasc Med 5:22–29
17. Lee JW, Kim JY (2011) Stress-induced cardiomyopathy: the role of echocardiography. J Cardiovasc Ultrasound 19:7–12
18. Kurisu S, Kihara Y (2012) Tako-tsubo cardiomyopathy: clinical presentation and underlying mechanism. J Cardiol 60:429–437
19. Ramaraj R, Movahed MR (2010) Reverse or inverted takotsubo cardiomyopathy (reverse left ventricular apical ballooning syndrome) presents at a younger age compared with the mid or apical variant and is always associated with triggering stress. Congest Heart Fail 16:284–286
20. Kurisu S, Inoue I, Kawagoe T et al (2011) Incidence and treatment of left ventricular apical thrombosis in Tako-tsubo cardiomyopathy. Int J Cardiol 146:e58–e60

21. Gianni M, Dentali F, Grandi AM et al (2006) Apical ballooning syndrome or takotsubo cardiomyopathy: a systematic review. Eur Heart J 27:1523–1529
22. Izumo M, Nalawadi S, Shiota M et al (2011) Mechanisms of acute mitral regurgitation in patients with takotsubo cardiomyopathy: an echocardiographic study. Circ Cardiovasc Imaging 4:392–398
23. Elesber AA, Prasad A, Bybee KA et al (2006) Transient cardiac apical ballooning syndrome: prevalence and clinical implications of right ventricular involvement. J Am Coll Cardiol 47:1082–1083
24. Kumar S, Kaushik S, Nautiyal A et al (2011) Cardiac rupture in takotsubo cardiomyopathy: a systematic review. Clin Cardiol 34:672–676
25. Shah BN, Simpson IA, Rakhit DJ (2011) Takotsubo (apical ballooning) syndrome in the recovery period following dobutamine stress echocardiography: a first report. Eur J Echocardiogr 12:E5
26. Choi JH, Nam JH, Son JW et al (2012) Clinical usefulness of myocardial contrast echocardiography to detect stress-induced cardiomyopathy in the emergency department. Circ J 76:1393–1398
27. Meimoun P, Malaquin D, Benali T et al (2009) Transient impairment of coronary flow reserve in tako-tsubo cardiomyopathy is related to left ventricular systolic parameters. Eur J Echocardiogr 10:265–270
28. Abdel-Aty H, Cocker M, Friedrich MG (2009) Myocardial edema is a feature of Tako-Tsubo cardiomyopathy and is related to the severity of systolic dysfunction: insights from T2-weighted cardiovascular magnetic resonance. Int J Cardiol 132:291–293
29. Joshi SB, Chao T, Herzka DA et al (2010) Cardiovascular magnetic resonance T2 signal abnormalities in left ventricular ballooning syndrome. Int J Cardiovasc Imaging 26:227–232
30. Neil C, Nguyen TH, Kucia A et al (2012) Slowly resolving global myocardial inflammation/oedema in Tako-Tsubo cardiomyopathy: evidence from T2-weighted cardiac MRI. Heart 98:1278–1284
31. Eitel I, Lucke C, Grothoff M et al (2010) Inflammation in takotsubo cardiomyopathy: insights from cardiovascular magnetic resonance imaging. Eur Radiol 20:422–431
32. Ferreira VM, Piechnik SK, Dall'Armellina E et al (2012) Noncontrast T1-mapping detects acute myocardial edema with high diagnostic accuracy: a comparison to T2-weighted cardiovascular magnetic resonance. J Cardiovasc Magn Reson 14:42
33. Gerbaud E, Montaudon M, Leroux L et al (2008) MRI for the diagnosis of left ventricular apical ballooning syndrome (LVABS). Eur Radiol 18:947–954
34. Mitchell JH, Hadden TB, Wilson JM et al (2007) Clinical features and usefulness of cardiac magnetic resonance imaging in assessing myocardial viability and prognosis in Takotsubo cardiomyopathy (transient left ventricular apical ballooning syndrome). Am J Cardiol 100:296–301
35. Eitel I, Behrendt F, Schindler K et al (2008) Differential diagnosis of suspected apical ballooning syndrome using contrast-enhanced magnetic resonance imaging. Eur Heart J 29:2651–2659
36. Eitel I, von Knobelsdorff-Brenkenhoff F, Bernhardt P et al (2011) Clinical characteristics and cardiovascular magnetic resonance findings in stress (takotsubo) cardiomyopathy. JAMA 306:277–286
37. Nakamori S, Matsuoka K, Onishi K et al (2012) Prevalence and signal characteristics of late gadolinium enhancement on contrast-enhanced magnetic resonance imaging in patients with takotsubo cardiomyopathy. Circ J 76:914–921
38. Naruse Y, Sato A, Kasahara K et al (2011) The clinical impact of late gadolinium enhancement in Takotsubo cardiomyopathy: serial analysis of cardiovascular magnetic resonance images. J Cardiovasc Magn Reson 13:67
39. Ito K, Sugihara H, Kawasaki T et al (2001) Assessment of ampulla (Takotsubo) cardiomyopathy with coronary angiography, two-dimensional echocardiography and 99mTc-tetrofosmin myocardial single photon emission computed tomography. Ann Nucl Med 15:351–355

40. Abe Y, Kondo M, Matsuoka R et al (2003) Assessment of clinical features in transient left ventricular apical ballooning. J Am Coll Cardiol 41:737–742

41. Ito K, Sugihara H, Katoh S et al (2003) Assessment of Takotsubo (ampulla) cardiomyopathy using 99mTc-tetrofosmin myocardial SPECT – comparison with acute coronary syndrome. Ann Nucl Med 17:115–122

42. Kurisu S, Inoue I, Kawagoe T et al (2003) Myocardial perfusion and fatty acid metabolism in patients with tako-tsubo-like left ventricular dysfunction. J Am Coll Cardiol 41:743–748

43. Owa M, Aizawa K, Urasawa N et al (2001) Emotional stress-induced 'ampulla cardiomyopathy': discrepancy between the metabolic and sympathetic innervation imaging performed during the recovery course. Jpn Circ J 65:349–352

44. Sato A, Aonuma K, Nozato T et al (2008) Stunned myocardium in transient left ventricular apical ballooning: a serial study of dual I-123 BMIPP and Tl-201 SPECT. J Nucl Cardiol 15:671–679

45. Pessoa PM, Xavier SS, Lima SL et al (2006) Assessment of takotsubo (ampulla) cardiomyopathy using iodine-123 metaiodobenzylguanidine scintigraphy. Acta Radiol 47:1029–1035

46. Cimarelli S, Sauer F, Morel O et al (2010) Transient left ventricular dysfunction syndrome: patho-physiological bases through nuclear medicine imaging. Int J Cardiol 144:212–218

47. Burgdorf C, von Hof K, Schunkert H et al (2008) Regional alterations in myocardial sympathetic innervation in patients with transient left-ventricular apical ballooning (Tako-Tsubo cardiomyopathy). J Nucl Cardiol 15:65–72

48. Bybee KA, Murphy J, Prasad A et al (2006) Acute impairment of regional myocardial glucose uptake in the apical ballooning (takotsubo) syndrome. J Nucl Cardiol 13:244–250

49. Feola M, Chauvie S, Rosso GL et al (2008) Reversible impairment of coronary flow reserve in takotsubo cardiomyopathy: a myocardial PET study. J Nucl Cardiol 15:811–817

50. Yoshida T, Hibino T, Kako N et al (2007) A pathophysiologic study of tako-tsubo cardiomyopathy with F-18 fluorodeoxyglucose positron emission tomography. Eur Heart J 28:2598–2604

51. Kwon SW, Kim BO, Kim MH et al (2013) Diverse left ventricular morphology and predictors of short-term outcome in patients with stress-induced cardiomyopathy. Int J Cardiol 168:331–337

52. Lee PH, Song JK, Sun BJ et al (2010) Outcomes of patients with stress-induced cardiomyopathy diagnosed by echocardiography in a tertiary referral hospital. J Am Soc Echocardiogr 23:766–771

53. Elesber AA, Prasad A, Lennon RJ et al (2007) Four-year recurrence rate and prognosis of the apical ballooning syndrome. J Am Coll Cardiol 50:448–452

54. Ellis ER, Josephson ME (2013) Heart failure and tachycardia-induced cardiomyopathy. Curr Heart Fail Rep 10:296–306

55. Jeong YH, Choi KJ, Song JM et al (2008) Diagnostic approach and treatment strategy in tachycardia-induced cardiomyopathy. Clin Cardiol 31:172–178

56. Fujino T, Yamashita T, Suzuki S et al (2007) Characteristics of congestive heart failure accompanied by atrial fibrillation with special reference to tachycardia-induced cardiomyopathy. Circ J 71:936–940

57. Selby DE, Palmer BM, LeWinter MM et al (2011) Tachycardia-induced diastolic dysfunction and resting tone in myocardium from patients with a normal ejection fraction. J Am Coll Cardiol 58:147–154

58. Paelinck B, Vermeersch P, Stockman D et al (1999) Usefulness of low-dose dobutamine stress echocardiography in predicting recovery of poor left ventricular function in atrial fibrillation dilated cardiomyopathy. Am J Cardiol 83:1668–1671, A1667

59. Ferguson JD, Helms A, Mangrum JM et al (2009) Catheter ablation of atrial fibrillation without fluoroscopy using intracardiac echocardiography and electroanatomic mapping. Circ Arrhythm Electrophysiol 2:611–619

60. Tibayan FA, Lai DT, Timek TA et al (2002) Alterations in left ventricular torsion in tachycardia-induced dilated cardiomyopathy. J Thorac Cardiovasc Surg 124:43–49

61. To AC, Flamm SD, Marwick TH et al (2011) Clinical utility of multimodality LA imaging: assessment of size, function, and structure. JACC Cardiovasc Imaging 4:788–798
62. Schneider C, Malisius R, Krause K et al (2008) Strain rate imaging for functional quantification of the left atrium: atrial deformation predicts the maintenance of sinus rhythm after catheter ablation of atrial fibrillation. Eur Heart J 29:1397–1409
63. Faletra FF, Ho SY, Regoli F et al (2013) Real-time three dimensional transoesophageal echocardiography in imaging key anatomical structures of the left atrium: potential role during atrial fibrillation ablation. Heart 99:133–142
64. Hasdemir C, Yuksel A, Camli D et al (2012) Late gadolinium enhancement CMR in patients with tachycardia-induced cardiomyopathy caused by idiopathic ventricular arrhythmias. Pacing Clin Electrophysiol 35:465–470
65. Matsumoto K, Takahashi N, Ishikawa T et al (2006) Evaluation of myocardial glucose metabolism before and after recovery of myocardial function in patients with tachycardia-induced cardiomyopathy. Pacing Clin Electrophysiol 29:175–180
66. Khasnis A, Jongnarangsin K, Abela G et al (2005) Tachycardia-induced cardiomyopathy: a review of literature. Pacing Clin Electrophysiol 28:710–721
67. Watanabe H, Okamura K, Chinushi M et al (2008) Clinical characteristics, treatment, and outcome of tachycardia induced cardiomyopathy. Int Heart J 49:39–47
68. Aretz HT, Billingham ME, Edwards WD et al (1987) Myocarditis. A histopathologic definition and classification. Am J Cardiovasc Pathol 1:3–14
69. Kindermann I, Barth C, Mahfoud F et al (2012) Update on myocarditis. J Am Coll Cardiol 59:779–792
70. Anzini M, Merlo M, Sabbadini G et al (2013) Long-term evolution and prognostic stratification of biopsy-proven active myocarditis. Circulation 128:2384–2394
71. Imazio M, Trinchero R (2008) Myopericarditis: etiology, management, and prognosis. Int J Cardiol 127:17–26
72. Buiatti A, Merlo M, Pinamonti B et al (2013) Clinical presentation and long-term follow-up of perimyocarditis. J Cardiovasc Med (Hagerstown) 14:235–241
73. Pinamonti B, Alberti E, Cigalotto A et al (1988) Echocardiographic findings in myocarditis. Am J Cardiol 62:285–291
74. Felker GM, Boehmer JP, Hruban RH et al (2000) Echocardiographic findings in fulminant and acute myocarditis. J Am Coll Cardiol 36:227–232
75. Lieback E, Hardouin I, Meyer R et al (1996) Clinical value of echocardiographic tissue characterization in the diagnosis of myocarditis. Eur Heart J 17:135–142
76. Hiramitsu S, Morimoto S, Kato S et al (2001) Transient ventricular wall thickening in acute myocarditis: a serial echocardiographic and histopathologic study. Jpn Circ J 65:863–866
77. Ong P, Athansiadis A, Hill S et al (2011) Usefulness of pericardial effusion as new diagnostic criterion for noninvasive detection of myocarditis. Am J Cardiol 108:445–452
78. Imazio M, Brucato A, Barbieri A et al (2013) Good prognosis for pericarditis with and without myocardial involvement: results from a multicenter, prospective cohort study. Circulation 128:42–49
79. Di Bella G, Coglitore S, Zimbalatti C et al (2008) Strain Doppler echocardiography can identify longitudinal myocardial dysfunction derived from edema in acute myocarditis. Int J Cardiol 126:279–280
80. Hsiao JF, Koshino Y, Bonnichsen CR et al (2013) Speckle tracking echocardiography in acute myocarditis. Int J Cardiovasc Imaging 29:275–284
81. Di Bella G, Gaeta M, Pingitore A et al (2010) Myocardial deformation in acute myocarditis with normal left ventricular wall motion – a cardiac magnetic resonance and 2-dimensional strain echocardiographic study. Circ J 74:1205–1213
82. Escher F, Kasner M, Kuhl U et al (2013) New echocardiographic findings correlate with intramyocardial inflammation in endomyocardial biopsies of patients with acute myocarditis and inflammatory cardiomyopathy. Mediators Inflamm 2013:875420

83. Afonso L, Hari P, Pidlaoan V et al (2010) Acute myocarditis: can novel echocardiographic techniques assist with diagnosis? Eur J Echocardiogr 11:E5

84. Skouri HN, Dec GW, Friedrich MG, Cooper LT (2006) Noninvasive imaging in myocarditis. J Am Coll Cardiol 48:2085–2093

85. Mahrholdt H, Goedecke C, Wagner A et al (2004) Cardiovascular magnetic resonance assessment of human myocarditis: a comparison to histology and molecular pathology. Circulation 109:1250–1258

86. Friedrich MG, Strohm O, Schulz-Menger J et al (1998) Contrast media-enhanced magnetic resonance imaging visualizes myocardial changes in the course of viral myocarditis. Circulation 97:1802–1809

87. Abdel-Aty H, Simonetti O, Friedrich MG (2007) T2-weighted cardiovascular magnetic resonance imaging. J Magn Reson Imaging 26:452–459

88. Friedrich MG, Sechtem U, Schulz-Menger J et al (2009) Cardiovascular magnetic resonance in myocarditis: a JACC White Paper. J Am Coll Cardiol 53:1475–1487

89. De Cobelli F, Pieroni M, Esposito A et al (2006) Delayed gadolinium-enhanced cardiac magnetic resonance in patients with chronic myocarditis presenting with heart failure or recurrent arrhythmias. J Am Coll Cardiol 47:1649–1654

90. Gutberlet M, Spors B, Thoma T et al (2008) Suspected chronic myocarditis at cardiac MR: diagnostic accuracy and association with immunohistologically detected inflammation and viral persistence. Radiology 246:401–409

91. Lurz P, Eitel I, Adam J et al (2012) Diagnostic performance of CMR imaging compared with EMB in patients with suspected myocarditis. JACC Cardiovasc Imaging 5:513–524

92. Iles L, Pfluger H, Phrommintikul A et al (2008) Evaluation of diffuse myocardial fibrosis in heart failure with cardiac magnetic resonance contrast-enhanced T1 mapping. J Am Coll Cardiol 52:1574–1580

93. Dambrin G, Laissy JP, Serfaty JM et al (2007) Diagnostic value of ECG-gated multidetector computed tomography in the early phase of suspected acute myocarditis. A preliminary comparative study with cardiac MRI. Eur Radiol 17:331–338

94. Grun S, Schumm J, Greulich S et al (2012) Long-term follow-up of biopsy-proven viral myocarditis: predictors of mortality and incomplete recovery. J Am Coll Cardiol 59:1604–1615

95. Mahrholdt H, Wagner A, Deluigi CC et al (2006) Presentation, patterns of myocardial damage, and clinical course of viral myocarditis. Circulation 114:1581–1590

96. Maya JD, Orellana M, Ferreira J et al (2010) Chagas disease: present status of pathogenic mechanisms and chemotherapy. Biol Res 43:323–331

97. Nunes MCP, Dones W, Morillo CA, Encina JJ, Ribeiro AL (2013) Chagas disease. An overview of clinical and epidemiological aspects. J Am Coll Cardiol 62:767–776

98. Andrade JP, Marin Neto JA, Paola AA et al (2011) Latin American Guidelines for the diagnosis and treatment of Chagas' heart disease: executive summary. Arq Bras Cardiol 96:434–442

99. Acquatella H (2007) Echocardiography in Chagas heart disease. Circulation 115:1124–1131

100. Viotti RJ, Vigliano C, Laucella S et al (2004) Value of echocardiography for diagnosis and prognosis of chronic Chagas disease cardiomyopathy without heart failure. Heart 90:655–660

101. Garcia-Alvarez A, Sitges M, Regueiro A et al (2011) Myocardial deformation analysis in Chagas heart disease with the use of speckle tracking echocardiography. J Card Fail 17:1028–1034

102. Rochitte CE, Oliveira PF, Andrade JM et al (2005) Myocardial delayed enhancement by magnetic resonance imaging in patients with Chagas' disease: a marker of disease severity. J Am Coll Cardiol 46:1553–1558

103. Regueiro A, Garcia-Alvarez A, Sitges M et al (2011) Myocardial involvement in Chagas disease: insights from cardiac magnetic resonance. Int J Cardiol 165:107–112

104. Nunes MC, Barbosa MM, Ribeiro AL et al (2009) Left atrial volume provides independent prognostic value in patients with Chagas cardiomyopathy. J Am Soc Echocardiogr 22:82–88

105. Nunes MP, Colosimo EA, Reis RC et al (2012) Different prognostic impact of the tissue Doppler-derived E/e' ratio on mortality in Chagas cardiomyopathy patients with heart failure. J Heart Lung Transplant 31:634–641

106. Albini A, Pennesi G, Donatelli F et al (2010) Cardiotoxicity of anticancer drugs: the need for cardio-oncology and cardio-oncological prevention. J Natl Cancer Inst 102:14–25

107. Ky B, Vejpongsa P, Yeh ET et al (2013) Emerging paradigms in cardiomyopathies associated with cancer therapies. Circ Res 113:754–764

108. Sawaya H, Sebag IA, Plana JC et al (2011) Early detection and prediction of cardiotoxicity in chemotherapy-treated patients. Am J Cardiol 107:1375–1380

109. Yeh ET, Tong AT, Lenihan DJ et al (2004) Cardiovascular complications of cancer therapy: diagnosis, pathogenesis, and management. Circulation 109:3122–3131

110. Lipshultz SE, Adams MJ, Colan SD et al (2013) Long-term cardiovascular toxicity in children, adolescents, and young adults who receive cancer therapy: pathophysiology, course, monitoring, management, prevention, and research directions: a scientific statement from the American Heart Association. Circulation 128:1927–1995

111. Oreto L, Todaro MC, Umland MM et al (2012) Use of echocardiography to evaluate the cardiac effects of therapies used in cancer treatment: what do we know? J Am Soc Echocardiogr 25:1141–1152

112. Drafts BC, Twomley KM, D'Agostino R Jr et al (2013) Low to moderate dose anthracycline-based chemotherapy is associated with early noninvasive imaging evidence of subclinical cardiovascular disease. JACC Cardiovasc Imaging 6:877–885

113. Armstrong GT, Plana JC, Zhang N et al (2012) Screening adult survivors of childhood cancer for cardiomyopathy: comparison of echocardiography and cardiac magnetic resonance imaging. J Clin Oncol 30:2876–2884

114. Ylanen K, Poutanen T, Savikurki-Heikkila P et al (2013) Cardiac magnetic resonance imaging in the evaluation of the late effects of anthracyclines among long-term survivors of childhood cancer. J Am Coll Cardiol 61:1539–1547

115. Neilan TG, Coelho-Filho OR, Pena-Herrera D et al (2012) Left ventricular mass in patients with a cardiomyopathy after treatment with anthracyclines. Am J Cardiol 110:1679–1686

116. Tham EB, Haykowsky MJ, Chow K et al (2013) Diffuse myocardial fibrosis by T1-mapping in children with subclinical anthracycline cardiotoxicity: relationship to exercise capacity, cumulative dose and remodeling. J Cardiovasc Magn Reson 15:48

117. Neilan TG, Coelho-Filho OR, Shah RV et al (2013) Myocardial extracellular volume by cardiac magnetic resonance imaging in patients treated with anthracycline-based chemotherapy. Am J Cardiol 111:717–722

118. Fallah-Rad N, Lytwyn M, Fang T et al (2008) Delayed contrast enhancement cardiac magnetic resonance imaging in trastuzumab induced cardiomyopathy. J Cardiovasc Magn Reson 10:5

119. de Geus-Oei LF, Mavinkurve-Groothuis AM, Bellersen L et al (2011) Scintigraphic techniques for early detection of cancer treatment-induced cardiotoxicity. J Nucl Med 52:560–571

120. Valdes Olmos RA, ten Bokkel Huinink WW, ten Hoeve RF et al (1994) Usefulness of indium-111 antimyosin scintigraphy in confirming myocardial injury in patients with anthracycline-associated left ventricular dysfunction. Ann Oncol 5:617–622

121. Elliott P, Andersson B, Arbustini E et al (2008) Classification of the cardiomyopathies: a position statement from the European Society of Cardiology Working Group on Myocardial and Pericardial Diseases. Eur Heart J 29:270–276

122. Chin TK, Perloff JK, Williams RG et al (1990) Isolated noncompaction of left ventricular myocardium. A study of eight cases. Circulation 82:507–513

123. Oechslin EN, Attenhofer Jost CH, Rojas JR et al (2000) Long-term follow-up of 34 adults with isolated left ventricular noncompaction: a distinct cardiomyopathy with poor prognosis. J Am Coll Cardiol 36:493–500
124. Oechslin E, Jenni R (2011) Left ventricular noncompaction revisited: a distinct phenotype with genetic heterogeneity? Eur Heart J 32:1446–1456
125. Aras D, Tufekcioglu O, Ergun K et al (2006) Clinical features of isolated ventricular noncompaction in adults long-term clinical course, echocardiographic properties, and predictors of left ventricular failure. J Card Fail 12:726–733
126. Pignatelli RH, McMahon CJ, Dreyer WJ et al (2003) Clinical characterization of left ventricular noncompaction in children: a relatively common form of cardiomyopathy. Circulation 108:2672–2678
127. Jenni R, Goebel N, Tartini R et al (1986) Persisting myocardial sinusoids of both ventricles as an isolated anomaly: echocardiographic, angiographic, and pathologic anatomical findings. Cardiovasc Intervent Radiol 9:127–131
128. Thavendiranathan P, Dahiya A, Phelan D et al (2013) Isolated left ventricular noncompaction controversies in diagnostic criteria, adverse outcomes and management. Heart 99:681–689
129. Paterick TE, Tajik AJ (2012) Left ventricular noncompaction: a diagnostically challenging cardiomyopathy. Circ J 76:1556–1562
130. Boyd MT, Seward JB, Tajik AJ et al (1987) Frequency and location of prominent left ventricular trabeculations at autopsy in 474 normal human hearts: implications for evaluation of mural thrombi by two-dimensional echocardiography. J Am Coll Cardiol 9:323–326
131. Jenni R, Oechslin E, Schneider J et al (2001) Echocardiographic and pathoanatomical characteristics of isolated left ventricular noncompaction: a step towards classification as a distinct cardiomyopathy. Heart 86:666–671
132. Stollberger C, Finsterer J, Blazek G (2002) Left ventricular hypertrabeculation/noncompaction and association with additional cardiac abnormalities and neuromuscular disorders. Am J Cardiol 90:899–902
133. Stollberger C, Finsterer J (2004) Left ventricular hypertrabeculation/noncompaction. J Am Soc Echocardiogr 17:91–100
134. Finsterer J, Stollberger C (2011) No rationale for a diagnostic ratio in left ventricular hypertrabeculation/noncompaction. Int J Cardiol 146:91–92
135. Frischknecht BS, Attenhofer Jost CH, Oechslin EN et al (2005) Validation of noncompaction criteria in dilated cardiomyopathy, and valvular and hypertensive heart disease. J Am Soc Echocardiogr 18:865–872
136. Belanger AR, Miller MA, Donthireddi UR et al (2008) New classification scheme of left ventricular noncompaction and correlation with ventricular performance. Am J Cardiol 102:92–96
137. Kohli SK, Pantazis AA, Shah JS et al (2008) Diagnosis of left-ventricular noncompaction in patients with left-ventricular systolic dysfunction: time for a reappraisal of diagnostic criteria? Eur Heart J 29:89–95
138. Saleeb SF, Margossian R, Spencer CT et al (2012) Reproducibility of echocardiographic diagnosis of left ventricular noncompaction. J Am Soc Echocardiogr 25:194–202
139. Gati S, Chandra N, Bennett RL et al (2013) Increased left ventricular trabeculation in highly trained athletes: do we need more stringent criteria for the diagnosis of left ventricular noncompaction in athletes? Heart 99:401–408
140. de Groot-de Laat LE, Krenning BJ, ten Cate FJ et al (2005) Usefulness of contrast echocardiography for diagnosis of left ventricular noncompaction. Am J Cardiol 95:1131–1134
141. Maltagliati A, Pepi M (2000) Isolated noncompaction of the myocardium: multiplane transesophageal echocardiography diagnosis in an adult. J Am Soc Echocardiogr 13:1047–1049
142. Bellavia D, Michelena HI, Martinez M et al (2010) Speckle myocardial imaging modalities for early detection of myocardial impairment in isolated left ventricular noncompaction. Heart 96:440–447

143. van Dalen BM, Caliskan K, Soliman OI et al (2008) Left ventricular solid body rotation in noncompaction cardiomyopathy: a potential new objective and quantitative functional diagnostic criterion? Eur J Heart Fail 10:1088–1093

144. van Dalen BM, Caliskan K, Soliman OI et al (2011) Diagnostic value of rigid body rotation in noncompaction cardiomyopathy. J Am Soc Echocardiogr 24:548–555

145. Peters F, Khandheria BK, Libhaber E et al (2014) Left ventricular twist in left ventricular noncompaction. Eur Heart J Cardiovasc Imaging 15:48–55

146. Niemann M, Liu D, Hu K et al (2012) Echocardiographic quantification of regional deformation helps to distinguish isolated left ventricular noncompaction from dilated cardiomyopathy. Eur J Heart Fail 14:155–161

147. Caselli S, Autore C, Serdoz A et al (2012) Three-dimensional echocardiographic characterization of patients with left ventricular noncompaction. J Am Soc Echocardiogr 25:203–209

148. Bodiwala K, Miller AP, Nanda NC et al (2005) Live three-dimensional transthoracic echocardiographic assessment of ventricular noncompaction. Echocardiography 22:611–620

149. Petersen SE, Selvanayagam JB, Wiesmann F et al (2005) Left ventricular noncompaction: insights from cardiovascular magnetic resonance imaging. J Am Coll Cardiol 46:101–105

150. Kawel N, Nacif M, Arai AE et al (2012) Trabeculated (noncompacted) and compact myocardium in adults: the multi-ethnic study of atherosclerosis. Circ Cardiovasc Imaging 5:357–366

151. Korcyk D, Edwards CC, Armstrong G et al (2004) Contrast-enhanced cardiac magnetic resonance in a patient with familial isolated ventricular noncompaction. J Cardiovasc Magn Reson 6:569–576

152. Jacquier A, Thuny F, Jop B et al (2010) Measurement of trabeculated left ventricular mass using cardiac magnetic resonance imaging in the diagnosis of left ventricular noncompaction. Eur Heart J 31:1098–1104

153. Grothoff M, Pachowsky M, Hoffmann J et al (2012) Value of cardiovascular MR in diagnosing left ventricular noncompaction cardiomyopathy and in discriminating between other cardiomyopathies. Eur Radiol 22:2699–2709

154. Captur G, Flett AS, Jacoby DL et al (2013) Left ventricular nonnoncompaction: the mitral valve prolapse of the 21st century? Int J Cardiol 164:3–6

155. Nucifora G, Aquaro GD, Pingitore A et al (2011) Myocardial fibrosis in isolated left ventricular noncompaction and its relation to disease severity. Eur J Heart Fail 13:170–176

156. Dodd JD, Holmvang G, Hoffmann U et al (2007) Quantification of left ventricular noncompaction and trabecular delayed hyperenhancement with cardiac MRI: correlation with clinical severity. AJR Am J Roentgenol 189:974–980

157. Dursun M, Agayev A, Nisli K et al (2010) MR imaging features of ventricular noncompaction: emphasis on distribution and pattern of fibrosis. Eur J Radiol 74:147–151

158. Junqueira FP, Fernandes FD, Coutinho AC et al (2009) Case report. Isolated left ventricular myocardiumnoncompaction: MR imaging findings from three cases. Br J Radiol 82:e37–e41

159. Melendez-Ramirez G, Castillo-Castellon F, Espinola-Zavaleta N et al (2012) Left ventricular noncompaction: a proposal of new diagnostic criteria by multidetector computed tomography. J Cardiovasc Comput Tomogr 6:346–354

160. Sidhu MS, Uthamalingam S, Ahmed W et al (2014) Defining left ventricular noncompaction using cardiac computed tomography. J Thorac Imaging 29:60–66

161. Jenni R, Wyss CA, Oechslin EN et al (2002) Isolated ventricular noncompaction is associated with coronary microcirculatory dysfunction. J Am Coll Cardiol 39:450–454

162. Stanton C, Bruce C, Connolly H et al (2009) Isolated left ventricular noncompaction syndrome. Am J Cardiol 104:1135–1138

163. McMahon CJ, Pignatelli RH, Nagueh SF et al (2007) Left ventricular noncompaction cardiomyopathy in children: characterisation of clinical status using tissue Doppler-derived indices of left ventricular diastolic relaxation. Heart 93:676–681

164. Wald R, Veldtman G, Golding F et al (2004) Determinants of outcome in isolated ventricular noncompaction in childhood. Am J Cardiol 94:1581–1584

165. Punn R, Silverman NH (2010) Cardiac segmental analysis in left ventricular noncompaction: experience in a pediatric population. J Am Soc Echocardiogr 23:46–53
166. McMurray JJ, Adamopoulos S, Anker SD et al (2012) ESC Guidelines for the diagnosis and treatment of acute and chronic heart failure 2012: The Task Force for the Diagnosis and Treatment of Acute and Chronic Heart Failure 2012 of the European Society of Cardiology. Developed in collaboration with the Heart Failure Association (HFA) of the ESC. Eur Heart J 33:1787–1847

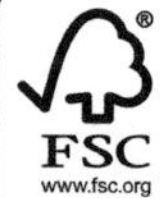